AF745967

NOVEL ASPECTS ON CYSTICERCOSIS AND NEUROCYSTICERCOSIS

Edited by **Humberto Foyaca Sibat**

Novel Aspects on Cysticercosis and Neurocysticercosis
http://dx.doi.org/10.5772/3311
Edited by Humberto Foyaca Sibat

Contributors

Humberto Foyaca Sibat, Lourdes de Fátima Ibañez Valdés, Karen Nava-Castro, Romel Hernández-Bello, Saé Muñiz-Hernández, Lorena López-Griego, Jhonatan A. Hernández-Valdés, Valeria López-Salazar, Nelly Tiempos-Guzmán, Jorge Morales-Montor, Rachana Bhattarai, Hélène Carabin, Christine Budke, Helena A. Ngowi, Samson Mukaratirwa, Faustin P. Lekule, Ndichu Maingi, Charles Waiswa, Chummy Sikasunge, Sonia Afonso, Julienne Sumbu, Sylvia Ramiandrasoa, Mary Louise Penrith, Arve Lee Willingham, Agnès Fleury, Edda Sciutto, Aline S. de Aluja, Carlos Larralde, Sonia Agudelo, Gisela Maria Garcia, Jaime Fandiño, Randy Guerra, Cáris Nunes, Samuel Carvalho de Aragão, Marcello Sato, Ronaldo Abraham, Arturo Carpio, Franklin Santillan, Maria Milagros Cortez A., Glenda Rojas, Elizabeth Ferrer, Cruz Manuel Aguilar, Juan Carlos Durán, R. Michael E. Parkhouse, María Carolina Salazar Campos, Ana Flisser, Arturo Carpio, Andrea Sylvia Winkler, Alejandro L. Escalaya, Jorge G. Burneo, Kelesidis Theodoros

Published by InTech

Janeza Trdine 9, 51000 Rijeka, Croatia

Copyright © 2012 InTech

All chapters are distributed under the Creative Commons Attribution 3.0 license, which allows users to download, copy and build upon published articles even for commercial purposes, as long as the author and publisher are properly credited, which ensures maximum dissemination and a wider impact of our publications. However, users who aim to disseminate and distribute copies of this book as a whole must not seek monetary compensation for such service (excluded InTech representatives and agreed collaborations). After this work has been published by InTech, authors have the right to republish it, in whole or part, in any publication of which they are the author, and to make other personal use of the work. Any republication, referencing or personal use of the work must explicitly identify the original source.

Notice

Statements and opinions expressed in the chapters are these of the individual contributors and not necessarily those of the editors or publisher. No responsibility is accepted for the accuracy of information contained in the published chapters. The publisher assumes no responsibility for any damage or injury to persons or property arising out of the use of any materials, instructions, methods or ideas contained in the book.

Publishing Process Manager Dragana Manestar
Technical Editor InTech DTP team
Cover InTech Design team

Additional hard copies can be obtained from orders@intechopen.com

Novel Aspects on Cysticercosis and Neurocysticercosis, Edited by Humberto Foyaca Sibat
p. cm.
ISBN 978-953-51-0956-3

We are IntechOpen, the world's leading publisher of Open Access books

Built by scientists, for scientists

4,100+
Open access books available

116,000+
International authors and editors

120M+
Downloads

151
Countries delivered to

Our authors are among the
Top 1%
most cited scientists

12.2%
Contributors from top 500 universities

CLARIVATE ANALYTICS BOOK CITATION INDEX INDEXED

WEB OF SCIENCE™

Selection of our books indexed in the Book Citation Index
in Web of Science™ Core Collection (BKCI)

Interested in publishing with us?
Contact book.department@intechopen.com

Numbers displayed above are based on latest data collected.
For more information visit www.intechopen.com

For EU product safety concerns:
IN TECH d.o.o., Prolaz Marije Krucifikse Kozulić 3, 51000 Rijeka, Croatia,
info@intechopen.com or visit our website at intechopen.com.

Meet the editor

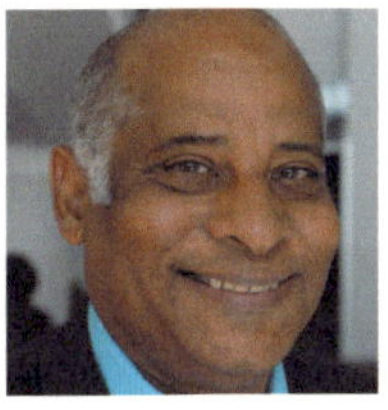

Professor H. Foyaca Sibat, born on May 03, 1948 in Havana City, Republic of Cuba, graduated as a Medical Doctor in Havana University in 1971. He became specialist in neurology in 1975 and got a higher degree level specialist in 1984. He also got a degree of PhD, Master of Sciences in Infectology, and an Associate Research Scientist. Currently Dr Foyaca has been working as an Associate Professor of Neurology at Walter Sisulu University (South Africa) for more than 15 years. He is a member of 15 Medical Societies from all over the world; he presented more than 350 papers in different scientific events and he published more than 70 manuscripts in peer-reviewed journals. He is the Editor-in-Chief of The Internet Journal of Neurology. He received and delivered many short and long training courses and organized many National and International Medical conferences.

Contents

Preface

Cysticercosis continues to be a gradually increasing health problem affecting millions of people all over the world, mainly in developing countries where parasitic zoonoses are more common and cysticercosis, as a leading cause, is endemic. Despite cysticercosis is a potential eradicable disease, there is epidemiological evidence for an increasing prevalence of cysticercosis throughout the world, and evidence of increasing morbidity and mortality in many countries as a consequence of higher incidence of parasitic zoonotic diseases, migration and globalization. Apart from that, in some countries of Sub-Saharan Africa, Asia and Latin America, there are communities who live, or have lived, either by choice (peoples living in voluntary isolation) or by circumstance, without significant contact with globalized civilization, therefore their current epidemiological situation is unknown and currently we don't even know how many people are infected by parasites.

At the present moment, there is a significant number of available books on cysticercosis. However, we decided to edit this book to introduce novel aspects on cysticercosis/neurocysticercosis which were not published before. Therefore, apart from the classic issues that cannot be missing in any book about this topic, we introduced novel aspects related with cysticercosis and neurocysticercosis as a leading cause of epilepsy in developing countries. Of course, the publication of this book could not have been possible without the ungrudging efforts put in by a large number of individuals working in this field and people from many countries as well as ethnic, religious and socioeconomic groups that coincidentally confluence in this publication.

In this book we focus on novel aspects of the historical background of this zoonotic parasitic disease, we highlight that *T solium* infested man long before there was any evidence of animal domestication which also served to declare that pigs are not guilty of human cysticercosis. We also delivered new hypotheses, and novel clinical descriptions and surgical ways of management. Because of the fact that the uncommon clinical presentations of cysticercosis and *orbital cysticercosis* are probably currently underestimated, and thus represent an area of legitimate concern, we dedicated two chapters these topics. Other chapters written by well known researchers were dedicated to the burden of cysticercosis, the control of *T solium* transmission of taeniosis and cysticercosis in endemic countries including the roles of continental networks of specialists and of local health authorities. The control of *T solium* transmission of taeniosis and cysticercosis in endemic countries, the roles of continental networks of specialists and of local health authorities and the agricultural impact of porcine cysticercosis in Africa which were never discussed in previous text book on cysticercosis and neurocysticercosis. In this book we also bring all our readers up to date with the impact and the latest scientific information in regard to epidemiology of neurocysticercosis, clinical diagnoses of neurocysticercosis and epilepsy including our experience in Sub-Saharan Africa, extraparenchymal neurocysticercosis addressed to health professionals working in the more disadvantage places. Finally we discuss about a novel surgical treatment of neurocysticercosis-related epilepsy.

Some chapters and the edition job were entirely made in a rural setting with a lot of inconvenience but this edition is aimed at health care professionals including general practitioners, family doctors, internists, neurologists, epileptologists, neurosurgeons, psychiatrists, medical students, nursing students, and students of the professions allied to medicine, among others.

Many abstracts were submitted for review from different parts of the world; about 25 % were selected for the first phase of this editorial process but unfortunately most of abstracts related to neurocysticercosis and written by peoples do not specialized in this field were rejected because of lack of basic and novel information. All material for this first edition has been thoroughly revised, and updated. Many specialists have provided expert advice on changes in their field and their help has been invaluable to us in our efforts to keep the relevance of the book for our readership community. All chapters were revised again by each author after submission; the final version was peer-reviewed by experts and recommendations were implemented. Nevertheless, some advices of contributors may differ from the approach of the editors or can be even different from the medical community. However, we kept and supported it as a part of our policy of respecting all scientific criteria, mainly for that work which still remains controversial. On the other hand, we also encouraged each author as an expert in the field, straight from the beginning to report their personal experience, expertise, and results.

Knowing that authors from many countries may have different experience and scientific results, in order to achieve a high degree of scientific content with a standard level of acceptance, we took a detailed overview of all important novel information. We all tried to keep the high prestige of our Editorial Company as a main priority and we declare our happiness in writing this book in the electronic era with a full-text website allowing us to display our scientific messages to an even larger global readership, apart from all benefits of print format.

Our aim has been to produce a reference book in which this information would be presented in an integrated and rapidly accessible format. With regards to pharmacological treatment of cysticercosis/neurocysticercosis we agree that medical treatment should be driven by "evidence-based" clinical-imagenologic and serological approach, but we did not exclude any "experience-based" approach from expert contributors and from the disadvantaged regions.

Every effort has been made to check the drug dosages given in this book. Despite dosages from all medication were double checked, it is important for our readership to scrutinize last information sheets about new dosages, side-effects, contraindications before administering any of the drugs listed. We all attempted to bring in valuable updated information about the treatment of cysticercosis/taeniosis/neurocysticercosis and other related problems to our readership.

ACKNOWLEDGEMENTS

We sincerely thank INTECH Open Access Publisher that unconditionally supported our initiative in editing this book. Special thanks should be given to my editorial process managers and beautiful friends Ms Dragana Manestar and Natalia Reinic for their kind attention, great inspiration, constant encouragement, and professional support which are highly appreciated. For understanding my long nights at the computer, I'd like to thank my wife Lourdes de Fátima, who was worked with me on this project; to my first daughter Zayra Susana and my Mon whom died long ago but they continue inspiring me from wherever they are; to my second daughter Lorna Maria who is a good lawyer and encourages me all the time to continue moving forward, and to my children Fatima Susana Adolfina (3 years old) and Thabo Humberto Jorge (4 years old) for helping me to find peace of mind, persistence and hope every time I needed. Their request to me for playing games at home also helped me to relax and later to find new ideas. My father, my sisters, nephews, nieces, aunts, uncles, cousins and almost all members of my family contributed to this project in one way or another - to all of them: Thanks a lot.

Many thanks also to family, relatives, and friends of all the collaborators for their patience and tolerance of the lost evenings, nights, weekends, and holidays.

Of course, without financial support most of medical studies are not possible. Therefore, I am very grateful from Ms. Noluntu Funani representing The Medical Research Council of South Africa.

A special thanks goes to Walter Sisulu University (WSU) which was established on 1 July, 2005 in terms of the Higher Education Act No 101 of 1997, as amended. WSU, a comprehensive university, resulted from the merger of the former University of Transkei (Unitra); Border Technikon and Eastern Cape Technikon. The new university was named in honour of an icon of the South African liberation struggle and close comrade of Nelson Mandela, the late Walter Max Ulyate Sisulu. Special thanks to Professor LR van Staden, Administator of WSU, Prof Kaya Mfenyana, Head: Office of Vice Chancellor and member of the Joint Technical Task Team of the Department of Higher Education and Training and the Department of Health, Prof. SVS Ngubentombi, Acting Deputy Vice Chancellor Academic Affairs & Research. Dr CA van der Merwe, Interim Deputy Vice Chancellor Planning, Quality Assurance & Development, Prof. GE Ekosse Director: Research Development (WSU), Prof. NE Sokhela, Dean of Faculty of Health Sciences (WSU), Prof JE Iputo Director of the School of Medicine (WSU), Prof. A Awotedu Chairman of the Department of Medicine (WSU), and Dr. TM Madiba Head: Clinical Governance of Mthatha Hospital Complex. A biggest special thanks should be given to Dr. M. Xamlashe the Chief Executive Officer of Mthatha Hospital Complex for his personal support, and his dedication to our hospital and all peoples working here.

In the end, I extend my deepest sense of appreciation to Dr. Roberto Morales Ojeda, Minister of Public Health of Cuba, Dr. Roberto Gonzalez Martin Vice-Minister of the Cuban Ministry of Health, Dr. Luisa Maria Diaz National Director of Postgraduate and Dr. Jorge Delgado Bustillo Deputy Head of National Unit of International Collaboration (CMH), Prof. PhD Nereyda Cantelar de Francisco, Prof. Susana Vázquez PhD, DrSc PAHO/WHO Collaborating Center for Dengue and its Vector "Pedro Kourí" Tropical Medicine Institute, Dr. PhD Reinaldo Menendez and Lic. Maribel Chao also from the National Institute of Tropical Medicine "Pedro Kouri.

Finally, I would like to highlight my deepest sense of appreciation to all my friends, colleagues, collaborators and patients.

Prof. Humberto Foyaca Sibat
Walter Sisulu University, Mthatha
South Africa

Section 1

Cysticercosis

Chapter 1

Introduction to Cysticercosis and Its Historical Background

Humberto Foyaca Sibat and Lourdes de Fátima Ibañez Valdés

Additional information is available at the end of the chapter

http://dx.doi.org/10.5772/50318

1. Introduction

In this chapter we are going to introduce some relevant aspects on neurocysticercosis (NCC) and it's background history in a sequence no previously reported in the medical literature.

Neurocisticercosis is a parasitic infection of central nervous system (CNS) caused by the larval stage (Cysticercus cellulosae) of the pig tapeworm *Taenia solium*. This is the most common helminth to produce CNS infection in human beings. The occurrence of acquired epilepsy or the syndrome of raised intracranial pressure in a person living in or visiting a region where tenacious is endemic or even in one living in close contact with people who have taeniasis should suggest a diagnosis of cysticercosis [1-4].

Neurocysticercosis may remain asymptomatic for months to years and sometimes its diagnosis is made incidentally when neuroimaging is performed. Symptoms and signs are related both: the parasite and the inflammatory-immunological response of the host. NCC is the most common cause of acquired epilepsy worldwide and most of the patients taking valproate acid, sodium valproate or carbamazepine for a proper control of their seizures, respond very well [2,5].

Neurocysticercosis is also an important cause of ischemic stroke secondary to infectious vasculitis [4]. The most common cause of epilepsy due to NCC is a calcified lesion with or without evidence of perilesional edema. The prognosis of this situation is worse when there is an associated intraventricular cyst that usually does not respond well to praziquantel and then Albendazole should be prescribed [6].

Parasitic diseases have occurred through the times and they caused more deaths and economic damage to humanity that all the genocidal wars together. Generally in countries with little socioeconomic development is where parasitic diseases occur more frequently, still favored this due to the climatic conditions (warm or temperate) and by the lack of

INTECH
open science | open minds

© 2013 Foyaca Sibat and de Fátima Ibañez Valdés, licensee InTech. This is a paper distributed under the terms of the Creative Commons Attribution License (http://creativecommons.org/licenses/by/3.0), which permits unrestricted use, distribution, and reproduction in any medium, provided the original work is properly cited.

health education in the population; as in the developed countries social, medical and economic, the parasitic diseases have been eradicated or have very little significance [4,7].

The NCC is a disease closely related to poverty in general, and in particular with a poor personal hygiene and lack of food hygiene, sociocultural and environmental factors, education for health in the community, and also very closely related to the sanitary conditions of each region. This is a preventable disease and able to be eradicated [8], which currently affects more than 50 million people around the world, of which 400 thousand lives in Latin America [9].

According to WHO figures confirmed by Roman and collaborators [10] around 50 thousand people die each year as a result of the NCC and epilepsy secondary to NCC (ESNCC).

The infection by *T solium* produces two different diseases: taeniasis (TE) and/or cysticercosis (CC). When humans eat eggs of *T. solium* they acquire CC that can be found in any tissue including heart, liver, lungs, and peritoneal cavity [11-16]. The location of the cysticercus (CT) in the CNS and in the retina (considering the retina as an extension of the CNS) is called NCC and is considered the most important neurological disease of parasitic origin in humans and the main cause of late-onset epilepsy [16-18]. Cysts of NCC are located mainly at the distal vascular territory in the cortical gray substance or at the level of the connection between substance gray and white where the blood supply is remarkable including in HIV patients [19].

It is considered that the CC is an important health problem in several developing countries where the social, economic and cultural conditions favor the maintenance of this zoonotic disease and it is seen as a growing community problem in those developed countries with a high rate of immigrants from endemic areas. WHO includes the NCC between neglected diseases or forgotten that cause a significant impact on the economy in several regions from all over the world. It affects 4% of the population in endemic areas [20, 21] where hygiene, habits-food and sometimes religious trends can determine the incidence and prevalence of the disease, for example: The Islam [4].

Islam was not the first religion to prohibit the consumption of pork, before the made Judaism with perhaps less severe restrictions, of all forms no ingestion of pork is not a defense to acquire the NCC, in fact have been reported cases in the Jewish community in New York [22].

Due to globalization, a growing number of uncontrolled immigrants coming from an endemic area of Latin America come to the USA every day, significantly increasing the number of cases of the NCC in the country especially in Texas and California. [11-13, 17,18,22-27]

In total 1494 patients with NCC were confirmed between 1980 and 2004 of which 66% suffered from epilepsy, 16% had an obstructive hydrocephalus and 15% headache due to NCC (91 %), intraventricular (6 %) or subarachnoid (2 %) either because travelled to endemic areas, were of Hispanic origin or had any contact with carriers of the parasite. (Wallin & Kurtzke, 2004; Uddin et al. , 2010)

In Latin America has been described the existence of the NCC in 18 countries with an estimated 350,000 patients infected by the complex CC/TE. In the year 2008, Pawlowski stipulated that in the world would have approximately 2.5 million people infected *T solium* and at least 20 million with CC. In his manuscript, Hotez [9] reported that in the United States were documented between one and two cases of NCC per year, considering that in the growing Latin population could have more than 41,000 Hispanics suffer from NCC [9, 28, 29].

The NCC is also frequent in certain countries in Europe such as Romania, Poland and even Portugal. In Spain the growing vogue of the migration of individuals coming from endemic areas has conditioned an increase in the frequency of this entity [30]. Apart from intraparenhymal NCC (NCCIp), there are some uncommon locations in the NCC that can be divided into: ventricular NCC (NCCiv), subarachnoid NCC (NCCSa), intraspinal NCC (NCCIs), and intraocular NCC (NCCIo) and there many well documented cases reported in the international medical literature [3,4, 31-59]. Some authors report a list of frequencies for these presentations including combinations among them, that we reproduce as follow: NCCIp (55.23 %), NCCIv (15.69 %), NCCSa (11.63 %), NCCIm (3.4 %), NCCIo (0.58 %), and insular neurocysticercosis (NCCI) (0.68 %) and the frequency of demonstrations combined in the following manner: Iv-IP (6.98 %), SA-IP (3.49 %) and SA-Iv (2.32 %) [4, 38].

In a hospital-based study conducted in Mexico, a rate of up to 8.6 cases of NCC for each 100 hospitalized is reported, and in the series of autopsies performed on up to 2 453 per 100 000 inhabitants and it is pointed out that 43.3 % of the cases were asymptomatic [34] and 80% were autopsy findings [60]. Official statistics report an annual average of 500 cases of NCC, with a national rate of raw 0.6 per 100,000 inhabitants [61-63] this report does not include cases uncovered by the health personnel or that were not included in the study for other reasons, it does not include the extra– parenchymal presentations, or other forms of CC as well. In Brazil, the prevalence in autopsies varies from 0.12 to 9%, in the series of clinical cases varies from 0.03 to 7.5 %, and in sero-epidemiological studies from 0.6 to 5.2 %. [64] In Colombia there is not much information on the NCC, only some work in the departments of Antioquia and Santander that reported the 1 and 2% of affectation to the population, and 2% in Ecuador. [65,66] On the other hand, has been estimated that over 50 million people are infected with the complex TE/CC in the world, of which 350 thousand lives in Latin America [67] especially in those countries that do not have an adequate infrastructure and the level of education for an appropriate health. [18, 68] The main risk factors associated with the CC are the presence of TE in members of the community, free-range pigs ingesting contaminated human feces [69] and the use of infested feces as agricultural fertilizer.[70] The NCC has become a public health problem in different countries of Africa, Asia and Latin America. [18, 71-78] Patients presenting NCC in Dominican Republic are located in the southern region and most of then are admitted with epilepsy. [79] In Venezuela the characteristics of the disease are also known and in spite of the fact that there are not many articles published in indexed journals, it was able to obtain some information from summaries of medical congresses [80,81], brochures for teaching purposes [82] and other printed materials [83-85]. In a study conducted in the Teaching Hospital of Maracaibo

(Zulia state), patients diagnosed with CTs or MRI in a period of 10 years, they reported clinical features of 15 patients with NCC. In this study, data obtained were recorded in a protocol sheet with 30 different aspects and analysis of the data is reported with absolute numbers or percentages. The most frequent clinical manifestations were the following: headache (27 %), seizures (20 %), blurred vision (13 %), nausea and vomiting (13 %), dizziness and vertigo (13 %), loss of consciousness (7 %) and in a 7% loss of muscle strength. [86]

Headache (hemicranial or bilateral) is a common symptom to almost all forms of NCC and it is often confused with migraine without aura or tension headaches. This aspect has been disseminated through the popular television program "Dr. House" by what is known by a large audience [87], however in the rest of the studies analyzed the convulsive manifestations were the most frequent clinical manifestation of the NCC and it was observed in 50% to 80% of cases, particularly in patients with lesions in the brain parenchyma for both: children and adults. [4,5 13, 18, 23,24, 34, 61, 67,70,86, 88- 105]

The prevalence of epilepsy has been studied in several African countries. In a rural area of northern Tanzania , 7,399 people were surveyed and found a prevalence for the epilepsy of a 11.2 /1.000 [95% CI 8.9 -13.9/1.000] prevalence for the active epilepsy was: 8.7 /1.000 (95% CI 6.7 -11/1.000) with a predominance of females, the average incidence in the last five years was 81.1 /100,000 (95% CI 65- 101/100,000), 54% (45 of 83) of the respondents were widespread attacks of unknown cause. The 71% (59 of 83) of the epileptic seizures had not been dealt with in an institution of public health and 76% (63 of 83) had never received treatment with DAE [106]. In 2005, de Preux & Druet-Cabanac [107] reported that studies on the incidence and prevalence of epilepsy in the sub-Saharan Africa is very scarce but the prevalence of epilepsy is two or three times higher in tropical countries compared with highly developed countries. Very few cases-control studies have been conducted on the African continent in search of the most common causes of epilepsy but all authors agree that the NCC is without doubt the most frequent cause of epilepsy in the sub-Saharan Africa. [107]

2. Background information

A known scientist said: "The past is the key to the present. Historical studies involving tapeworms contribute to a predictive foundation for understanding today's environments and communities of living things. Besides telling us something about their hosts, parasites can tell us about their geographical links to long ago. They're both the products of a current environment and, at the same time, of a long ancestry reflecting millions of years of association with their hosts." [108].

Homo ergaster is represented by fossils such as "Nariokotome Boy" (Figure 1). They lived during the Lower Pleistocene epoch (dated at between 1.51 and 1.56 million years old), with fossils dated between 1.8 and 1.2 million years old. Some scientists have split *H. erectus* into three separate species, based on the geographic region in which specimens have been found: *H. ergaster* (Africa), *H. erectus* (Asia), and *H. heidelbergensis* (Europe). However, the discovery of *H. ergaster* fossils outside Africa are forcing a reanalysis of this species. *H. ergaster* has thinner cranial bones, a higher cranial vault, a less robust face and lighter frame than *H. erectus.* [109] For the case made in this listing, all *erectus*like specimens from African will fall under the classification of *Homo ergaster*.

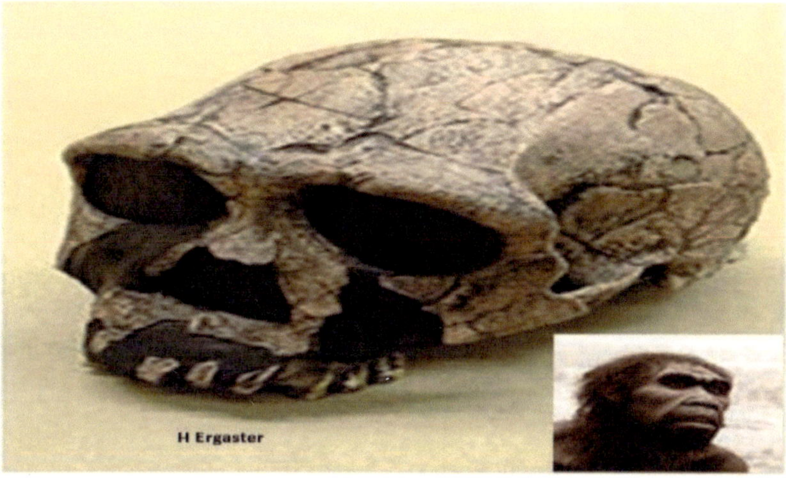

Figure 1. Shows shape of the face and skull of the H Ergaster who is the ancestor of later Homo populations [109].

The use and control fire, a milestone in human development, occurred 1 to l. 5 million years ago. Control of fire may have enabled *Homo erectus* to migrate out of Africa. *H. ergaster* fossil finds are not associated with evidence of fire use. Modern humans share the same differences as *H. ergaster* with the Asian *H. erectus,* leading to the possibility that *H. ergaster* is the ancestor of later Homo populations. [109]

As a clue to a part of our evolutionary history, scientists have studied the evolutionary relationships of our host-specific taeniid tapeworms: *Taenia saginata, T. asiatica* and *T. solium* and those of other species. [108]

This is done by looking at genetic and host differences among tapeworm species. A tapeworm's life cycle is adapted to its parasitic existence. For taeniids, this center upon a predator-prey relationship, with a carnivore carrying the adult tapeworm and a herbivore hosting the infective larvae. Evolutionary relatives of our tapeworm are usually found in the intestines of carnivores such as lions, hyenas or African wild dogs.

Tapeworms that plague humanity originated in carnivores such as lions and hyenas, and jumped to humans after we began eating their prey animals on the African savannah.

This contradicts the long-held view that humans acquired tapeworms from our domesticated livestock, cattle and swine, following the agricultural revolution around 10,000 years ago.

In a 2001 published paper by Eric Hoberg [108] and his collaborators about the origins of the Taenia tapeworms in humans based on genetic analysis of a wide variety of tapeworm species they found that the human-infecting varieties were most closely related to those that infect modern lions and hyenas. According to Hoberg and his colleagues, tapeworms probably jumped from predators to humans between 2 and 2.5 Mya, when hominids inhabited savannah environments in sub-Saharan Africa and were likely hunting or scavenging the same prey favored by hyenas and lions. Of the three tapeworms that infect people today, the researchers linked one, *T solium,* closer to a species that uses hyenas and African hunting dogs as its hosts. The other two, *T. saginata* and *T. asiatica,* are linked more closely to a species with lions as its host. Because *T. solium* and the pair *T. saginata/T. asiatica* are only distantly related, it appears that two tapeworms independently made the jump to hominids: the ancestor of *T. solium,* and a single parent species of both *T. saginata* and *T. asiatica.* The hyenas in a group are more dangerous than the lions but easier to repel what may have favored a preference for food hunted by hyenas. The amount of genetic difference between *T. saginata* and *T. asiatica* suggests that they split from a single human-adapted species by 160,000 years ago. [108] Worm-carrying human populations may have migrated out of Africa at or before this time, leading to the separation of parasite populations that evolved into the two species. Cattle eventually became the intermediate host in T. saginata, pigs in T. asiatica.

In 2001, Hoberg [108] said: "Surprisingly, rather than humans' acquiring *Taenia* from cattle and pigs, we believe man gave tapeworms to these domestic animals, because the association between *tuna* and hominids was established before the domestication of these food animals" and second because humans are the most important element in the *T solium* transmission. Of course, if we take into account that the process of domestication of animal begins some 10 000 years ago and even many of them do not hates in sub-Saharan Africa then it is easy to understand that it was the man who infested cattle and pigs and not in the opposite direction. Probable we owe an apology to the porcine population because we have been blaming something whose responsibility was our ancestors, we think.

Tapeworms are a large group from the so-called 'flatworm' family (known technically as the Platyhelminthes), which are relatively simple creatures with no body cavity, heart, circulatory system or lungs. They are evolutionary simpler than the unrelated but misleadingly similarly named 'roundworms' (also called nematodes), which also parasites humans and animals. Like most tapeworms, these parasites have a relatively simple life cycle involving a definitive predator host in which the adults live, and an intermediate host in which juveniles reside as tissue cysts called cysticerci. When the predatory definitive host eats (undercooked) meat infected with cysticerci, the cysts hatch and adult worms can grow to meters in size in the definitive host's intestines, producing eggs which pass in the feces and are eaten by the herbivorous intermediate hosts, where upon cysticerci form in the tissues and the life cycle is completed. [108]

Scientists have traditionally adopted an 'anthropophilic' view in which humans acquired *T. saginata* and *T. asiatica* from ancestors of cows, and *T. solium* from ancestors of pigs, following the domestication of these species. But Hoberg's work turns this on its head: one of the closest relatives of *T. saginata* and *T. asiatica* is *T. simbae.* As you might guess from the name, this is a tapeworm whose definitive host is the African lion ('Simba' is Swahili for lion). *T. simbae* cycles between antelope and lions in a typical predator-prey lifecycle.

Similarly, the closest relative of *T. solium* is *T. hyaenae*, which cycles between the predatory hyena and various prey species including Impala and the Sable antelope [108], examination of the evolutionary histories of hosts and parasites and DNA (Shampa, 2009) evidence shows that over 10,000 years ago, ancestors of modern humans in Africa became exposed to tapeworm when they scavenged for food or preyed on the antelopes and bovids, and later passed the infection on to domestic animals such as pigs.

It is assumed that early human ancestors generally had parasites, but until recently there was no evidence to support this claim. Generally, the discovery of parasites in ancient humans relies on the study of feces and other fossilized material. The earliest known parasite in a human was eggs of the lung fluke found in fossilized feces in northern Chile and is estimated to be from around 5900BC. There are also claims of hookworm eggs from around 5000BC in Brazil and large roundworm eggs from around 2330BC in Peru. Tapeworm eggs have also been found present in Egyptian mummies dating from around 2000BC, 1250BC, and 1000BC along with a well preserved and calcified female worm inside of a mummy. [112]

Medical researchers at the Pasteur Institute of Madagascar have travelled around the country, gathering tapeworm from different regions. They isolated DNA from 13 of the samples and then compared their genetic sequences to see how they were related from one to another and to tapeworms from other parts of the world. The family tree of tapeworms they got was strangely ancient and alien. In many cases, the closest relatives of tapeworms on Madagascar are not other tapeworms. The tapeworms that live in the southwest part of the island are closely related to tapeworms hundreds of miles away, in Africa. The tapeworms in other parts of the island are more closely related to tapeworms thousands of miles away, in south Asia.

The scientists then tallied up the mutations in each lineage of tapeworm to figure out how long ago they had split off from a common ancestor. All the *T. solium* tapeworms the scientists studied descend from a common ancestor that lived about 680,000 years ago. The southwest Madagascar tapeworms and the tapeworms of Africa share a common ancestor that lived 235,000 years ago. All of the Madagascar and Asian tapeworms share a common ancestor that lived about 260,000 years ago. The Madagascar tapeworms and their very closest Asian relatives share an ancestor that lived 85,000 years ago. [113]

Pigs and cows were only domesticated within the past 11,000 years or so. The best way to find clues to how these tapeworms colonized us is to compare them to the 39 species of *Taenia* tapeworms that infect wild animals. Eric Hoberg, found that most *Taenia* tapeworms form cysts in wild ungulates, such as antelopes, and then become adults in the carnivores that eat their intermediate hosts. The closest relatives of all three human tapeworms live in Africa. Hyenas are the hosts of the closest relatives of pork tapeworms, while lions are the hosts of the closest relative to the other two species, T. saginata and T. asiatica. Hoberg and his colleagues compared the mutations in the DNA of T. *saginata* and T. asiatica and found that their common ancestor lived somewhere between 780,000 and 1.71 Mya. [108]

The new results from Madagascar fit in nicely with Hoberg's results. Hundreds of thousands of years ago, our ancestors lived in Africa, where they scavenged meat from ungulates. In so doing, it appears, they stepped into the life cycle of *Taenia* tapeworms. Tapeworms that might have ended up in the gut of a hyena or a lion ended up in the gut of our ancestors instead. Over thousands of years, some populations of these tapeworms adapted to our scavenger ancestors. These were the common ancestors of today's human tapeworms, whose great antiquity is now recorded in the DNA of living tapeworms.

The genealogy of the tapeworms also matches up nicely with the human history of Madagascar. People only arrived on the island 2000 years ago. They came from two directions. Bantu farmers sailed from the west of Africa across the Mozambique channel. Asians came from the east, traveling thousands of miles across the Indian Ocean from Indonesia. Malagasy culture emerged from the mingling of these two origins. That culture also includes the livestock that the Bantu and Indonesians brought to the island. And those animals brought parasites with them that had been separated for almost 700,000 years, reaching back to a time when our ancestors had yet to invent fire or spoken language. [113]

In the other hand Hoberg says: "Pathogenic macro parasites, like tapeworms, have parasitized the world's vertebrates and invertebrates for millions of years," "And although they remain a constant threat to economically important fisheries, livestock, and wildlife, only about one-third have been described or named". "Our incomplete knowledge and understanding of taxonomy and species-level relationships of these parasites have hindered our full understanding of their host associations—final and intermediate—and their potential for causing disease." [108]

Southern Africa has provided scientists with a steady flow of Australopithecines, from its numerous caves and quarries. The geological structures here differ quite differently from those in Eastern Africa, in ways that are not as productive to the paleoanthropologist. Although it is not flat by any means, Southern Africa does not have the ground exposure in the form of gorges and ancient river beds, as is the case in the east.

These are phylogenetic studies based on comparative morphology. There is also ongoing research dealing with molecular data, primarily with a research group in Finland. The current hypothesis under examination is that T. solium is related to an assemblage of species that circulate in hyenas, and that *T. saginata* + *T. asiatica* (which are sister species) are related to parasites in lions. Both appear to have emerged from Africa. The implication was that the origins of those species now host-specific in humans is related to host switches driven by ecological connections established prior to the origins of modern humans. Current studies suggest that it may be more complicated as the molecular data still support a host switch from carnivores to hominids, but the context may be somewhat different, some papers by Laivikainen, Haukisalmi and their colleagues in Helsinki are exploring Taenia phylogeny. (Dr. Hoberg, personal communication on March, 16, 2012)

3. Ancient times

The Biblical Hebrews may have inherited a number of their beliefs from ancient Mesopotamian cultures, among them a conviction that the disease was divine punishment and therefore a mark of sin. This belief was passed on as a basic concept to Christian Medieval Europe. Assyro-Babylonian taboos against close proximity to the sick were also continued by the Hebrews in their isolation of the unclean, who, in addition to the diseased, included the dead, a potential source of soul transference among the Mesopotamian peoples. [114]

The first written records of what are almost certainly parasitic infections come from a period of Egyptian medicine from 3000 to 400 BC, particularly the Ebers papyrus of 1500 BC discovered at Thebes (Bryan, 1930).

In the writings of Greek physicians between 800 to 300 BC, such as the collected works of Hippocrates, known as the *Corpus Hippocratorum,* and from physicians from other civilizations including China (3000 to 300 BC), India (2500 to 200 BC), Rome (700 BC to 400 BC), and the Arab Empire in the latter part of the first millennium, we can find information about parasites as well. As time passed, the descriptions of parasitic infections became more accurate and Arabic physicians, particularly by Rhaze. [112]

Hippocrates was the first physician to systematically classify diseases based on points of similarity and contrast between them. He virtually originated the disciplines of etiology and pathology. By systematically classifying diseases, Hippocrates placed their diagnosis and treatment on a sounder footing. Hippocrates lived a very long life and died at a ripe old age in the town of Larissa in Thessaly. [115]

Hippocrates, Aristotle and Theophrastus called flatworms to worms responsible, either from its resemblance with tapes or ribbons, that Paracelso and Pliny the Elder poured into the Latin and the expression "lubricious latus", worm width. The Arabic medicine, with Serapione also to the head, thought that each proglottid was a worm different. Muslims imposed owning restricted the name "cucurbitineos", not only for its resemblance to the owning miles of the pumpkin, but also because these were one of the oldest remedies against tenacious, still in use. Is attributed to Arnau de Vilanova, at the beginning of the 14th century, the first description of the species. Reflected the old error that only had one parasite per person. [116]

Rhazes was one of the most prolific Muslim doctors and probably second only to Ibn Sina in his accomplishments. He born at Ray, Iran and became a student of Hunayn ibn Ishaq and later a student of Ali ibn Rabban. He wrote over 200 books, including Kitab al-Mansuri, ten volumes on Greek medicine, and al-Hawi, an encyclopedia of medicine in 20 volumes where some advices about the management of parasitic diseases are given [117].

Dioscorides was the first to organize the *material medica* into therapeutic groupings of drugs, based on similarities of medicinal action [118]. We have strong reasons to think that Dioscorides contributed remarkably to the pharmacological treatment of parasitic diseases in ancient times [118]. If we consider that even the traditional Chinese herbal *materia medica* is organized according to similar therapeutic groupings of herbs, we can see exactly how influential and far-reaching were Dioscorides' revolutionary new ideas.

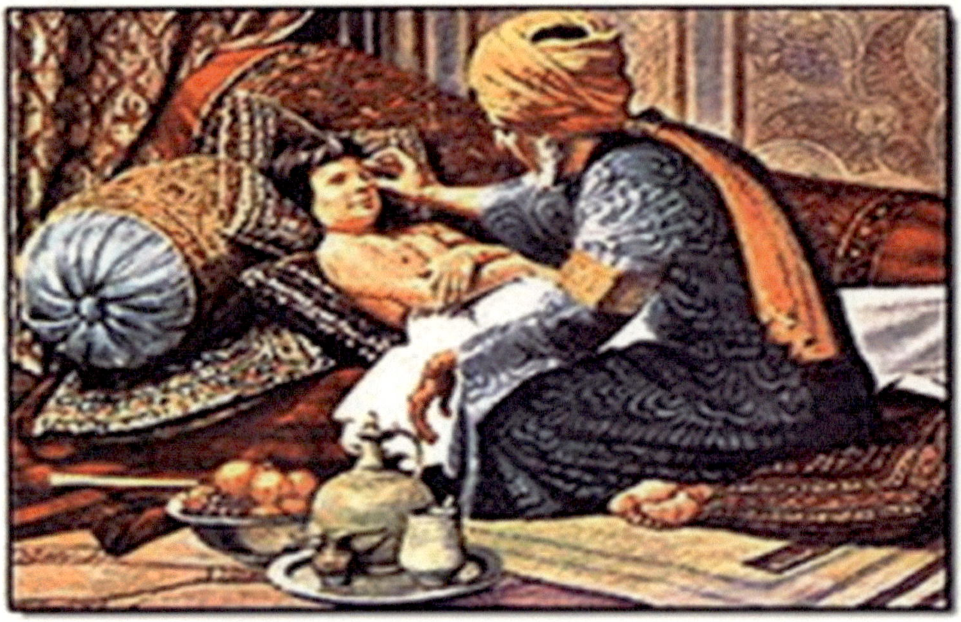

Figure 2. Abu Bakr Muhammad Ibn Zakariya al-Razi (865-925 AD) , known as Rhazes.

Dioscorides' therapeutic groupings by medicinal action have a dynamic, kinetic character: warming, binding, softening, drying, cooling, concocting, relaxing, nourishing and the like.

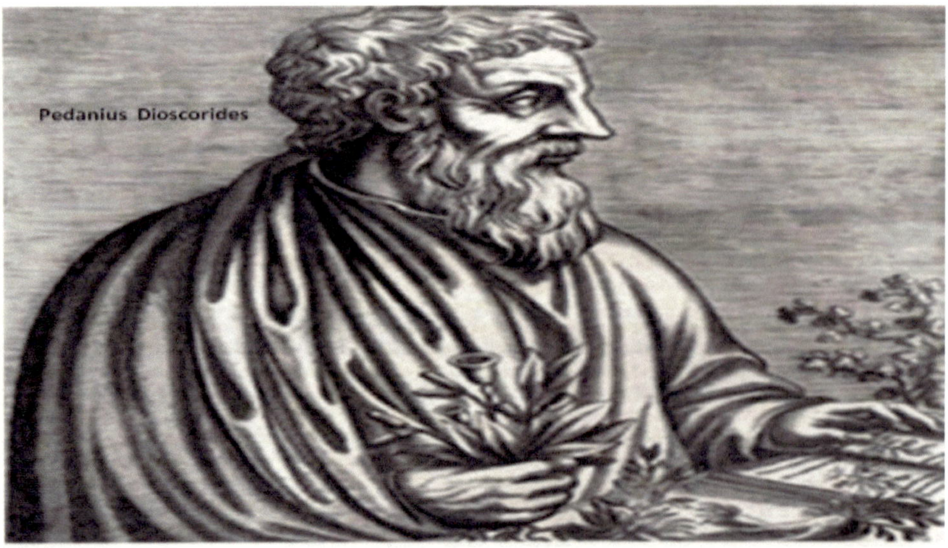

Figure 3. Pedanius Dioscorides was born around 30 A.D. at Anazarbius (Turkey) in Asia Minor.

The hallmark of infection with the adult worm has been the release of proglottids in the stool. They are also considered symptoms of taeniosis: discomfort abdominal, flatulence, weight loss, and other gastrointestinal disturbances. However, the field research reveals that patients with taeniosis tended to be asymptomatic; not even half the who claim to have past proglottids with bowel movements, however some author reported that the earliest clinical references to tapeworms were found in the works of the ancient Egyptians that date back to *almost 2000 BC.* The background of Cysticercosis as a disease of pigs goes back in ancient times. In the 3th century BC, Aristotle was an epileptic patient probable due to cysticercosis of his brain and in his work "The history of animals", describes the presence of cysticercosis in the tongue and muscles of pigs. Afterwards Plinio (25-79 BC) names the adult form of the parasite *Taenia* (from the Greek *tainia,* which means "lace" or "strip" The background of cysticercosis as a disease of pigs goes back in ancient times.[119]

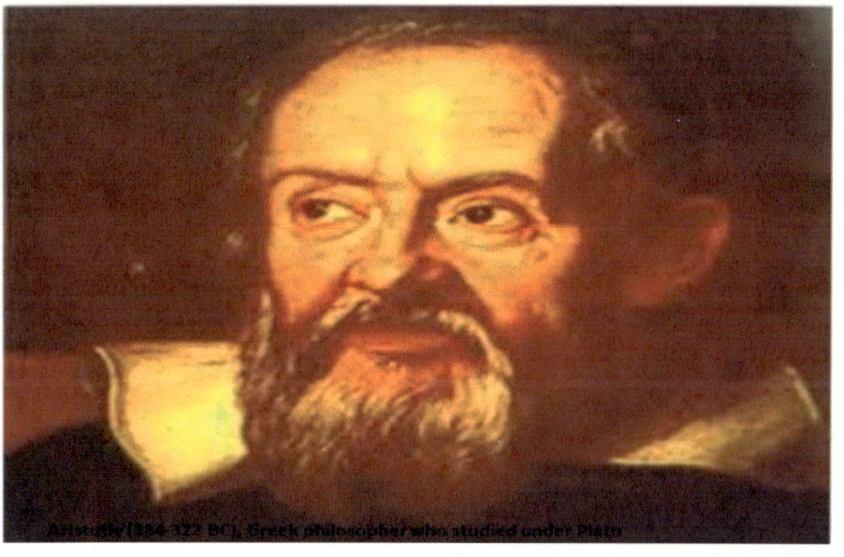

Figure 4. Aristotle (384–322 BC), the greatest and most influential of all the Greek philosophers. Aristotle was born at the town of Stageira in the year 384 B.C. His father, Nikomachus, was the friend and physician of Amyntas II, king of Macedonia, father of Philip II and grandfather of Alexander the Great. The description of measles pork in the History of Animals written by Aristotle in the 4th century showed that the infection of pork with tapeworm was known to ancient Greeks at that time [120]. In his treatise "History of animals" Aristotle accurately describes the presence of parasitic larvae in the musculature of the pig: "... The pigs with the soft meat have bladders that are like snowflakes hailing in the region of the thighs, neck and loins; these are the areas that are normally displayed. If there are few, meat is lean; if there are many, meat becomes soft and filled with serous fluid. The pigs that are suffering from this disease are easily recognized, the bladders can be seen on the inner surface of the tongue where they are particularly abundant"; this reference reports clearly pictures of porcine cysticercosis and its main location on the tongue and muscles of the pig. [120]

We could not find enough information to confirm what role Galen played in the management of patients with NCC despite he was the greatest physician of ancient Rome. Whereas Hippocrates laid the foundation of Greek Medicine, Galen further developed its theory and practice, and carried Greco-Roman medicine to its zenith. Galen became the personal physician to the emperor Marcus Aurelius. [121]

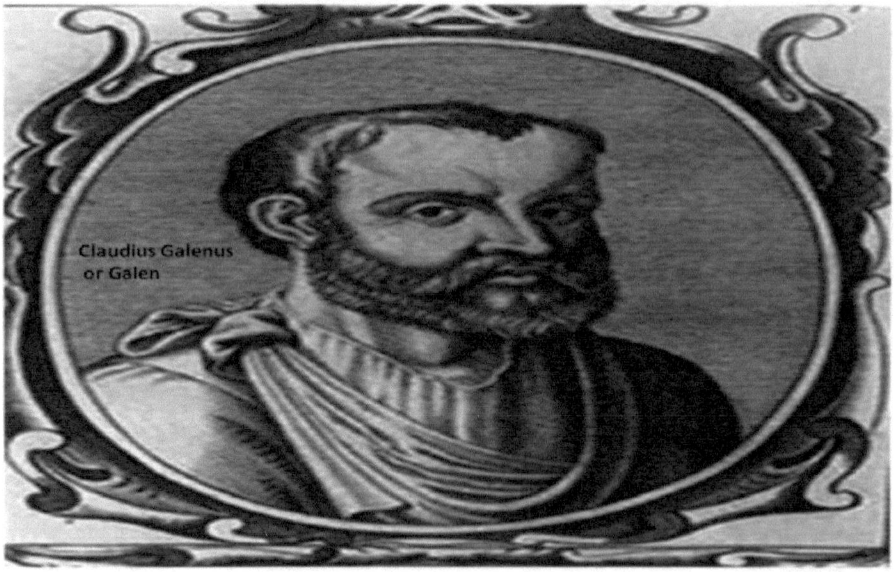

Figure 5. Claudius Galenus, or Galen, was born in Pergamum, an old Greek city on the Aegean coast of Asia Minor, or present day Turkey, in the year 130 A.D.

Theraric was an herbal jam or electuary with some 64 different ingredients that was a virtual panacea or cure-all for many diseases, and an antidote to many poisons made by Galen. Theriac's use and manufacture continued until the late 19th century. Since Venice was a key center for its manufacture, it is sometimes called Theriac Venezian, or Venice Treacle. Today, Theriac Venezian is a key ingredient in Swedish Bitters, an herbal elixir popularized by the Austrian herbalist Maria Treben. [121] We strongly suspect that Theriac was a medication of choice for many patients presenting parasitic diseases inlcuding *T solium* but we found no way to probe it, and unfortunately most of the 80 Galen's treatises are missing.

At this time, there was strong suspicion about contaminated food and parasitic diseases, it was also known to Jewish [114] and later to early Muslim physicians and has been proposed as one of the reasons for pork being forbidden by Jewish and Islamic dietary laws but most probable they had other reasons. Much has been made of a presumably medical basis for the food prohibitions in Jewish tradition, but there may be other explanations. One recent suggestion is that the taboo against pigs was originally related to their competition with humans for water and grain (scarce commodities in a barren land), in contrast to cattle and sheep which consume relatively little water and graze on forage inedible to man.

The rules prohibiting the intake of pork in the religions that have appeared in the Hellenistic period such as the Judaic and later the Muslim possibly related to this and other parasite in muscles. Some of the rules of the Koran are clear indications hygienic aimed at the prevention: "believers brush your arms up to the elbow ... And brush your feet until the ankle. If one of you comes to make their needs recourse than to clean sand, in has revealed to me there is nothing that prohibits eating, except dead meat, bloodshed, or pork that is a diet ... " (Koran 6, 145).

In the Bible also makes reference to dietary measures that can be taken as a standard of prevention for different types of zoonoses including the cysticercosis: "between the animals and everyone who has-hoofed and that chews the eat. But rumian or have hoof, not to eat these: the camel, because he chewed but does not have-hoofed, I shall unclean. Also, because he chewed but does not have hoof, you will have him unclean. Also the hare, because ruminating but does not have hoof, you will have as unclean. Also the pig, because has a split hoof, and is-hoofed, but not chew the cud, what ye shall "unclean" [Leviticus 11.3 -7].

The contribution from the Islamic world cannot be ignored. Abu Ali al-Husayn ibn Abd Allah ibn Sina, known in the West as Avicenna, was a highly respected Persian physician whose medical treatise, the *Canon of Medicine,* influenced medical practice for centuries. At the age of 16, he already had a reputation as an authority in legal and medical matters [123]

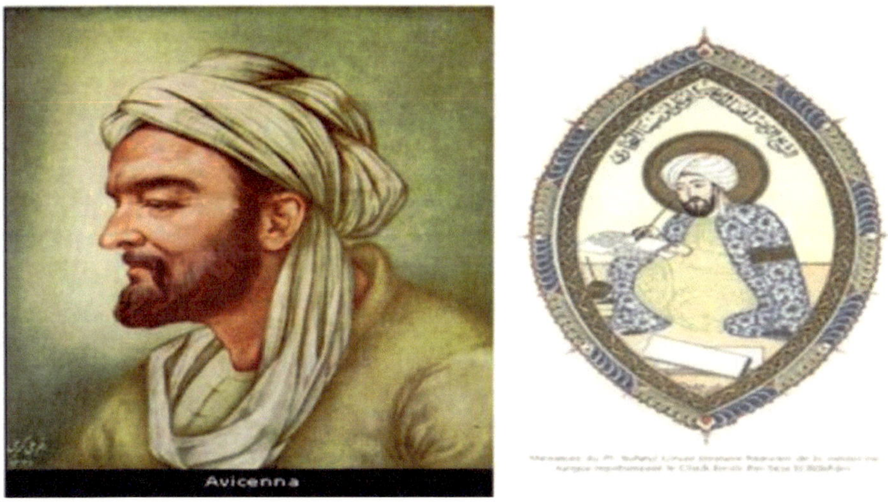

Figure 6. Avicenna was born in 980 A.D. near Bokhara, an ancient center of culture and learning in Persia.

For centuries, Avicenna's Canon was a standard textbook in many European medical schools. Even today, it is the standard reference manual for practitioners of Umami Medicine where some guidelines on management of parasitic diseases were included. [124] In 1524, Paracelsus returned home to Europe. He lectured and wrote in German instead of Latin. His classes were filled to overflowing.

In 1536 Paracelsus published his masterwork *Der grossen Wundartzney,* which restored his reputation virtually overnight. Paracelsus (name modified by himself) suspected that epilepsy of a sick priest derived from the presence of brain cysts. After Paracelsus first suspicion of epilepsy secondary to parasitic disease of the brain, it is not well elucidated exactly when the NCC was really confirmed for the first time in the history of medicine. As a general agreement it is accepted that NCC is a millennial disease about which there is an early description made Paracelsus and another three centuries later on its relationship with the parasitic infection by T solium. [125, 126]

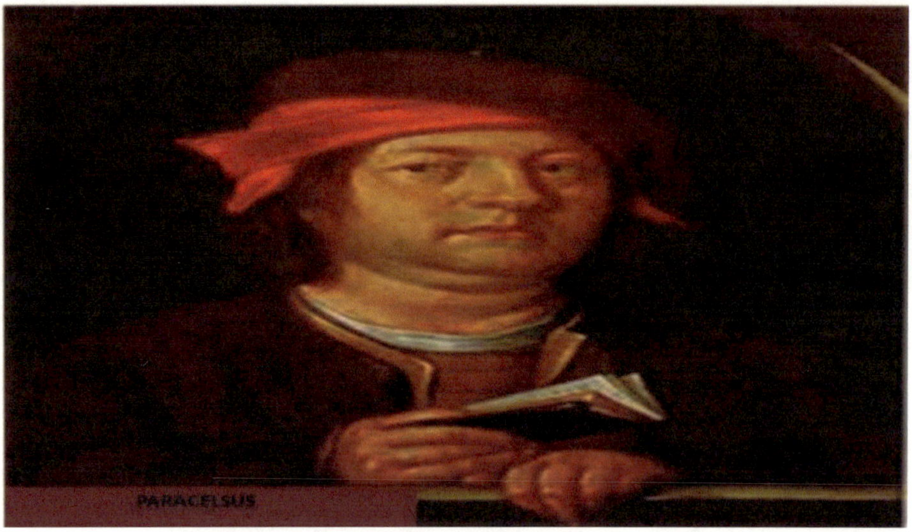

Figure 7. Paracelsus' reputation as a great doctor preceded him.

The first reference to a case of human cysticercosis we owe it to Johannes Udalric Rumler in 1558, who attributed it to a tumor of the dura mater of an epileptic patient but better description was made by Celsus however, the connection between tapeworms and cysticercosis had not been recognized at that time. [112, 127]

Some authors have raised the NCC helped change the history of the ancient world in the person of Julius César whose epilepsy late-onset (54 years old) greatly influenced their behavior. [128] Domenico Panarolus in 1652 noted similar cysts in the corpus callosum of the brain of another epileptic seizure. But not alludes to its parasitic character up to 1697, when Marcello Malpighi discovered the animal origin of these cysts and described the scolex. [129]

In 1784, Johann August Ephraim Goeze, alien to the work of the Malpighi re-examined in the cysticerci pork and identified its nature helminthic owning. Two years later, P. C. Werner rediscovered the human cysticercosis owning an in the autopsy of a soldier; found two cysts in the pectoral muscle that reminded him they observed in porcine cysticercosis. [129]

In this same period Morgagni determines the similarities between the cysticerci of pork and those found in human musculature. The "had hidatogena was described by Fischer in 1789. In 1818 it gives you the name of "cysticerci fisherianus" attributed to Laenec on the basis of "kistis" bladder, "kestus tail, and "fisherianus" in honor of its discoverer. Was Laenec who first introduced the term "cellullosae" [130].

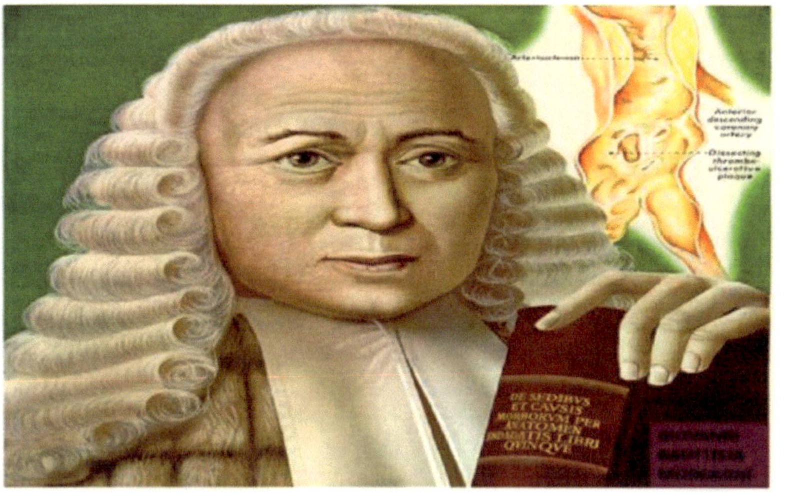

Figure 8. Giovanni Battista Morgagni: Italian anatomist and pathologist, born in February 25, 1682, Forlì; died December 5, 1771, Padua.

In 1829, the first description of the infestation of cysticercus to the anterior chamber of the eye is made [130] being it the first report about active cysticercus in living people. He believed in contagion and would not dissect patients with tuberculosis or smallpox. Virchow considered that Morgagni introduced modern pathology, «with him begins modern medicine» in summary he made discoveries similar to those of Paracelsus [132].

Abraham Gottlob Werner (German geologist) was born in Wehrau, Upper Lusatia, now Polish Osiecznica, on 25 September 1749. In 1786, Werner determines the similarities between the cysticerci of pork and those found in human musculature. That controversy was the focus of much geological activity through the end of the 18th century, and well into the 19th centure and although at the end of the 18th century taeniosis and cysticercosis were well known by him because the biological cycle of the parasite is ignored, the association between them was not identified among the greatest scientific at that time [133]. Goes in 1784 and Felix Dujardin in 1845 noted similarities in the shape of the scolex of the adult worms with the cysticerci and suspected a relationship between the two [129].

A first step was taken in the discovered owning of the eggs of flatworms. Some were raised then the formation of the adult worm. The "taenia hidatigena" was brought by Fischer in 1789. René-Théophile-Hyacinthe Laennec invented the stethoscope in 1816, while working at the Hôpital Necker and pioneered its use in diagnosing various chest conditions [134].

Laennec was a gifted student, he learned English and German, and began his medical studies under his uncle's direction. Laennec studied medicine in Paris under several famous physicians, including

Dupuytren and Nicolas Corvisart des Marest [130]. He was trained to use sound as a diagnostic aid. Corvisart advocated the re-introduction of percussion during the French Revolution. Laennec was a devout Catholic. He was noted as a very kind man and his charity to the poor became proverbial [134]. In 1818 the name "cysticerci fisherianus" was given by Laenec based on "kistis" bladder, "kestus queue, and "fisherianus" in honor of its discoverer. Was Laenec who first introduced the term "cellullosae" [131].

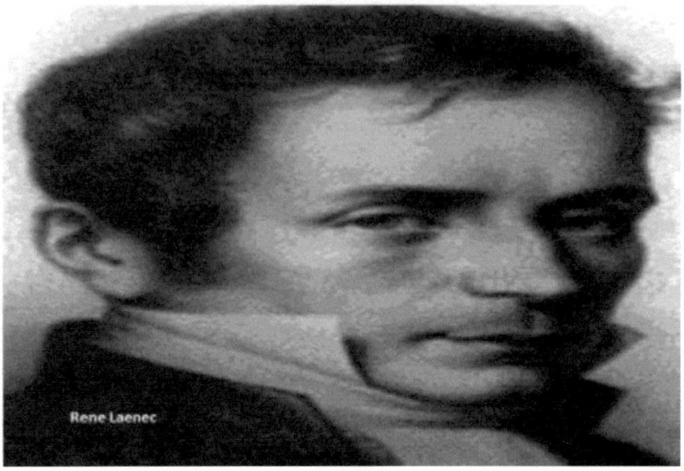

Figure 9. Laennec (17 February 1781 – 13 August 1826) was a French physician.

The first description of the infestation of cysticercus to the anterior chamber of the eye is made in 1829 [130].

The development of cysticerci in pigs has been demonstrated in 1853 when Pierre Joseph Van beneden fed to a pig with T. solium eggs and found cysticerci in the muscles during necropsy. Van beneden used as animal control to another pig that was kept in the same conditions, but without giving eggs; in this found no cysticerci. At this time Van Manedem sets out the "law of the transmigration of the tapeworms" [130].

Two years later, in a controversial study, Friedrich Kuchen showed that tapeworms are developed from cysticerci.

Around 1850, Kuchenmeister fed pig meat containing cysticerci of T. solium to humans awaiting execution in a prison, and after they had been executed, he recovered the developing and adult tapeworms in their intestines. By the middle of the 19th century, it was established that cysticercosis was caused by the ingestion of the eggs of T. solium (Shampa, 2009)

In December 1854, Aloys Humbert is auto infected eating 13 cysticerci; toward March of the following year began to expel segments of T. solium [129].

The first pathological descriptions and their respective clinical correlations were made by Virchow in 1860, who also identified the location basal meningeal of this parasite calling cysticerci multilocularis" [130].

Leuckart earned his degree from the University of Göttingen, where he was a student of Rudolf Wagner (1805-1864). Leuckart is remembered for his work in Parasitology, particularly research regarding tapeworm and trichinosis. He was the first to prove that *Taenia saginata* occurs only in cattle (and humans), and *Taenia solium* occurs only in swine (and humans). His study of *Trichina* helped support Rudolf Virchow's campaign to create meat inspection laws in Germany. With Virchow and von Zenker , he was the first to document the life cycle of the parasite *Trichinella spirals* in swine and humans.

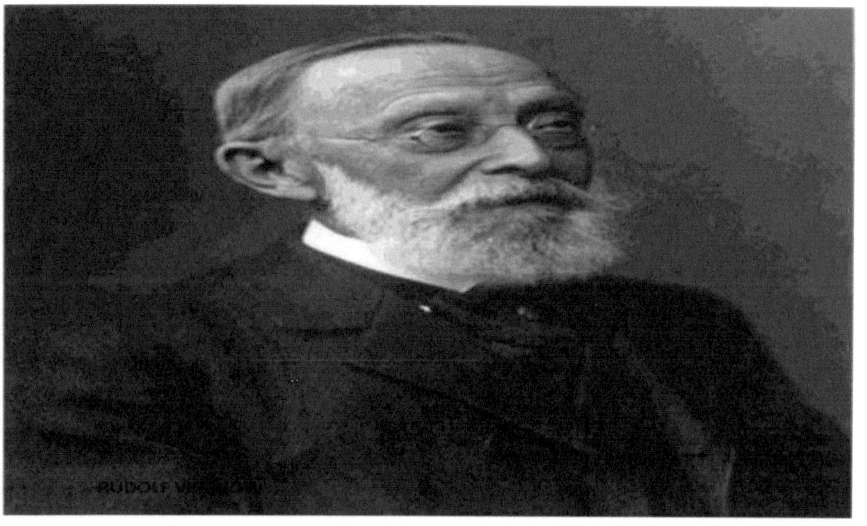

Figure 10. Rudolph Carl Virchow (13 October 1821 – 5 September 1902) was a German doctor who made many great discoveries.

He also made important studies of the sheep liver fluke. Leuckart is credited with splitting George Cuvier's Radiate into two phyla; Coelenterata and Echinodermata. Today the "Rudolf-LeuckartMedaille" is an annual award given for research in Parasitology by the Deutschen Gesellschaft für Parasitologie (German Society of Parasitology). [138]

Zenker was born in Dresden, and was educated in Leipzig and Heidelberg. His important discovery of the danger of trichinae dates from 1860 he made studies on *T solium* but his results are not well documented. In that season he published "Ueber die Trichinenkrankheit des Menschen" (in volume xviii of Virchow's *Archiv.* [139]

Also in 1862, Griesinger analyzes a series of 86 patients, and it establishes a direct relationship between cerebral cysticercosis and epilepsy, and proposes a first classification of disease. The term "cysticerci multilocularis by cysticercus racemose" was permanently changed by Zenker in 1882 [130] and three years later Kuchenmeister discovers that the cysticercus is the larval stage of Taenia solium. [131] Askanzazy discovers the arterial lesions: "temporal arteritis obliterant disease" and it was attributed to cysticercosis in 1890. [140]

In the 19th century some people attributed the pig taboo in the Middle East to the danger of the parasite trichina. Marvin Harris posited that pigs are not suited to being kept in the Middle East on an ecological and social-economic level; for example, pigs are not suited to living in arid climates and thus require far more water than other animals to keep them cool, and instead of grazing they compete with humans for foods such as grains. As such, raising pigs was seen as a wasteful and decadent practice. A common explanation to the fact that pigs have widely been considered unclean in the Middle East is that they are omnivorous, not discerning between meat or vegetation in their natural dietary habits. The willingness to consume meat sets them apart from most other domesticated animals which are commonly eaten (cattle, horses, goats, etc.) who would naturally eat only plants [139]. At the end of the XIX century cysticercosis was already spread on all over the Europe until 1900 when Germany began an effective fight against CC/TE creating a law for the obligatory inspection of the porcine population confirming a decrease in the frequency of cysticercosis of the 2% to 0.1 %. [130]

In Ecuador the first descriptions were carried out by the Dr. Valenzuela (1901) who reported the first case of NCC in Guayaquil [141]. Doctor Valenzuela from Ecuador made the first descriptions on CC in 1901 and reported the first case of NCC in Guayaquil [141]. In 1906, Hennenberg performs a comprehensive review of the topic and modifies the first classification proposed by Grisinger and Hennenberg. [130] Between 1909 and 1911, Moses and Wimberg began serologic studies for diagnostic purposes using complement fixation in serum. [131]

In 1932, Heinert describes 11 patients diagnosed with *T solium* in Ecuador [130]. Salazar-Viniegra describes in Mexico for the first time (1936) the CC of the CNS in deceased from the bedlam of the Mexico City [142]. Spider and Asenjo by means of the gaseous ventriculography diagnosed a case with NCC in the posterior fossa (1945) and one year later in Chile Coastal publishes its findings in the General Hospital of Social Security in Mexico, finding evidence of CC in the 3.6 % of autopsy material. In this same year Robles published 47 cases treated surgically. In Argentina, Dickmann was the first to communicate their results on NCC in the child population from that same year. [143]

In 1948 Nieto [144], reported that 11% of the Mexican patients admitted to the neurology service of a general hospital, and 0.8 % of the internees in a psychiatric hospital presented NCC, while Stepien and Choroboski a year after reporting a series of patients treated surgically with success, an opinion not shared by the great neurosurgeons of the era; on that date Arseni reported 65 patients with NCC verified in a period of 20 years (1935-19550) by highlighting that it was hereditary or affecting other countries. Returning to Latin America, it is reported that in Mexico the 3.6 % of the hospital autopsy showed evidence of CC. [140] In the year 1965 in Ecuador the first findings of autopsies are attributed to Guerrero. In Brazil, the prevalence of NCC increased up to 2.9 % in that same year and in 1970 the prevalence of the NCC in the hospitals of neurosurgery and neurology in Colombia was 0.9 %. [130] Mora-Rubio (1971) in Colombia reported 114 confirmed cases of NCC. In 1972 there was a cooperative study in Latin American countries, remain at the forefront of this research Sixto Obrador who found a decrease in the CC with tumor presentations "intracranial lesions expansionary" of 3% in 1950 to 0.6 % in 1960 [145] his work is considered a classic monograph on this topic. [146] The first reports on the treatment of the CC on the American continent were reported in 1983 (Andrews & Thomas) followed by the publication of a guide for the management, prevention and control of the complex CC/TEA prepared by the WHO. In 1985 was a collaborative study of the NCC in the hospitals of the city of Los Angeles that grouped 497 patients (Richards et al. ,) while Sotelo (1985) in Mexico publishes a new classification for the NCC based on the presence of active and inactive forms. In 1987-1989, Sotelo proposes a plan for management of NCC according to the characteristics and tomographic studies of CSF. An episode recorded in 1934 enabled us to establish the time of appearance of the symptoms of the disease. In that year, British soldiers stationed in India returned to their country and some of these soldiers were diagnosed as NCC, for which they were subjected to a strict medical follow-up. Seizures, as the main symptom, took on average two years to appear, although there were cases where the epilepsy has lasted up to 20 or more years since their return. [129]

Over 1973, as a result of the increase in technology and the onset of the CT scan that it would be in the long run the fundamental pillar of the diagnosis and treatment of the cysticercosis increases the number of publications with respect to the topic and in Mexico, the frequency of the NCC in the specialized hospitals was 4%. [130]

The frequency of the NCC in the hospitals of Neurology and Neurosurgery in México (1973) increased up to 10 %; while in the general hospitals of Ecuador it was 2.6%. [130]

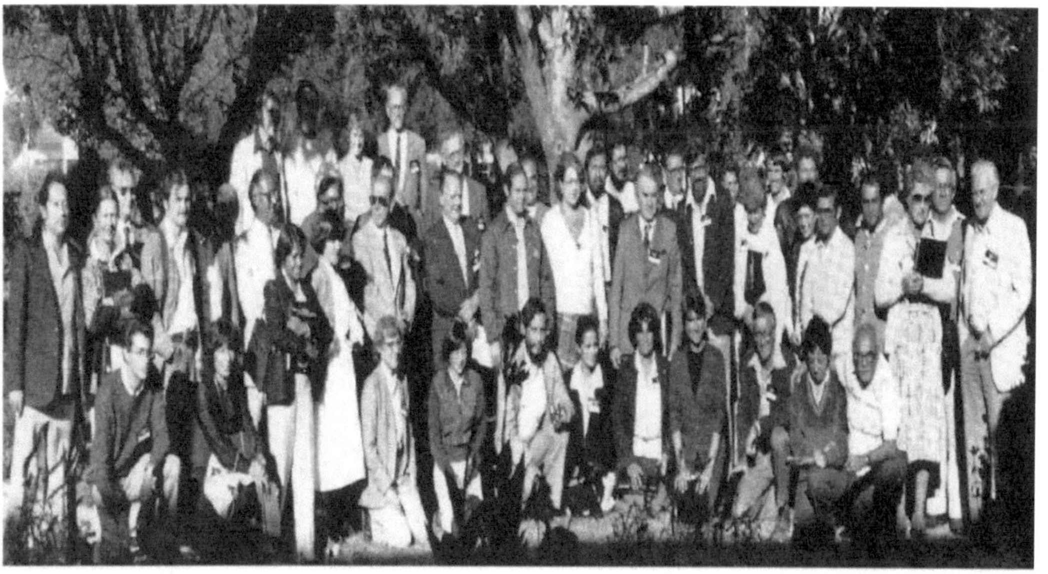

Figure 11. First International Congress on Cysticercosis, San Miguel Allende, Mexico, November 1981 (Source: Cysticercosis Present State of Knowledge and Perspective. Edited by Ana Flisser, Kaethe Willms, Juan Pedro Laclette, Carlos Larralde, Cecilia Ridaura; Fernando Beltran. Red Book, was published in 1982. (Courtesy of Dr. Flisser)

The First International Meeting on Cysticercosis was held in Mexico in 1981 with a good participation of international scientists. (Figure 16)

In 1982, Zenteno publishes a classification of human cysticercosis and in 1983 appear the first reports of treatment of the cysticercosis. The World Health Organization published a guide for the management, prevention and control of the complex taeniasis/cysticercosis (WHO, 1983). One year later The World Health Organization, indicates that the world's population already was 5,000 million inhabitants and that the taeniasis were 1.5 % [130].

1985 Was conducted a collaborative study of the NCC in the hospitals in the city of Los Angeles that grouped 497 patients (Richards, 1985). Sotelo in Mexico publishes a new classification of NCC based on the presence of active forms and inactive (Sotelo, 1985) and two years later he proposes a management scheme about NCC with categorization tomographic and studies of cerebro-spinal fluid. [146]

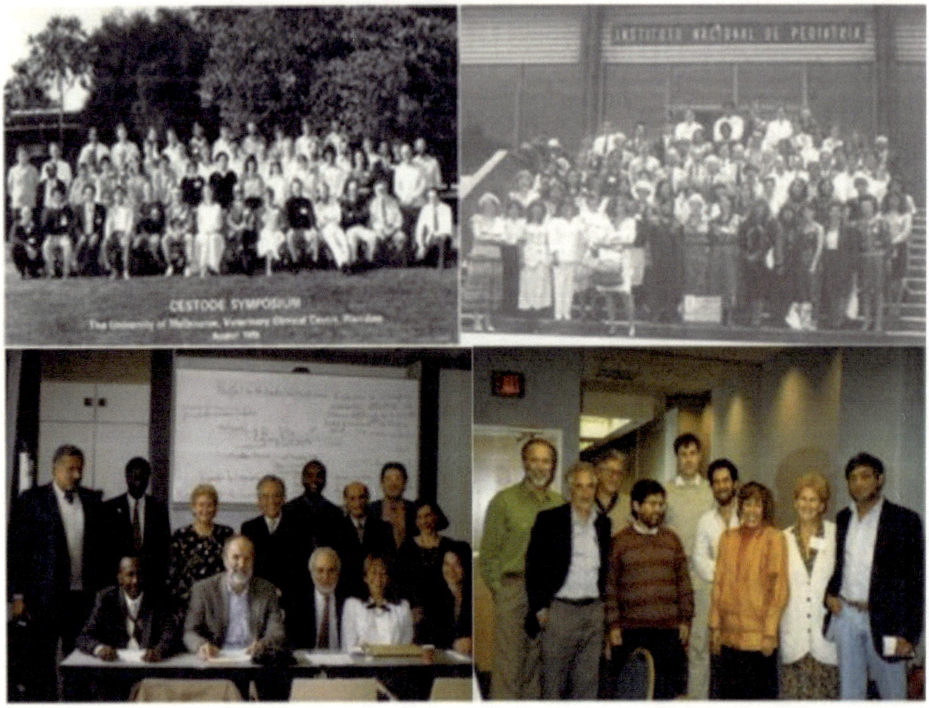

Figure 12. Upper left, Cestodes Symposium held in Australia, 1986 . Upper right, Neurocysticercosis Symposium in Mexico. Lower left: Cysticercosis meeting in France, 1994. Lower left: Cysticercosis meeting in Perú, 1993 (Courtesy of Dr. Flisser)

In 1988, Italy has been carrying out a review of all published cases of NCC since the beginning of the century and 11 cases were reported, most of them in Sicily. [130] Figueredo de Coimbra warned of an increase in the incidence of NCC in Portugal by the presence of population from African colonies. [130] Stanol and collaborators propose a new prognostic classification of NCC (Español, 1986). Madrazo and Sandoval published a new classification of neurocysticercosis in 1989. [146] In the 1980s there was much emphasis on the immunological diagnosis of the NCC existed a large number of publications highlighting mainly studies on the enzyme linked immunosorbent assays [147-155] and immunoelectron transfer (EITB) by Tsang and collaborators [156-159] and Wilson [160] plus other contributions made by Flisser a little bit later. [161,162]

In 1990, Medina et al. studied 100 consecutive Mexican patients with epilepsy that started after the age of 25 years. All patients underwent clinical evaluation, computed tomography, and electroencephalography; additionally, cerebro-spinal fluid analysis was performed in 82 of them.

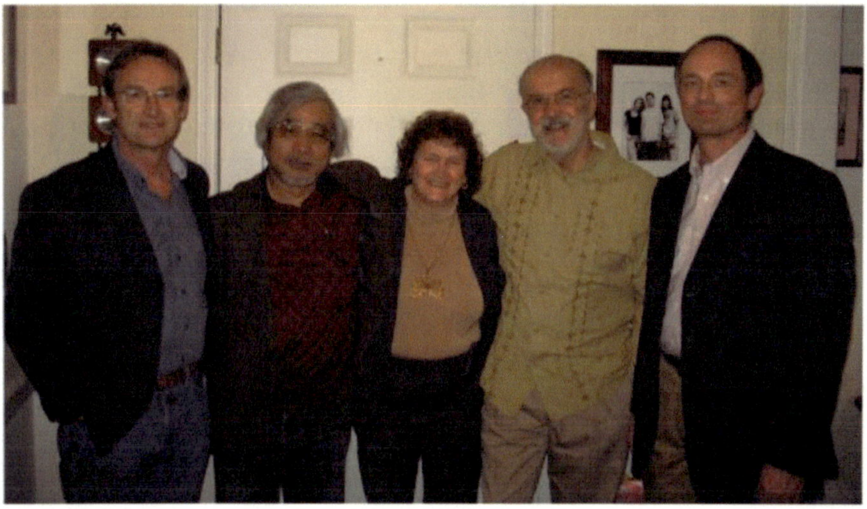

Figure 13. Shows some of most relevant scientists in the field of cysticercosis who attended to the meeting in Atlanta, Georgia on February 24, 2008. From left to right: Phillip S Craig, Akira Ito, Ana Flisser, Peter Schantz and Lee Willigham III (Courtesy of Dr Flisser).

The volume of research and publications on cysticercosis, taeniosis and NCC increased gradually in this decade reaching a large number therefore it is not possible sum it up in the limited space we have but we should not conclude this historical review without prior highlight the meritorious work performed by some prominent researchers in this stage such as: Ana Flisser, Peter Schantz, Julio Sotelo, Hugo García, Oscar del Bruto, Akira Ito, Jefferson Proaño, Vedantam Rajshekhar, Ravindra Kumar Garg, Ted Nash, Carlton Evans, Osvaldo Takayanagui, Clinton White, Lee Willingham, Phillip S Craig, Gagandeep Singh, Sudesh Prabhakar, Hélène Carabine, Andrea Wrinkle, Arturo Carpio, Agnes Fleury, David Botero, Svetlana Agapejev, Gustavo Román, P Dorny, M Raghava, V Prabhakaran, Victor Tsang, Jorge Morales-Montor, Tetsuya Yanagida, Marshall Lightowlers, Elsa Sarti, Joachim Blocher, Yasuhito Sako, Minoru Nakao, Feng Zheng, Kazuhiro Nakaya, Jim Allan, Dolores Correa, Armando Gonzalez, Robert Gilman, García E, Márquez C, Fragoso G, Sciutto E, Cuetter A, Andrews R. Ferrer E., Cabrera Z., T Kelesidis, Tony Velasco, Cortés M, Alain Dessein, Pierre-Marie Preux PM, Jose A Serpa, Linda S Yancey, Pratibhasinghi Singhi, Dumas M, Carlos Larralde, Tapia G, Eon Keeseon, Carlos Larralde, Tammi Krecek, M Gupta, P Agarwal, GA Khwaja, P Sharma, R Shukla, D Singh, MV Padma, NK Misra, GK Ahuja, IK Phiri, Helena Ngowi, Sam Mukaratirwa, LM Michael, S Siziya, Humberto Foyaca, Emilia Noormahomed, Aline S de Aluja, Molina Alvarez, J Lasso, F Quet, M Guerchet, EB

Ngoungou, A Nicoletti, N Wadia, Jorge Burneo, Tonicarlo Velasco, Theodoros Kelesidis, P Huc, M Druet-Cabanac, M Strobel, Li T, Phil Craig, X Chen, D Qiu, J Qiu, MO Sato, T Wandra, H Bradshaw, L Li, N Nakao, J Waikagul, D Wattanakulanich, W Maipanich, K Nakaya, MO Sato, Y Sako, M Okamoto, K Swastika, C I Dewiyani, T Yanagida, K Nakaya, Hiroshi Yamasaki, James C. Allan, Marcello Otake Sato, Minoru Nakao, Yasuhito Sako, Kazuhiro Nakaya, Dongchuan Qiu, S Desai, A Cuetter, AE Gonzalez, S. Geerts, NC Kyvsgaard, DP McManus, ZS Pawlowski. However over this relationship there are still a significant number of researchers that do not appear in the listing.

Most of these scientists have been grouped to work together on the same objective: *Taenia solium*. Some have more than 20 years of experience and more than 20 publications. Among the groups with better results are the groups in México, Perú, and the three groups from Ecuador (Quito, Cuenca, and Guayaquil). There are other groups from the Eastern and Southern Africa (CWGESA), Asia and Oceania, and the group of Europe of recent constitution (Willingham LA III et al., 2008).

The CWGESA was established in 2002 to promote communication, collaboration and coordination of integrated research and control activities to combat cysticercosis, a serious and sometimes fatal disease transmitted between pigs and people by the zoonotic tapeworm, Taenia solium.

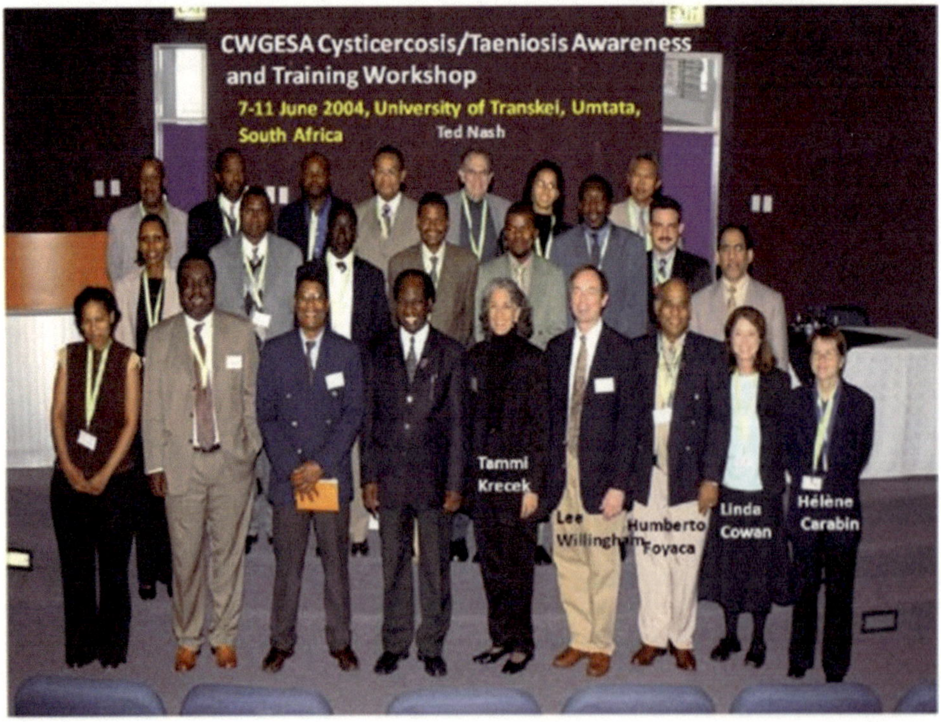

Figure 14. Cysticercosis Working Group for Eastern and Southern Africa International Training Workshop organized by CWGESA and held on June 2004 Mthatha where delegates from 11 African countries participated.

The 7th General Assembly on cysticercosis/taeniosis was held at the Faculty of Health Sciences, Walter Sisulu University, Mthatha, South Africa, from 20 – 22 July 2011. The meeting was organized by the Cysticercosis Working Group in Eastern and Southern Africa (CWGESA) in collaboration with the Faculty of Health Sciences of Walter Sisulu University. Veterinary, medical, agricultural and socioeconomic researchers met in Mthatha to discuss the Roadmap for Elimination of *Taenia solium* cysticercosis/taeniosis (TSCT) in Eastern and Southern Africa and to evaluate progress and make recommendations on intervention research for the elimination of the disease.

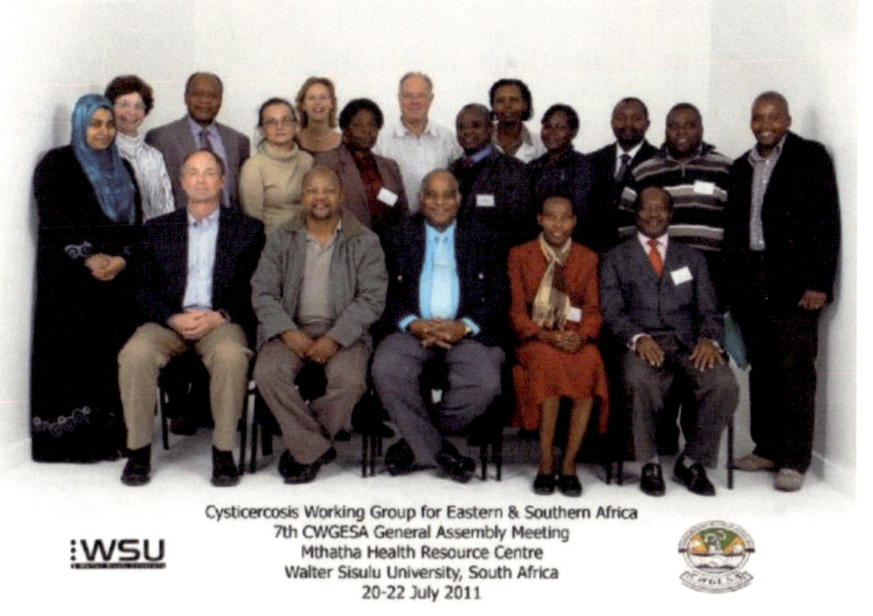
WSU
Cysticercosis Working Group for Eastern & Southern Africa
7th CWGESA General Assembly Meeting
Mthatha Health Resource Centre
Walter Sisulu University, South Africa
20-22 July 2011

Figure 15. Members of the CWGESA attended to this meeting. Seated from left to right: Lee Willigham III, Samson Mukaratirwa, Humberto Foyaca, Helena Ngowi and Faustin Lekule.

We have the advantage that the disease has been virtually isolated in the communities around Mthatha where there are also human and material resources needed to eradicate the cysticercosis if we receive the necessary support of governmental institutions and non-governmental organizations committed to this goal. Eradicating the cysticercosis of the surrounding area of Mthatha is equivalent to delete the T solium in South Africa and this could be the first country in the world to achieve it.

Mexico is the country that more progress has been achieved in this regard and their doctors and researchers take pride that flag.

4. Honor to honor deserves

For prevention and eradication of cysticercosis are needed peoples dedicated and committed to this cause, which should be headed only by honorable scientists stripped of any trait of hubris, arrogance and self-sufficiency.

In our opinion, the person who has been most prominent in the research work related to the tapeworm *Taenia solium* is the Dr. Ana Flisser as shown below; she is a full time, upper rank, senior scientist at the National Autonomous University of Mexico, UNAM since 1972.

The authors of this chapter believe that in order to be considered a researcher whose example should be followed by the younger generations are they must comply with certain requirements among which protrude the modesty, honesty, solidarity and a desire to help the younger generations of researchers to its best development unconditionally. In our opinion that example is Dr. Ana Flisser.

5. Recent awards and distinctions received:

Dr. Ana Flisser won the University Award 2011 in Research in Natural Sciences.

Coordinator of the first MD/PhD Program in Mexico, UNAM, 2011.

First Vice-President of the World Federation of Parasitologists and President of the XIII International Congress of Parasitology to be held in Mexico City in August 2014

Award Ciudad Capital "Heberto Castillo Martínez" Research in Health and Environment, 2008 President, From Alaska to Chiapas: The First North American Parasitology Congress, Merida, Yucatan, June 21-25, 2007

Director of Research, Hospital General "Dr. Manuel Gea Gonzalez" SSA, 2001-2005.

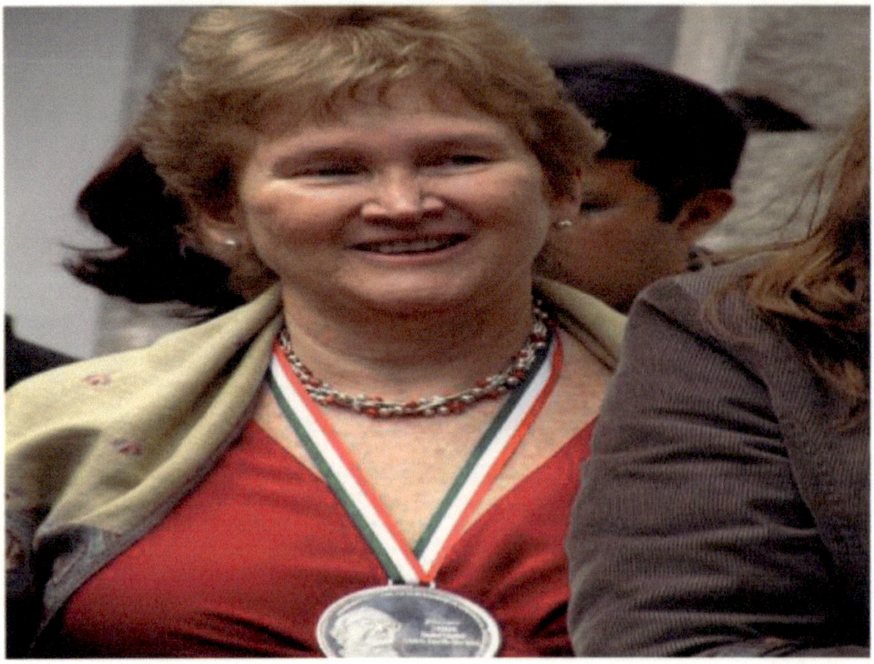

Figure 16. Dr. Ana Flisser Department of Microbiology and Parasitology, Faculty of Medicine, National Autonomous University of Mexico.

PAHO Award for Administration 1999. For her work to transform the network of public health laboratories in her country to support priority health programs, including administration, teaching, and research. Director, National Institute for Epidemiology Diagnosis and Reference (INDRE), SSA, 1995-2000.

Research area

Cysticercosis and taeniosis due to *Taenia solium*

Publications

128 original articles in international and Mexican refereed journals. 60 reviews or invited articles

62 book chapters (two chapters in this book are not included). 8 books as editor or coeditor. 3 books as author or coauthor

Advisor of thesis

11 for doctor in science, 12 for master in science, 12 as member of advisory committee, 2 for medical specialties, 15 at the bachelor level

Financial support

20 research projects from: DGAPA/UNAM, CONACYT, European Community, IDRC/Ottawa, WHO/PAHO, Merck-Darmstadt/Merck-México.

Recent teaching activities

Immunoparasitology since 2004, Faculty of Sciences, UNAM. Immunoparasitology in graduate programs since 2005, Faculty of Medicine, UNAM.

Academic activities

483 papers in national and international congresses. 182 national and international invited lectures 44 graduate and bachelor courses. 52 lectures at different graduate courses and various memberships of Societies of Parasitology, Tropical Medicine and Immunology of Mexico, USA and Great Britain, as well as of the International Federations in these areas. (Source: World Federation of Parasitology). Again, we want to emphasize that not only fatten the results to the person, other qualities such as modesty, friendship, solidarity, honesty, and the desire to selflessly help young researchers are also qualities that make an example to follow that I wish to report to the new generations of scientists worldwide.

We would like to make it very clear that we have received from Dr. Flisser some photos to illustrate this chapter but that the decision to include this modest but deserved tribute to her maintained and hard work, is ours. Therefore she had no role in chapter design, information collection, decision to publish, or preparation of the manuscript. By her modesty, we know that she will not fully agree with this decision but we could not ignore her history. To pay a tribute to their achievements including her personal contribution to the reduction of the morbidity and mortality of the cysticercosis in Mexico and everything she has done by and for the rest of humanity, is right.

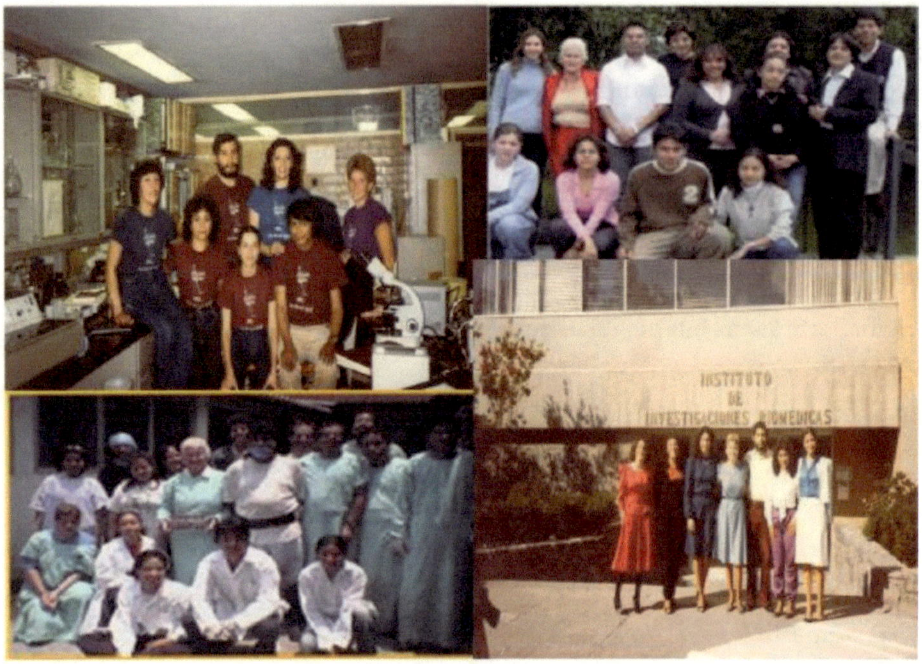

Figure 17. Dr. Ana Flisser: Always surrounded by talented young people who receive her teachings, experience and wisdom.

Author details

Humberto Foyaca Sibat and Lourdes de Fátima Ibañez Valdés

Walter Sisulu University, Faculty of Health Sciences, Nelson Mandela Academic Hospital Division of Neurology., Mthatha,South Africa

Acknowledgement

Special thanks are due to the Cuban Ministry of Health and the Institute of Tropical Medicine "Pedro Kouri", and authorities of Nelson Mandela Academic Hospital, School of Medicine, Faculty of Health Sciences and Directorate: Research Development from Walter Sisulu University for their kind support. Finally, we wish to declare publicly our eternal and deepest gratitude to Lorna María Foyaca García, Fátima Susana Foyaca Ibañez and Thabo Humberto Foyaca Ibañez for their delight support. We like to thank to Dr Ana Flisser for her contribution to this chapter.

6. References

[1] Foyaca-Sibat H, Ibañez-Valdés LdeF & J. Moré-Rodríguez : Parasitic Zoonoses Of The Brain: Another Challenger?. The Internet Journal of Neurology. 2010 Volume 12 Number 2.

http://www.ispub.com/journal/the_internet_journal_of_neurology/volume_12_number_2_4/article/par asitic-zoonoses-of-the-brain-another-challenger.html. (Accessed 22 January 2012).
[2] Foyaca-Sibat H, editor. Treatment of Epilepsy Secondary to Neurocysticercosis, Novel Treatment of Epilepsy. Rikeja; InTech, 2011.
[3] Foyaca-Sibat H editor.Clinical Features of Epilepsy Secondary to Neurocysticercosis at the Insular Lobe, Novel Aspects on Epilepsy; InTech,2011.
[4] Foyaca-Sibat H. editor. Epilepsy Secondary to Parasitic Zoonoses of the Brain, Novel Aspects on Epilepsy, Humberto Foyaca-Sibat. Rikeja; InTech,2011.
[5] Foyaca-Sibat H, Ibañez-Valdés L de F. Clinical trial of praziquantel and prednisone in rural patients with neurocysticercosis presenting recurrent epileptic attacks The Internet Journal of Neurology 2002;2):41-50. http://www.ispub.com/journal/the_internet_journal_of_neurology/volume_1_number_2_39/article/cli nical_trial_of_praziquantel_and_prednisone_in_rural_patients_with_neurocysticercosis_presenting_w ith_recurrent_epileptic_attacks.html. (accessed 22 January 2012).
[6] Foyaca-Sibat H Ibañez-Valdés L de F. Intraventricular neurocysticercosis in HIV patients. The Internet Journal of Neurology 2003;2(1):23-31. http://www.ispub.com/journal/the_internet_journal_of_neurology/volume_2_number_1_37/article/int raventricular_neurocysticercosis_in_hiv_positive_patients.html. (ac es sed 22 January 2012).
[7] Bautista IR. Neurocisticercosis una realidad y sus limitantes en el diagnóstico. SIRIVS. Curso: Investigación II . Maestría en Salud Animal. Universidad Nacional Mayor de San Marcos Facultad de Medicina Veterinaria.2008
[8] Sotelo J. Eradication of cysticercosis is an attainable goal. BMJ 2003;326(7388):511-512.
[9] Hotez PJ; Bottazi ME, Franco-Paredes C, Ault SK, Periago MR. The Neglected Tropical Diseases of Latin America and the Caribbean: A Review of Disease Burden and Distribution and a Roadmap for Control and Elimination. *PLoS Neglected Tropical Diseases* 2008; 2: e300 doi:10.1371/journal.pntd.0000300.
[10] Román G, Sotelo J, Del Brutto O, Flisser A, Dumas M, Wadia N. et al. A proposal to declare neurocysticercosis an international reportable disease. *Bull World Health Organ* 2000; 78: 399-406.
[11] Shanley JD, Jordan MC: Clinical aspects of CNS cysticercosis. *Arch Inter Med* 1980;140:1309- 1315.
[12] Loo L, Braude A: Cerebral cysticercosis in San Diego: a report of 23 cases and review of the literature. *Medicine* (Baltimore) 1982;61:341-350.
[13] McComick G, Zec Chi-S, Heiden J. Cysticercosis Cerebri. Review of 127 cases. *Arch Neurol* 1982; 39:534-539.
[14] McCormick GF. Cysticercosis: review of 230 patients. *Bull Clin Neurosci.* 1985;50:76–76.
[15] Carpio A. Neurocysticercosis: an update. *Lancet Infect Dis* 2002;2:751-62.
[16] Uddin J, Gonzalez AE, Gilman RH, Thomas LH, Rodriguez S, Evans CA, Remick DG, Garcia HH, Friedland JS. Mechanisms regulating monocyte CXCL8 secretion in

neurocysticercosis and the effect of antiparasitic therapy. J Immunol. 2010 Oct 1;185(7):4478-84. Epub 2010 Sep 8.

[17] White AC Jr. Neurocysticercosis: a major cause of neurological disease worldwide. *Clin Infect Dis* 1997;24:101-106.

[18] White AC Jr. Neurocysticercosis: updates on epidemiology, pathogenesis, diagnosis and management. *Ann Rev Med* 2000;51:187-206.

[19] Foyaca-Sibat H, Ibañez-Valdés LdeF "Neurocysticercosis in HIV-positive patients" The Internet Journal of Infectious Diseases 2003:2(2):15-23. http://www.ispub.com/ostia/index.php?xmlFilePath=journals/ijn/current.xml (accessed 25 January 2012).

[20] Sarti E, Schantz PM, Plancharte A, Wilson M, Gutierrez R, Lopez AS, Roberts J, Flisser A. Prevalence and risk factor for *Taenia solium* taeniasis and cysticercosis in humans and pigs in a village in Morelos, Mexico. *Am J Trop Med Hyg* 1992; 46:677-684.

[21] Garg RK. Neurocysticercosis. *Postgrad Med J* 1998; 74(872):321-326.

[22] Schantz PM, Moore AC, Muñoz JL, et al.: Neurocysticercosis in an Orthodox Jewish community in New York City. *N England J Med* 1992;327:692-696.

[23] Rousseau MC, Guillotel B, Delmont J. Neurocysticercosis in the South-East of France 1988- 1998. *Presse Med* 1999;28(39):2141-2144.

[24] García HH, Del Brutto OH; Cysticercosis Working Group in Peru. Neurocysticercosis: updated concepts about an old disease. *Lancet Neurol.* 2005; 4:653-661.

[25] O'Neal S, Noh J, Wilkins P, Keene W, Lambert W, Anderson J, Compton Luman J, Townes J. Taenia solium Tapeworm Infection, Oregon, 2006-2009. *Emerg Infect Dis.* 2011 Jun;17(6):1030-1036.

[26] Kelesidis T, Tsiodras S. Extraparenchymal neurocysticercosis in the United States. *J Med Case Reports.* 2011;5:359.

[27] Serpa JA, Graviss EA, Kass JS, White AC Jr. Neurocysticercosis in Houston, Texas: an update. *Medicine* (Baltimore). 2011;90(1):81-86.

[28] Takayanagui O, Leite J. Neurocisticercose. *Revista da Sociedades Brasileira de Medicina tropical* 2000;34:283–290.

[29] Pawlowski ZS. Control of neurocysticercosis by routine medical and veterinary services. *Trans R Soc Trop Med Hyg* 2008;102:228-232.

[30] García Albea E., Cisticercosis en España. Algunos datos Epidemiológicos. Rev Clin Esp.184:15- 18, 1989.

[31] [31]Sánchez L, Abad L, Lozano E, Maldonado G. Neurocisticercosis intraventricular. Presentación de un caso localizado en el tercer ventriculo. *Radiologia.* 2002;44:309-313.

[32] Sandeep GJ, Vipul CC, Bhakti SY, Himanshu VB. Imaging Findings of Disseminated Cysticercosis with Unusual Involvement of Spleen and Pancreas. *J Glob Infect Dis.* 2011;3(3):306– 308.

[33] Sang-Wook K, Moon-Kyu K, Sae-Moon Oh, Se-Hyuck P. Racemose Cysticercosis in the Cerebellar Hemisphere. *J Korean Neurosurg Soc.* 2010; 48(1):59–61.

[34] Sarti E. La taeniasis y cisticercosis en México (revisión bibliográfica). *Salud Pública Mex* 1986; 28:556-563.

[35] Sawhney IM, Singh G, Lekhra OP, Mathuriya SN, Parihar PS, Prabhakar S. Uncommon presentations of neurocysticercosis. *J Neurol Sci.* 1998;154(1):94-100.

[36] Seo HJ, Seo JH, Kim SW, Shin H. Isolated Spinal Neurocysticercosis : Unusual Ocular Presentation Mimicking Pseudotumor Cerebri. *J Korean Neurosurg Soc.* 2011 May; 49(5): 296–298.

[37] Ahmad FU, Sharma BS. Treatment of intramedullary spinal cysticercosis: report of 2 cases and review of literature. *Surg Neurol.* 2007;67(1):74–77.

[38] Amaral L, Maschietto M, Maschietto R, Cury R, Ferreira NF, Mendonça R, et al. Unusual manifestations of neurocysticercosis in MR imaging : analysis of 172 cases. *Arq Neuropsiquiatr.* 2003;61:533–541.

[39] Amaya MA, Roa JL. Neurocisticercosis raquídea: Reporte de caso. *Rev Colomb Radiol.* 2011;22(1):3134-3137.

[40] Delobel P, Signate A, Guedj M, Couppie P, Gueye M, Smadja D, Pradinaud R. Unusual form of neurocysticercosis associated with HIV infection. *European Journal of Neurology.*2004; 11(1):55-58.

[41] Dewan P, Shankar J, Sunil S, Gupta A Uncommon presentation of neurocysticercosis. *South African Journal of Child Health,* 2011;5(2):12-13.

[42] Dickmann, G.H. Cisticercosis de la fosa craneana posterior. *Rev. Neurol.*1946;15:160-179.

[43] Figueroa JJ, Davis LE, Magalhaes A. Extraparenchymal neurocysticercosis in Albuquerque, New México. *J Neuroimaging.* 2011;21(1):38–43

[44] Flisser A, Madrazo I, Plancarte A, Schantz P, Allan J, Craig P, Sarti E. Neurological symptoms in occult neurocysticercosis after single taeniacidal dose of praziquantel. Lancet.1993;18:342-348.

[45] Flisser A, Madrazo I. Evagination of Taenia solium in the fourth ventricle. N Engl J Med. 1996 Sep 5;335(10):753-754

[46] Flisser A. Cisticercosis subcutáneo. *Ciencias,* UNAM 2011. http://hydra.fciencias.unam.mx:8080/xmlui/handle/123456789/62343?show=full

[47] Foyaca-Sibat H, Ibañez-Valdés LdeF: "Generalized Cysticercosis With Cardiac Involvement". The Internet Journal of Neurology. (ISSN: 1531-295X). 2007;7(2):6-11. http://www.ispub.com/journal/the_internet_journal_of_neurology/volume_7_number_2_5/article/gen eralized_cysticercosis_with_cardiac_involvement.html

[48] Ibañez-Valdés LdeF, Foyaca-Sibat H. Neurogenic heart secondary to insular stroke and neurocysticercosis. International Journal of Stroke (ISSN 1747-4930) 2006;1(1):68.

[49] Lamejjati M, Aniba K, Haddi M. et al. Spinal Intramedullary arachnoid cyst in children. *Pediatr Neurosurg.* 2008;44(3):243–246.

[50] Leite CC, Jinkins JR, Escobar BE, et al. MR imaging of intramedullary and intradural-extra medullary spinal cysticercosis. *AJR* 1997;169:1713-1717.

[51] Musumdar D, Nadkarni T, Desai K, Dindorkar K, Goel A. Thoracic intramedullary cysticercosis. *Neurol Med Chir* (Tokyo)2002; 42 :575-579.

[52] Neal JH. An endoscopic approach to cysticercosis cysts of the posterior third ventricle. *Neurosurgery* 1995;36(5):1040-1043.

[53] Park SY, Min HK, Jung HK, Kwan YS. Disseminated cysticercosis. *Journal of Korean Neurosurgical Society*. 2011;49(3):190-193.

[54] Ramírez-Ceballos JA, Marquéz RMC.Tratamiento endoscópico de la neurocisticercosis intraventricular. *Rev Neurocir* 2007;9(4):107-113.

[55] Razdan S, Pandita KK, Pandita S. Reversible hemifacial spasm due to neurocysticercosis. *Ann Indian Acad Neurol*. 2009 Jul-Sep; 12(3): 191–192.

[56] Ruangkanchanasetr P,Bangchuad T, Sithinamsuwan P, Benjasuratwong Y, Chuankrerkkul W, Ubolwatra S, Supaporn T. Hypothalamic neurocysticercosis presenting with polyuria: a first report of an unusual manifestation. *Nephrol. Dial. Transplant*. 2006;21 (8):2308-2310.

[57] Villanueva M, Alcocer JL, Martinez J, Horna A. Cisticercosis intramedular. Reporte de un caso. *Arch Neurocien* 2004;9(2):110-113.

[58] Wadia N, Desai S, Bhatt M: Disseminated cysticercosis. New observations, including CT scan findings and experience with treatment by praziquantel. *Brain* 1988, 111:597-614

[59] Xinou E, Lefkopoulous M, Gelagoti M, Drevelegas A, Diakou A, et al. Successful treatment of isolated cerebellar cysticercosis with albendazole. *Chin Med J* (Engl) 2003;116:637–638.

[60] Rabiela MT, Lombardo L, Flores F. Cisticercosis cerebral. Estudio de 68 casos de autopsia.Patología (Mex) 1972; 10:27-40.

[61] Lopez-Hernández A, Garaizar C. Childhood Cerebral Cysticercosis: clinical features and computed tomographic findings in 98 Mexican children. *Can J Neurol SC* 1982;9:401-407.

[62] Flisser A. Neurocysticercosis in Mexico. *Parasitol Today*1988; 4:131-137.

[63] Sotelo J, Penagos P, Escobedo F, Del Brutto OH: Short course of albendazole therapy for neurocysticercosis. *Arch Neurol* 1988;45:1130-1133.

[64] Agapejev S. Epidemiology of Neurocysticercosis in Brazil. *Rev Inst Med Trop Sao Paulo* 1996;38(3):207-216.

[65] Ramírez G, Pradilla G, Rodríguez M, González C. Cisticercosis. Estudio de 80 casos. *Acta Med Colombiana* 1986;11:62-73.

[66] Botero D. Cisticercosis en Colombia. Investigations realizadas hasta 1988. *An Acad Med Medellin* 1989;2(II):75-82.

[67] Takayanagui OM, Jardim E. Clinical aspects of nerocysticercosis: analysis of 500 cases. Arq Neuropsiquiatr 1983; 41(1):50-63.

[68] Gemmell M, Matyas Z, Pawloski Z, Soulsby EJL, Larralde C, Nelson G, Rosieky B. Guidelines for surveillance, prevention and control of taeniasis/cysticercosis. VPH/83.49. *World Health Organization*, Geneva, 1983:1.207.

[69] García HH, del Brutto OH. *Taenia solium* cysticercosis. *Infect Dis Clin North Am* 2000; 14(1):97-119.

[70] Turkulov V, madle-Samardzija N, Canak G, Vukadinov J, Aleksic-Dordevic M. Clinical and diagnostic approaches to neurocysticercosis. *Med Pregl* 2001; 54(7-8):353-356.

[71] Flisser A. Cisticercosis Humana: Epidemiología, diagnóstico e inmunología. Revista UIS Medicina Bucaramenga Colombia; 1986, 14(1):51-60.

[72] Flisser A. Cysticercosis and Taenia solium. J Clin Neuroophthalmol. 1986 Sep;6(3):200
[73] Flisser A. Taeniasis and cysticercosis due to Taenia solium. Prog Clin Parasitol. 1994;4:77-116
[74] Flisser A. Neurocysticercosis and epilepsy in developing countries. J Neurol Neurosurg Psychiatry. 2001 May;70(5):707-712
[75] Flisser A. Where are the tapeworms? Parasitol Int. 2006;55 Suppl:S117-20. Epub 2005 Dec 6.
[76] Flisser A, Madrazo I, Delgado H. Cisticercosis humana. ED. *El Manual Moderno*. RSC-048, ISO-90002:1994/NMX-CC-004:1998
[77] Chimelli L, Lovalho AF, Takayanagui OM. Neurocysticercosis: contribution of autopsies in the consolidated of mandatory notification in Ribeirao Preto-SP, *Brazil. Arq Neuropsiquiatr* 1998; 56(3B):577-584.
[78] Sanchez AL, Ljungstrom I, Medina MT. Diagnosis of human neurocysticercosis in endemic countries: clinical study in Honduras. *Parasitol Int* 1999;48(1):81-89.
[79] MedikaMag.com. 2011 Rep. Dom. http://www.medikamag.com/Page.asp?key=751&export=html
[80] Torres J. Recomendaciones para el tratamiento de la Neurocisticercosis. *Memorias 1as Jornadas Venezolanas de Medicina Tropical,* Caracas, 28 al 31 de julio de 1991.
[81] Torres J. Avances en el tratamiento de la neurocysticercosis. *Memorias 2das jornadas de Medicina Tropical,* Caracas, 26 al 29 de julio de 1994.Torres M, Pérez C, Galdámez E, Gabor M, Miranda C, Cofré X et al. Teniosis: serie clínica en 35 pacientes. *Parasitol día* 2001;25:55-59.
[82] Vera A. Prevalencia de teniasis por Taenia solium y riesgo epidemiológico de cisticercosis en las comunidades del Valle del Río Temerla, Estados Carabobo y Yaracuy. Curso Medio de Salud Pública, Dpto. de Medicina Preventiva y Social VII, Escuela de Medicina "Witremundo Torrealba", Facultad de Ciencias de la Salud, Universidad de Carabobo.1994.
[83] Ferrer E., Cabrera Z., Cortés M M, Lares M, Harrison L, Parkhouse RME. Inmunodiagnóstico de cisticercosis basado en la detección de antígenos en comunidades rurales alrededor de Canoabo. Ed. Carabobo. *Act. Cient. Venezolana, AsoVAC.* 1998;49(2): 297.
[84] Ferrer E., Cortés M. M, Rojas G., Lares M., Fernández I., Harrison L., Parkhouse R.M.E. y Cabrera Z. Seroprevalencia y factores de riesgo de cisticercosis en dos comunidades rurales, Sanare y Río Tocuyo Edo. Lara 1998. *Act. Cient. Venezolana, AsoVAC.* 1999;50(2): 345.
[85] Meza N., Rossi N., Sánchez N., Muñoz J., Hernández M. y Urdaneta H. Teniasis y cisticercosis humana en una población rural del Estado Táchira, Venezuela. *Act. Cient. Venezolana, AsoVAC.* 1999;50(2):265-267.
[86] Carpio A, Hauser WA. Prognosis for seizure recurrence in patients with newly diagnosed neurocysticercosis. *Neurology* 2002;59:1730–1734.
[87] David J. Neurocysticercosis. "Dr. House Series" .Martes 22 de febrero del 2011.(última revisión en septiembre 22, 2011).

http://mentiraomedicina.blogspot.com/2011/02/neurocisticercosis.html

[88] Lombardo L, Matheus J.H., Cerebral Cysticercosis in México, Neurology 1961;11:825-828.

[89] Takayanagui OM. Neurocysticercosis: I. Clinical and laboratory course of 151 cases. *Arq Neuropsiquiatr* 1990; 48(1):1-10.

[90] Takayanagui OM, Leite JP. Neurocysticercosis. *Rev Soc Bras Med Trop* 2001;34(3):283-290.

[91] Kalra V, Paul VK, Marwah RK, Kichhar Gs, Bhargava S. Neurocysticercosis in childhood. *Trans R Soc Trop Med Hyg* 1987;81(3):371-373.

[92] Scharf D. Neurocysticercosis. Two hundred thirty-eight cases from a California Hospital. *Arch Neurol* 1988; 45:777-780.

[93] Sotelo J, Guerrero V, Rubio F. Neurocysticercosis: a new classification based on active and inactive forms. *Arch Intern Med.* 1985;145:442–445.

[94] Villa AM, Monteverde DA, Rodríguez W, Boero A, Sica RE. Neurocysticercosis in a hospital of the city of Buenos Aires: study of 11 cases. *Arq Neuropsiquiatr* 1993;51(3):336-336.

[95] Singh G. Neurocystycercosis in South-Central America and the Indian subcontinent. A comparative evaluation. *Arq Neuropsiquatr* 1997; 55(3A):349-356.

[96] Singh G, Kaushal V, Ram S, Kaushal RK, Dhanuka AK, Khurana S. Cysticercus immunoblot assay in patients with single, small enhancing lesions and multilesional neurocysticercosis. *J Assoc Physicians India* 1999;47:476–479.

[97] Del Brutto OH. Neurocysticercosis in children: clinical and radiological analysis and prognostic factor in 54 patients. *Rev Neurol* 1997; 25(147):1681-1484.

[98] Del Brutto OH. Neurocysticercosis. *Rev Neurol* 1999; 29(5):4456-4466.

[99] Del Bruto OH, Santibáñez R, Rubio CA, Aguirre R, Diez E, Alarcón TA. Epilepsy due to neurocysticercosis: analysis of 203 patients. *Neurology* 1992; 42:389-392

[100] Del Bruto OH, Rajshekhar V, White AC Jr, Tsang VC, et al. Proposed diagnostic criteria for Neurocysticercosis. *Neurology* 2001; 57(2):177-183.

[101] Sanchez, A.L.; Lindback, J.; Schantz, P.M.; Sone, M.; Sakai, H.; Medina, M.T. & Ljungstrom I. A population based case-control study of *Taenia solium* taeniosis and cysticercosis. *Ann Tropical Medical Parasitology* 1999;93: 247-258.

[102] Varma A, Gaur KJ. The clinical spectrum of Neurocysticercosis in the Uttraranchal region. *Assoc Physicians India* 2002;50:1398-1400.

[103] García HH, Evans CA, Nash TE, Takayanagui OM, White AC jret al., Current Consensus Guidelines for Treatment of Neurocysticercosis. *Clin Microbiol Rev* 2002; 15(4)747-756.

[104] García HH, Gonzalez AE, Evans CA, Gilman RH; Cysticercosis Working Group in Peru. Taenia solium cysticercosis. *Lancet.* 2003; 362: 547-556.

[105] Uddin J, Garcia HH, Gilman RH, Gonzalez AE, Friedland JS. Monocyte-astrocyte networks and the regulation of chemokine secretion in neurocysticercosis. *J Immunol.* 2005;175(5):3273-3281.

[106] Winkler AS, Kerschbaumsteiner K, Stelzhammer B, Meindl M, Kaaya J, Schmutzhard E. Prevalence, incidence, and clinical characteristics of epilepsy--a community-based door-to-door study in northern Tanzania. *Epilepsia.* 2009;50(10):2310-2313.

[107] Preux P-M and Druet-Cabanac M. Epidemiology and aetiology of epilepsy in sub-Saharan Africa. *Lancet Neurol* 2005; 4:21-31.

[108] Hoberg EP, Alkire NL, de Queiroz A, and Jones A. Out of Africa: origins of the Taenia tapeworms in humans. *Proc. R. Soc.* Lond.B 2001;268:781–787.

[109] Heslip , S. 2001. Time-Space chart. ANP440. Hominid fossils. Spring Semester, 2001. http://www.msu.edu/~heslipst/contents/ANP440/index.htm (accessed 27 February 2012).

[110] Alles , D. 2001. Cenozoic. http://fire.biol.wwu.edu/trent/alles/Cenozoic.pdf (accessed 28 February 2012).

[111] Asfaw , B., White T, Lovejoy O, Latimer B, Simpson S, Suwa G. 1999. *Australopithecus garhi* : A New Species of Early Hominid from Ethiopia. SCIENCE 1999;284:629-635.

[112] Cox, F.E.G. History of Human Parasitology. Clinical Microbiology Reviews. 2002; 15(4):595- 612. http://cmr.asm.org/content/15/4/595 (accessed 05 March 2012).

[113] Discover magazine. http://blogs.discovermagazine.com/loom/2010/04/26/why-madag as carstapeworms-matter-to-you. (accessed 20 March 2012).

[114] Ancient Hebrew Medicine. http://www.healthguidance.org/entry/6309/1/Ancient-HebrewMedicine.html (accessed 07 March 2012).

[115] Greek Medicine. Hippocrates. Available at the URL: http://www.greekmedicine.net/whos_who/Hippocrates.html (accessed 27 February 2012).

[116] Flisser A, Espinoza B, Tovar A, Plancarte A, Correa D. Host--parasite relationship in cysticercosis: an immunological study in different compartments of the host. Vet Parasitol. 1986 Mar;20(1-3):95-102.

[117] Wikipedia- Muhammad ibn Zakariya al-Razi. http://en.wikipedia.org/wiki/Muhammad_ibn_Zakariya_al-Razi (accessed 10 March 2012).

[118] Wikipedia- Pedanius Dioscorides. http://en.wikipedia.org/wiki/Dioscorides. (accessed 10 March 2012).

[119] Cordero M, Hidalgo A, Cisticercosis (C. cellulosae). 1999. Parasitología Veterinarian. Edit. Cordero del Campillo M, and Rojo V. Ed Mc Graw Hill-Interamericana, Madrid. pages 493-495.

[120] Wadia, NH, Singh, G. "Taenia Solium: A Historical Note" Taenia Solium Cysticercosis: From Basic to Clinical Science CABI Publishing, 2002. 157-168.

[121] Great Medicine-Galen. http://www.greekmedicine.net/whos_who/Galen.html. (accessed 13 March 2012).

[122] Hort AF: Theophrastus (1916). ed. *Theophrastus: Enquiry into Plants.* 1, Book I-V. New York: Loeb Classical Library/G.P. Putnam's Sons. cited in: http://en.wikipedia.org/wiki/Theophrastus (accessed 15 March 2012).

[123] Greek Medicine-Avicenna. Available at the URL:

http://www.greekmedicine.net/whos_who/Avicenna.html accessed 15 March 2012).
[124] Umami Medicine. http://www.greekmedicine.net/whos_who/Avicenna.html (accessed 15 March 2012).
[125] Macias V, Maqueo M. Cisticercosis cerebral. *Rev Invest Clin.* 1958;4:443-454.
[126] Del Brutto O, Sotelo J. Neurocysticercosis Update. *Rev. Inf. Dis.*1988;10(6):1075-1087
[127] Olive J.L., Angulo, R.P. introduction and general aspects Panel discussion. Cysticercosis of the nervous system. J. Neurosurg 19:632-34, 1962.
[128] McLachlan RS. Julius Caesar's late onset epilepsy: a case of historic proportions. *Can J Neurol Sci.* 2010 Sep;37(5):557-561.
[129] Flisser A. Neurocysticercosis in Mexico. *Parasitol Today*1988; 4:131-137.
[130] García E, Cruz, Historia de la Cisticercosis. *Teniasis y Cisticercos en el Ecuador*, ed. MSP, Quito, 1991.
[131] Mora R, et al., "Neurocisticercosis" .En infecciones del sistema nervioso central. *Ed. Fondo Educativo Interamericano.* Págs.267-283, Bogotá 1978.
[132] Giovanni Battista Morgagni. http://en.wikipedia.org/wiki/Giovanni_Battista_Morgagni (accessed 25 March 2012).
[133] Abraham Gottlob Werner. http://en.wikipedia.org/wiki/Abraham_Gottlob_Werner (accessed 25 March 2012).
[134] René Laennec. http://en.wikipedia.org/wiki/Ren%C3%A9_Laennec (accessed 25 March 2012). [137]
[135] Rudolf Virchow. Wikipedia. http://creationwiki.org/Rudolf_Virchow (accessed 28 March 2012).[138] Rudolf Leuckart http://en.wikipedia.org/wiki/Rudolf_Leuckart (accessed 29 March 2012).
[136] Friedrich Albert von Zenker. http://en.wikipedia.org/wiki/Friedrich_Albert_von_Zenker(accessed 29 March 2012).
[137] Lasso J. Contribución a la historia de la cisticercosis cerebral.Vol XXXI, 1994 http://escuela.med.puc.cl/publ/cuadernos/1994/pub_02_94.html. (accessed 30 March 2012).
[138] Alarcón T. Cisticercosis cerebral en el Ecuador, revisión de 32 casos estudiados. *Revista Ecuatoriana de Ciencias Neurológicas.* 1978;1:13-25.
[139] Carvajal J. La cisticercosis humana en México (simposio),1988; 124 (5,6), 1988.
[140] Dickmann, G.H. Cisticercosis de la fosa craneana posterior. *Rev. Neurol* (B. Aires), 15:160-179, 1946.
[141] Nieto D. Cysticercosis of the nervous system. Diagnosis by mean of spinal fluid complement fixation test. Neurology 1956;6:725-737.
[142] Obrador S. Cysticercosis cerebri. Acta Neurochirurgica. 1962; 10(3): 320-364.
[143] Proaño J, Proaño J.V, Molina Alvarez, Lasso J. Guía de Intervención: normas técnicas, métodos y procedimientos para el programa de control y vigilancia epidemiológica del complejo teniasis/cisticercosis. Editorial Ministerio de Salud Pública, Quito-Ecuador 1993.
[144] Flisser A, Tarrab R, Willms K, Larralde C. Immunoelectrophoresis and double immunodiffusion in the diagnosis of human cerebral cysticercosis. Arch Invest Med (Mex). 1975;6(1):1-12.

[145] Flisser A, Pérez-Montfort R, Larralde C. The immunology of human and animal cysticercosis: a review. Bull World Health Organ. 1979;57(5):839-856

[146] Flisser A, Woodhouse E, Larralde C. Human cysticercosis: antigens, antibodies and non-responders. Clin Exp Immunol. 1980 Jan;39(1):27-37

[147] Flisser A, Laclette JP, Larralde C, Vogt M, Willms K. Integral study of cysticercosis. A summary of a scientific event.Bol Chil Parasitol. 1981 Jul-Aug;36(3-4):63-65.

[148] Flisser A. Immunology of human cysticercosis. Bol Estud MED Biol. 1983 Jul-Oct;32(7-8 Suppl 1):143-76

[149] Pérez Sánchez E., Zúñiga G, Sarmiento J, Hernández C. Correlaciones Preliminares entre Clínica, Escanografía e Inmunología. Rev. UIS-Medicina.Buaramanga (Colombia); 1986,14(1):115- 127.

[150] Vaz JA, Ferreira WA. Immunodiagnóstico da neurocisticircose: Teste inmunoenzimático com antigenos quimicamente ligados a suportes para pesquisa de anticorpos em soro e líquido cefalorraquiano. Rev. Inst. Med.Trop.Sao Paulo; 1988,30 (1)1-10.

[151] Gonzales Armando E., Cama Vialiano., Hilman Robert H., et al. Prevalence and comparisons of serologic assays, necropsy and tongue examination for the diagnosis of porcine cysticercosis in Perú. Am. Jour. Trop Med Hyg; 1990, 43(2):194-199.

[152] Foyaca-Sibat H, Cowan LD, Carabin H, Serrano-Ocaña G, , Krecek RC, Willingham A. "Accuracy of serological exam for the diagnosis of neurocysticercosis in outpatients with epilepsy, Eastern Cape Province, South Africa" PLOS Negleted Trop.Dis.Dec.2009;3(3):1-7.

[153] Tsang, Víctor C., Brand Joy ., Boyer Ann E., An Enzime Linked inmunoelectrotransfer Blot Assay and Glycoprotein Antigens for Diagnosing HumanCysticercosis (Taenia Soliu). Journal H of Infectous Diseases; 1989, 159 (1): 50-59.

[154] Tsang VCW, Brand AJ, Boyer AE. An Enzyme-linked immunoelectrotransfer blot assay by glycoprotein antigens for diagnosing human cysticercosis (*Taenia solium*). *J Infect Dis.*1989;159: 50– 59.

[155] Tsang C.W., and Brand A. Joy ., A rapid inmunoblot Assay (Western Blot), to Detected Taenia Solium (cysticercosis), Journal of Inmuno Assay; 1989, 10(2-3-:237.

[156] Tsang C W Víctor., Pilcher Joy A., Zhou Wei., et al Efficacy of the inmunoblot assay for cuysticercosis in pigs and in pigs and mpodiulated expression of distinct IgM, IgG activities to taennia solium antigens in exparimental infections. Veterinary Inmonology and Inmunopathology; 1991, 29:69-66.

[157] Wilson M., Bryan Ralph T., Fried Janet A., et al., Clinical evaluation of the cysticercosis Enzyme-Linked Inmunoelectrotransfer Blot in Patients with neurocysticercosis. The Journal of infectous Diseases; 1991, 164:1007-1009.

[158] Flisser A. Overview of immunology. Arch Med Res. 1997 Spring;28(1):145, 147

[159] Flisser A, Gyorkos TW. Contribution of immunodiagnostic tests to epidemiological/intervention studies of cysticercosis/taeniosis in Mexico. Parasite Immunol. 2007 Dec;29(12):637-649.

[160] Medina MT, Rosas E, Rubio-Donnadieu F, Sotelo J. Neurocysticercosis as the main cause of late-onset epilepsy in Mexico. Arch Intern Med. 1990 Feb;150(2):325-7.

Chapter 2

Neuroimmunoendocrine Interactions in Murine Cysticercosis: From the Lab Bench Work to Its Possible Applications in Controlling Porcine Cysticercosis and Human Neurocysticercosis

Karen Nava-Castro, Romel Hernández-Bello,
Saé Muñiz-Hernández, Lorena López-Griego,
Jhonatan A. Hernández-Valdés, Valeria López-Salazar,
Nelly Tiempos-Guzmán and Jorge Morales-Montor

Additional information is available at the end of the chapter

http://dx.doi.org/10.5772/50700

1. Introduction

The immune and neuroendocrine systems are interconnected by a network in which hormones, antigens, receptors, cytokines, antibodies and neuropeptides modulate immune response in connection with neuroendocrine changes while maintaining homeostasis (Besedovsky & del Rey, 1996). Two of the main components of this network are the hypothalamic-pituitary-adrenocortical (HPA) and the hypothalamic-pituitary-gonadal axes (HPG) (Besedovsky & del Rey, 2000; Rivier & Rivest, 1993).

Interactions between the immune system and both the HPA and HPG axes are characterized by their activation and starting of the stress response, which, in turn, has immunomodulating activities that are important in preventing excessive immune responses (Chikanza & Grossman, 2000; Morales-Montor *et al.*, 2004b). Furthermore, the important functions of both axes have been shown for adaptation and maintenance of homeostasis during critical illness and viral, bacterial, parasitic and autoimmune diseases (Besedovsky & del Rey, 1996). An important aspect of cell communication that has emerged as a result of studying neuro-endocrine-immune interactions is the redundancy of the use of some chemical messengers to communicate among them. As an example, neurotrophins are chemical messengers first identified and characterized in the nervous system. Members of this protein family are also expressed and secreted by immune and endocrine cells, and have immunological and endocrinological functions (Haddad *et al.*, 2002).

INTECH
open science | open minds

© 2013 Morales-Montor et al., licensee InTech. This is a paper distributed under the terms of the Creative Commons Attribution License (http://creativecommons.org/licenses/by/3.0), which permits unrestricted use, distribution, and reproduction in any medium, provided the original work is properly cited.

Thus, the lack ubiquitous use of some cellular messengers by different organic systems might be a rule, rather than an exception. Although strong evidence supports that neurons, endocrine and immune cells produce hormones, while neural, endocrine and immune cells synthesize and secrete neuroactive messengers (Ferone *et al.*, 2006), it remains somewhat controversial whether this network is involved in the final outcome of parasitic diseases, and, particularly in cysticercosis (natural and experimental) (Morales-Montor & Larralde, 2005).

Taeniids, particularly *Taenia solium,* the porcine cysticercosis (CC) and human neurocysticercosis (NCC) causal agent; and *Taenia crassiceps*, murine cysticercosis causal agent, are highly evolved parasites that have developed diverse mechanisms of survival that facilitate their establishment in the host. These mechanisms can be roughly grouped into two types: 1) evasion of the immune response by molecular mimicry or by inactivating effector immune processes (i.e, complement inhibition) (Baig *et al.*, 2005; Laclette *et al.*, 1989); and 2) by exploiting the host system to allow its establishment, growth or reproduction (Escobedo *et al.*, 2004). This exploitation mechanism provides parasites with a dual benefit: first, obtaining amino acids for metabolism, and second preventing the surface-bound antibody from interfering with cytotoxic cells interacting with the parasite (Damian, 1989; Locksley, 1997). A striking example of host's molecules exploitation is the ability of several taeniids to use host-synthesized cytokines as indirect growth factors for themselves and also exploit the hormonal microenvironment within the host in their favor (Escobedo *et al.*, 2005). Taeniids have evolved structures similar to the steroid and protein hormone receptors expressed in upper vertebrates, with binding properties and terminal effects similar to the hormonal metabolites synthesized by the host (Gomez *et al.*, 2000). Such cross regulation from host to parasite has been described in at least eight parasitic infections that are caused by parasitic cestodes, like schistosomiasis (LoVerde *et al.*, 1985), filariasis (Rajan *et al.*, 2005), hydatid disease (Brehm *et al.*, 2003) and murine cysticercosis (Escobedo *et al.*, 2004).

Understanding how the host's endocrine system can favor the establishment of taeniids under certain circumstances, led us to explore the parasite's hormone receptors that might be involved, designing hormonal analogs and drugs to specifically affect the parasite (Escobedo *et al.*, 2004). This review is focused on the literature concerning sex-steroids, adrenal steroids and other hormones and neurohormones that have been studied in regard to control parasite loads in experimental murine cysticercosis.

1.1. Experimental murine cysticercosis

Due to the intrinsic difficulties in working with the natural hosts (pigs and humans) of *T. solium* and the high costs of enough pigs plus the slowness in data retrieval, we have used an experimental cysticercosis approach to gain knowledge of the complex host (H) parasite (P) relationship in CC. Murine intraperitoneal cysticercosis is caused by the taeniid *T. crassiceps* and it has been useful to explore the physiological host factors associated with porcine cysticercosis, and to some degree, with human NCC (Larralde *et al.*, 1990). Intraperitoneal *T. crassiceps* cysticercosis of mice (Huerta *et al.*, 1992; Larralde *et al.*, 1990; Smith *et al.*, 1972) lends itself well to controlled and reproducible experimentation, generating numerical data of parasite loads in individual mice in a matter of weeks after infection. Its general representation of other forms of cysticercosis has later been strengthened by similar results in other mouse and parasite strains (Larralde *et al.*, 1986), by the parasite's extensive sharing of antigens with other taeniids and cestodes and by the DNA homology between *T. crassiceps and T. solium* (Larralde *et al.*, 1986; Larralde *et al.*, 1990). These characteristics have made murine cysticercosis a convenient instrument to test vaccine candidates (Sciutto *et al.*, 1990) and new drugs or treatments against CC. Several features of natural cysticercotic disease have been found by extrapolation from experimental murine cysticercosis (Morales-Montor *et al.*, 2002a; Sciutto *et al.*, 2007).

1.2. Immuno-endocrine interactions in the host

In order to figure out the effect of infection on the immune system, on the feminized male mice, thymic cell analysis performed by flow cytometry showed a diminution in the content of CD3+, CD4+, and CD8+ subpopulations in the infected mice. This suggest that the increase in estradiol levels of the host could change the expression pattern of several genes that participate in apoptosis regulation in the thymus of male mice during chronic infection with *T. crassiceps* cysticerci, by inhibiting the inhibit the specific cellular immune response to the parasite (Morales-Montor *et al.*, 1998). Previous immunological experiments had led to suspect that estradiol positively regulates parasite reproduction in hosts of both genders, presumably by interfering with the thymus-dependent cellular immune mechanisms that obstruct parasite growth (Th_1) and favoring those that facilitate it (Th_2) (Bojalil *et al.*, 1993; Terrazas *et al.*, 1994). A specific shift from Th_1 to Th_2 immune response in the course of infection was found that coincided with the initial low rate of reproduction that accelerates at later times of infection. The shift is characterized by a marked decrease of IL-2 and IFN-γ in both genders, while the secretion of cytokines involved in the specific humoral response (IL-6, IL-10 and IL-4) is enhanced (Terrazas *et al.*, 1998; Terrazas *et al.*, 1999). Thus, striking differences in susceptibility to cysticercosis between male and female mice may involve the joint action of the immune system and the gonads, both driven by a parasite, which is able to change the parasite´s restrictive male normal hormonal milieu during chronic infection to a more parasite´s permissive female environment.

To strengthen the above notions and in an effort to identify the sex steroids involved we studied the effects of testosterone (T_4), dihydrotestosterone (DHT), and 17β-estradiol (E_2) in castrated mice of both genders infected with *T. crassiceps* cysticerci (Morales-Montor *et al.*, 2002a). In this study, we found that castration and treatment with either T_4 or DHT before infection markedly decreased parasite loads in both gender mice, while the treatment with E_2 increased it in both genders (Morales-Montor *et al.*, 2002a). The specific splenocyte cell proliferation and IL-2 and IFN-γ production were depressed in infected-castrated mice of both genders, while treatment with T_4 or DHT produced a significant cell proliferation recovery and enhanced production of IL-2 and IFN-γ (Morales-Montor *et al.*, 2002a). An opposite effect of the same sex steroids was found on the humoral response: it was unaffected with T_4 or DHT restitution, while the treatment with E_2 in both genders augmented the levels of anti-cysticerci IgG, as well as IL-6 and IL-10 production. These results suggest androgens mediate immune functions, which protect mice from cysticercosis, possibly through the stimulation of the specific cellular immunity of the host (Morales-Montor *et al.*, 2002a).

Immunoendocrine interactions during cysticercosis are the cornerstone of the feminization of male mice. When the infected male mice have an intact immune system, there is an increase in serum estradiol levels and a decrease of those of T_4 and DHT. However, when the immune system is knocked down by total irradiation or neonatal thymectomy, there is no change in the levels of serum steroids in chronically infected male mice, and the levels remain steady between infected and uninfected male mice (Morales-Montor *et al.*, 2001). Interleukin-6 (IL-6) was demonstrated a key factor in this puzzle: IL-$6^{-/-}$ (KO) infected mice do not develop the feminization process, while the restitution with IL-6 again allows the feminization. The expression of IL-6 gene in the testes of parasitized mice was enhanced, a fact that can explain the primordial role of the testes in the feminization process produced by cysticercosis (Morales-Montor *et al.*, 2002a; Morales-Montor *et al.*, 2001). Thus, IL-6 activates aromatase expression in the testes of the cysticercotic mice and produces active aromatization from androgens to estrogens. The increased serum levels of follicle stimulating hormone (FSH), the natural activator of aromatase expression, found in the chronically infected mice, supports the notion that FSH could be also a factor involved in the feminization process in the male mouse (Morales-Montor *et al.*, 2001). Actually, macrophage-migration inhibitory factor (MIF) is known to be involved in immunoendocrinological processes during sex-associated susceptibility in cysticercosis. Thus, to determine the role of IL-6 and MIF during infection, knockout (KO) mice were used, and the number of parasites and serum sex-steroid levels were measured. It was found that IL-6 and MIF KO mice of both genders infected with *T. crassiceps* cysticerci harbor similar numbers of parasites, with no change in sex-hormone levels. However, in wild-type strains, the sex-associated susceptibility to infection is observed, concomitantly with the feminization process in the chronically infected mice (Morales-Montor *et al.*, 2002b). These results suggest a role for both IL-6 and MIF genes in sex-associated susceptibility in murine *T. crassiceps* cysticercosis.

The importance of sex hormones driving the specific immune response during cysticercosis was assessed by administration of fadrozole (a P450-aromatase inhibitor) in male and female mice to suppress the production of E_2 (Morales-Montor *et al.*, 2002c). A reduction was found in parasite loads (~ 70%) in infected mice treated with fadrozole. The protective effect of the P450-aromatase inhibitor was associated in male mice with a recovery of the specific cellular immune response. IL-6 serum levels, and its production by splenocytes were dramatically augmented, together with an increase in its expression in the testes of infected male mice. Fadrozole treatment returned these levels to baseline values. These results suggest that P450-ase and IL-6 are key molecules in feminization undergone by infected male mice and in regulating parasite loads. Fadrozole treatment appears as a possible new therapeutic approach to control murine cysticercosis (Morales-Montor *et al.*, 2002c) and perhaps other parasites with active asexual reproduction in intermediate hosts.

Progesterone (P_4) was recently tested and implicated in the regulation of the parasite loads during murine cysticercosis. P_4 treatment has a dichotomic effect: in non-gonadectomized (intact) of both genders, P_4 treatment increased parasite loads, while gonadectomized mice, P_4 completely decreases parasite loads, an impressive and unprecedented cysticidal effect. In the first case, the effect of P_4 is possibly associated to the manipulation of the specific cellular immune response, besides the steroid's promotion of parasite reproduction (Vargas-Villavicencio *et al.*, 2006). In a second analysis, it was demonstrated that infected mice that received P_4 treatment increased estrogen levels two-fold compared to infected control mice. (Vargas-Villavicencio *et al.*, 2005; Vargas-Villavicencio *et al.*, 2006). A flow chart of the main immunoendocrinological effects of *T. crassiceps* infection in male and female mice is depicted in Figure 1.

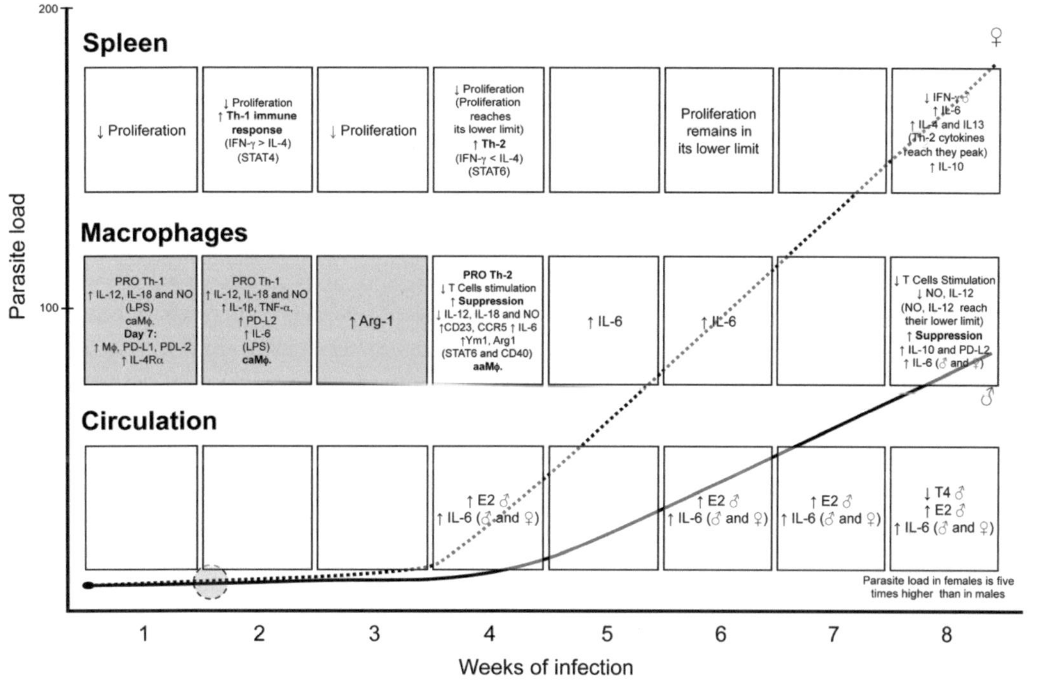

Figure 1. Early immune events during murine cysticercosis. During murine cysticercosis, there is a marked sexual dimorfism in parasite loads, having females, higher parasite loads than males, because of the effect of E_2 and T_4. These hormones also regulate immune responses. During the second week post infection, there is a clear Th1 response characterized by the expression of STAT4, high levels of IFN-γ and reduced levels of IL-4. After 4 weeks post-infection, immune response polarizes to a Th2 profile, in which STAT6, high levels of IL-4 and reduced levels of IFN-γ are observed. All these changes correlate to an overproduction of E_2. IL-6 levels are also increased as infection takes place. High levels of this cytokine are associated to a feminization process, as observed by the low levels of T_4. Doted line: Female parasitic load. Solid line: Male parasitic load. Signs (↑ and ↓) denote increase or decrease phenomena.

The major steroid produced by the adrenal gland is the androgen dehydroepiandrosterone (DHEA). So, another set of experiments showed DHEA effect on male and female infected mice. DHEA treatment reduced parasite loads by 70 and 80% respectively. In contrast with the common assumption of DHEA as an immune-stimulatory hormone, the immune responses of our mice, characterized by the expression of IL-2, IFN-γ, IL-4 or IL-10, was not affected by DHEA treatment (Vargas-Villavicencio *et al.*, 2008). *In vitro*, treatment of *T. crassiceps* cysticerci with DHEA induced 80% reduction in parasite reproduction, which may partially explain the reduction of parasite loads observed *in vivo* a partial effect suggesting the involvement of other unknown factors in the in vivo regulation of parasite loads (Vargas-Villavicencio *et al.*, 2008). In addition, the use of 16α-bromoepiandrosterone (EpiBr), a DHEA analog without significant androgenic activity, inhibited proliferation of cysticerci in vitro and decreased the *T. crassiceps* cysticerci load up to 50% in the peritoneal cavity of Balb/c mice (Carrero *et al.*, 2010).

1.3. Behavioral changes in the infected host

The hormonal changes in cysticercotic mice, profoundly affect their behavior, such as sexual activity (Morales *et al.*, 1996), aggressiveness (Gourbal *et al.*, 2001), social status (Gourbal *et al.*, 2002) prey/predator defense responses, and also cognitive functions. Male mice infected with *T. crassiceps* show remarkable changes in sexual behavior, characterized by a complete loss of the ejaculation response early at the infection (six weeks), followed by a gradual decrease in the number of mounts and intromissions, and their latencies increased, until none of the parasitized mice showed any sexual response toward female mice (Morales *et al.*, 1996). Moreover, it was demonstrated that changes in sexual behavior were due to the change in the normal production of sex-steroids by the mouse, since there was a complete restoration of their sexual behavior after T_4 or DHT restitution of the infected male mice (Gourbal *et al.*, 2001). Since *c-fos* and progesterone receptor gene (PGR), both are key E_2-regulated genes involved in the regulation of sexual behavior, we studied possible changes of *c-fos* and PGR expression in the central nervous system (CNS) of infected male mice. Indeed, *c-fos* and PGR expression oscillated with time of infection and to different magnitudes in hypothalamus, brain cortex and preoptic area but neither in other areas of the brain nor in several other organs of the host (Morales-Montor *et al.*, 2004a; Rodriguez-Dorantes *et al.*, 2007).

Furthermore, infection disrupts the dominant-subordinate status (Gourbal *et al.*, 2002). In infected male mice strong perturbations in territorial behavior and aggressiveness were found. In addition, during confrontation between naive infected and healthy mice, infected animals more often assumed a subordinate status than healthy ones. The effects of the infection by *T. crassiceps* were more likely to prevent adult male mice from becoming behaviorally dominant than to reverse existing dominance relationships (Gourbal *et al.*, 2001).

Significant CNS changes in *c-fos,* and PR expression during infection signifies the brain senses the infection episode and may be involved in the ensuing behavioral changes of the infected mice, as well as, through its connectivity, extend the effects of infection to other physiological systems under its influence. That these changes in CNS are beneficial to the host or parasite remains speculative (Klein, 2000). One could argue that feminization of male hosts favors the parasite by allowing reproduction in otherwise restrictive male mice, but equally arguable would be to consider feminization of the male host as deleterious to the parasite's completion of its cycle by reducing male exposure to its predators, the definitive hosts. Other similar mutually conflicting statements may be elaborated with the above premises, the true ones remain to be identified and could perhaps vary with each different host-parasite relationship.

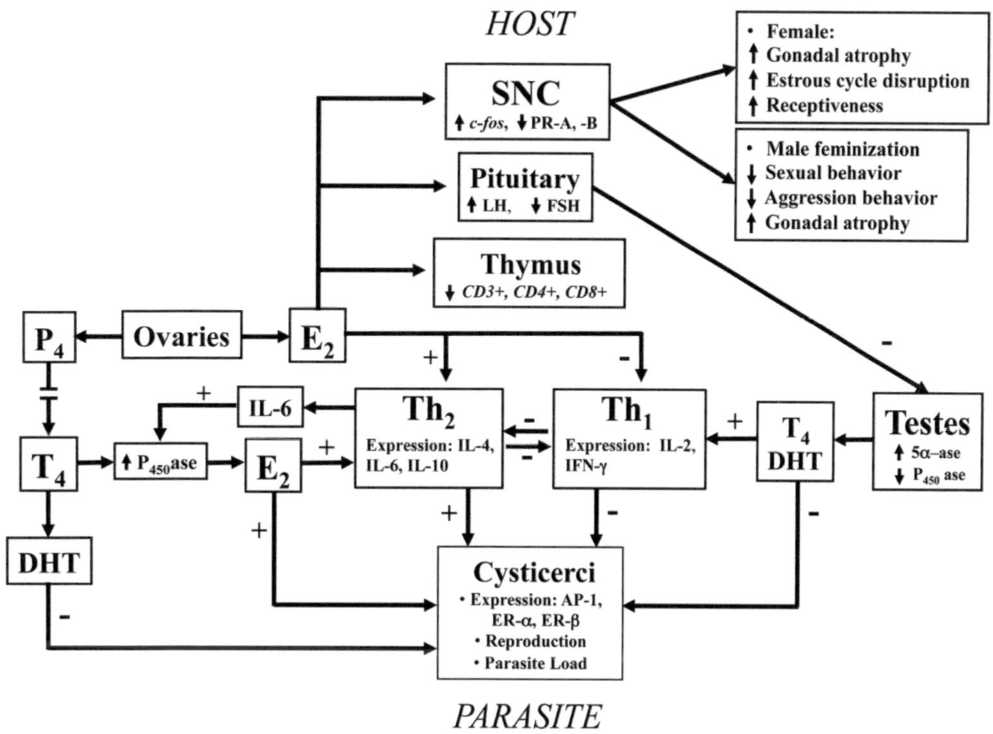

Figure 2. Neuroimmunoendocrine changes in host during murine cysticercosis. Infection with *Taenia sp*, leads to a Th2 response with high levels of IL-6 activating the P450-aromatase, which convert T_4 into E_2 increasing its level in the host. Estrogens are permissive for the infection while androgens (T_4, DHT) inhibit parasite reproduction and reduce parasite load. E_2 overproduction induces behavioral changes in male and female. Signs (+ and -) means induction and inhibition respectively; signs (↑ and ↓) denote increase or decrease phenomena.

However, not only male mice are behaviorally affected by CC, female mice also suffer perturbations in their sexual behavior. Infected females were less receptive to the male at 6 weeks post infection (p.i.) and until 12 weeks p.i.; and there was also an interruption in the estrous cycle that was clearly starting at 12 weeks of infection and remained until the 16th weeks. These changes were associated to the low levels of serum E_2 that were comparable to those found during the diestrus stage of control mice (Arteaga-Silva *et al.*, 2009). That sex steroids, particularly E_2 is very important to the host-parasite relationship in CC, was recently demonstrated by Guzman, *et al* (Guzman *et al.*, 2009). A single injection of E_2 administered to 4-day-old male and female mice increased the cellular immune response and induced resistance to *T. crassiceps* cysticercosis. At the same time, there are changes in the expression pattern of PR and estrogen receptor (ER) isoforms in the brain and splenocytes. Regardless of gender, when treated mice reached adulthood, they were highly resistant to infection. Female mice presented early vaginal opening and altered estrous cycles. In male and female mice, the expression of the PR and ER isoforms in the brain was differentially regulated after neonatal exposure to estradiol. Moreover, an increase in the expression of IL-4 and IFN-γ was found in the serum of experimentally infected neonatally estrogenized animals, which correlated with the observed protection against *T. crassiceps* infection. In conclusion, early exposure to E_2 permanently modifies immune system activity and sex steroid hormone receptors in the brain, and causes profound changes in sex-associated susceptibility, leading to resistance to helminthic infection (Guzman *et al.*, 2009). A chart of all neuroimmunoendocrine changes during murine cysticercosis is depicted in Figure 2.

1.4. *Taenia solium* cysticercosis, neurocysticercosis and taeniosis

As described for the mouse model of CC, host's biological factors such as genetic background, the innate and acquired immunity and gender can lead to resistance and/or susceptibility to cysticercosis/taeniosis by *Taenia solium*. It has been shown that sexual hormones play an important role in porcine CC. For instance, castrated male pigs increased by 30% the prevalence of naturally acquired CC, while pregnant sows doubled the prevalence, compared to non castrated males and non-pregnant sows (Morales *et al.*, 2002). Another interesting finding, was found when in experiments designed to explore the hormonal profiles of sex steroids, as well as DHEA in serum of boars that had naturally acquired CC, it was observed a significant reduction in the T_4 levels, change that was independent of the heterogeneous genetic background and large range of ages. These findings suggest that sex steroids can be associated to *T. solium* susceptibility and transmission dynamics of this parasite in natural conditions (Pena *et al.*, 2007).

Interestingly, sex steroids are not the unique hormones that can be useful to this parasite. It has been recently described that the *in vitro* culture of *T. crassiceps* with insulin stimulates parasite reproduction by two-fold and increased the average of the bud diameter. However, this hormone had no effect on *T. solium* cysticerci culture (Escobedo *et al.*, 2009). On the other hand, hamsters treated with P_4 and experimentally infected with *T. solium* showed an 80% reduction of anchored-*T. solium* tapeworms, a reduced growth of these parasites and a down-regulation of the PR expression in 50% duodenum associated tapeworms. Immune response of P_4 treated hamsters showed an increase in IL-4, IL-6 and TNF-α cytokines and an exacerbated inflammatory infiltrate located along the lamina propria, compared to infected non-progesterone treated controls (Escobedo *et al.*, 2011). These results clearly support the fact that P_4 protects against the *T. solium* adult tapeworm establishment by improving the immune system.

The studies in mice and pigs have already been scaled to the natural human disease. A recent study on human NCC, caused by larvae of *T. solium* infiltration in the CNS demonstrated a strong correlation between the endocrine, immune systems, gender and age during the clinical manifestation and susceptibility to the disease. Cardenas, *et. al*, designed a clinical study to evaluate the hormonal changes associated with NCC and the relationships between disease heterogeneity, endocrine and immunological status. Since the proper diagnostic of the disease was fundamental in this study, a precise clinical and radiological description of the disease and a complete hormonal and immunological profile was performed to 50 patients and 22 healthy subjects. Patients had lower DHEA levels compared to healthy subjects. Concerning to gender, male patients showed a clear decrease in 17β-estradiol serum levels and high levels of Luteinizing Hormone (LH), while female patients with clinically severe disease showed lower levels of progesterone and androstenedione. Higher concentrations of follicle stimulating hormone (FSH) and lower concentrations of testosterone (similar to those reported previously during murine cysticercosis) were found in male patients with severe disease, when compared with the less clinically severe patients. Significant correlations were found between E_2 and IL-10 in male patients, and between DHEA and IL-1β, and androstenedione and IL-17 in female patients, suggesting a possible immunoendocrine interaction. The study by Cardenas, *et. al.* in neurocysticercotic patients constitutes the first demonstration that the presence of *T. solium* larvae in the central nervous system, can modify the host environment by the induction of endocrine and immunological changes. As the authors point out, these results provide a stimulating background to analyze the repercussions of the hormonal changes during the course of disease and on patient reproductive health (Cardenas *et al.*, 2012). Taken together, the above-presented evidence open up the possibility of the use analogues of hormones, as novel anti-cysticercotic agents.

1.5. Direct effect of sex steroids on *Taenia crassiceps* and *Taenia solium* cysticercy

As described before, hormones play a significant role in murine *T. crassiceps* cysticercosis and participate in the susceptibility to *T. solium* cysticercosis. However, this effect is not only due to the regulation of the immune response by sex steroids, but also by acting directly upon cysticerci reproduction. For instance, it has been shown that *in vitro* treatment with E_2 and P_4 stimulates *T. crassiceps* reproduction. In contrast, T_4 or DHT inhibit and even exert a toxic effect on the parasite (Escobedo *et al.*, 2004). The possible molecular mechanisms by which sex-steroids affect *T. crassiceps* reproduction imply the presence of sex hormone receptors, since the use of tamoxifen, an anti-estrogenic compound (Escobedo *et al.*, 2005), decreases parasite reproduction *in vitro* and parasite loads *in vivo*, as described before (Vargas-Villavicencio *et al.*, 2007), we look for a estrogen receptor expressed by parasitic cells. As described by Ibarra, *et. al.* there is a molecule similar to the estrogen receptor alpha (ERα) identified by diverse methods such as western blot and PCR. This receptor is expressed exclusively by parasitic cells, as identified by the expression of a parasite-specific protein, paramyosin (Ibarra-Coronado *et al.*, 2011). Parasite cells expressing the ER-like protein were located by confocal microscopy in the subtegumental tissue exclusively. Sequencing of the spot produced a small fragment of protein similar to the mammalian nuclear ER. In addition to, once host's E_2 has bound to its parasite estrogen receptor, the dimeric complex would activate the transcription of several *T. crassiceps* proliferative genes, such as *c-fos*, *c-jun* and cyclin D1, directly or through the activation of the MAPK family of serine/threonine kinase, such as ERK, which has been also recently described in this parasite (Escobedo *et al.*, 2010). Since this hypothetical molecular mechanism could be *in vitro* interrupted by using tamoxifen, we suggest a genomic action mechanism for E_2 on the parasite.

On the other hand, the androgen mechanism might be different from the found for estrogens and progesterone. T_4 and DHT directly affect parasitic DNA integrity probably by activating apoptotic mechanism in the cysticercus cells. This experimental finding is not dependent of a nuclear receptor because flutamide (a well studied and used anti-androgen) did not have effects upon parasite reproduction *in vitro* (Escobedo *et al.*, 2005). These results demonstrate that sex steroids act directly upon parasite reproduction perhaps by binding to receptors closely resembling classic and specific sex-steroid vertebrate receptors (Escobedo *et al.*, 2005).

Furthermore, it has been shown that T. crassiceps cysticerci are able to metabolize sex steroids in vitro and, and that it possibly uses hosts hormones as positive or negative factors for its own reproduction (Gomez *et al.*, 2000). *T. solium* cysticercosis is a health problem in underdeveloped and developed countries. Sex hormones are involved in cysticercosis prevalence in female and male pigs. Interestingly, progesterone increased *T. solium* scolex evagination and worm growth, in a concentration-independent pattern. This effect could be mediated by the expression of a novel *T. solium* progesterone receptor (TsPR) since RU486 inhibits both scolex evagination and worm development induced by progesterone (Figure 3).

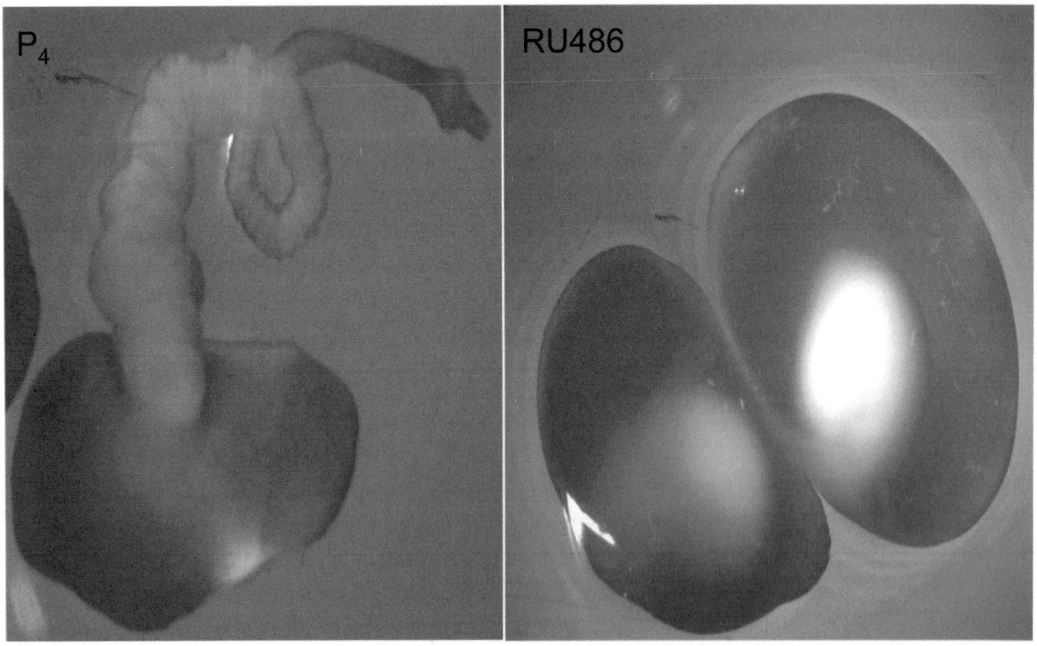

Figure 3. Effect of progesterone (P_4) and RU486 (progesterone analogue) in cultured cysts of *T. solium*. Progesterone promotes scolex evagination and worm growth while RU486 inhibit scolex evagination.

Using RT-PCR and western blot, sequences related to progesterone receptor were detected in the parasite. A phylogenetic analysis reveals that TsPR is highly related to fish and amphibian progesterone receptors, whereas it has a distant relation with birds and mammals. Conclusively, progesterone directly acts upon *T. solium* cysticerci, possibly by binding to a progesterone receptor synthesized by the parasite. The strong effects of sex steroids upon cysticercosis open new avenues for its control. In Table 1, there is a list of some hormone receptors reported in helminth parasites to date.

Hormone Receptor	Parasite	Ref/AC
Epidermal Growth Factor	*Schistosoma mansonii* *Echinococcus multilocularis*	(Ramachandran *et al.*, 1996) (Spiliotis *et al.*, 2003)
Insulin Receptor	*Schistosoma mansonii* *Schistosoma japonicum* *Echinococcus multilocularis*	(Khayath *et al.*, 2007) (You *et al.*, 2010) (Konrad *et al.*, 2003)
Retinoid X receptor	*Schistosomamansonii* *Brugia malayi*	(Freebern *et al.*, 1999) (Tzertzinis *et al.*, 2010)
Transforming growth factor-β	*Brugia pahangi*	(Gomez-Escobar *et al.*, 1997)
Retinoic acid-binding protein	*Onchocerca volvulus* *Onchocerca gibsoni,* *Dipetalonemaviteae* *Brugia pahangi* *Dirofilaria immitis*	(Sani *et al.*, 1985)
Estrogen Receptor	*Taenia crassiceps*	(Ibarra-Coronado *et al.*, 2011)
Constitutive androstane Receptor	*Schistosoma mansonii*	(Hu *et al.*, 2006)
Estrogen-related receptor-β	*Schistosoma japonicum*	(Wu *et al.*, 2012)
Putative Follicle-stimulating hormone receptor	*Trichinella spiralis*	XP_003375811
Ecdysone receptor	*Brugia malayi* *Dirofilaria immitis*	(Tzertzinis *et al.*, 2010) (Shea *et al.*, 2010)
Nuclear Hormone Receptors	*Brugia malayi* *Dirofilaria immitis* *Onchocerca volvulus* *Echinococcus multilocularis*	(Crossgrove *et al.*, 2002) (Crossgrove *et al.*, 2008) (Unnasch *et al.*, 1999) (Forster *et al.*, 2011)

Table 1. Principal hormonal receptors in parasites reported to date.

In vitro effects of human chorionic gonadotropin (hCG) on the larval stages of *T. crassiceps* (WFU strain) and *T. solium* have also been reported. As a matter of fact, these effects were correlated to the presence of receptors for hCG in different developmental phases of both cultured parasites. Authors argued that direct effect of hCG can be recognized as a factor contributing to the growth and development of *T. crassiceps* and *T. solium* cysticerci (Castellanos-Sanchez *et al.*, 2009). *T. crassiceps* and *T. solium* cysticerci have the ability to metabolize exogenous androstenedione to T_4, using different hormonal precursors (Jimenez *et al.*, 2006). A chart of all the immunoendocrine effects during *T. solium* cysticercosis is presented in Figure 2.

Finally, both *T. crassiceps* and *T. solium* expressed the insulin receptor, although insulin had effects only on *T. crassiceps.* Thus, insulin may be recognized by *T. crassiceps* cysticercus cells as a mitogenic factor, and contribute to parasite proliferation inside the host. This phenomenon has not been reported for cysticercosis caused by *T. solium*, which could, in part, be related to the poor effect of insulin upon the human parasite (Escobedo *et al.*, 2009).

1.6. Therapeutic applications of hormones in cysticercosis/taeniosis

The study and evaluation of new substances of hormonal nature and its analogues has emerged with great importance to develop a new generation of anti-parasitic drugs. In the case of *T. crassiceps*, the reconstitution and substitution (depending the host and hormone used) with sex steroids showed that T_4 or DHT treatment before infection decreased parasite loads by 50 and 70% respectively, suggesting a protective role for androgens (Morales-Montor *et al.*, 2002a). In contrast the treatment with E_2 increased it by three times in both genders as compared with controls. Even more, castrated mice of both genders treated with progesterone before infection, decreased parasite loads by 100% compared with intact uninfected mice. However the negative effects in the establishment, growth and reproduction of *T. crassiceps* was mediated by the metabolism of progesterone to DHEA in the adrenal gland of castrated animals (Vargas-Villavicencio *et al.*, 2006). To strength out the notion of DHEA as a protective agent, we designed experiments to test this hypothesis, by incubating *in vitro T. crassiceps* cysticerci with increasing concentrations of DHEA, and by *in vivo* treating male and female mice with DHEA and infecting them with *T. crassiceps* cysticerci. *In vitro*, DHEA has a strong cysticidal effect, being dose-dependent in physiological and pharmacological conditions. *In vivo* assays showed that DHEA reduce the viability of cysticerci in both male and female mice (Carrero *et al.*, 2006; Carrero *et al.*, 2010).

The use of EpiBr (analogue of DHEA) reduced the parasitic load in a major proportion in both male and female infected with *T. crassicepps* (Freilich *et al.*, 2000). Tamoxifen is an antiestrogen compound belonging to the group of Selective Estrogen Receptor Moduladors (SERM). Administration of tamoxifen in infected mice of both genders produced an 80% parasite load reduction in female mice, and a weaker effect of 50% in male mice. This protective effect was associated in both genders, with an increase in the mRNA levels of IL-2 (a cytokine associated with protection against cysticerci) and IL-4 (no effect on infection). Tamoxifen treatment modified E_2 production on females, whereas serum testosterone was not affected. However, the expression of the 2 types of ER, i.e., ER-α and ER-β in the spleen of infected mice of both genders, was decreased by tamoxifen treatment. *In vitro*, treatment of *T. crassiceps* with tamoxifen reduced reproduction and loss of motility. These results indicate that tamoxifen treatment is a new therapeutic possibility to treat CC, because it can act at both ends of the host–parasite relationship, i.e., by increasing the cellular immune response protective against the parasite and by directly affecting the parasite's reproduction and survival (Vargas-Villavicencio *et al.*, 2007). Table 2 has a summary of the above-mentioned therapeutic use of hormone analogue in *T. crassiceps* cysticercosis.

Compound	Infection	Reference
DHEA / DHEAS	*Cryptosporidium parvum*	(Rasmussen & Healey, 1992)
	Plasmodium falciparum	(Kurtis *et al.*, 2001)
	Entamoeba histolytica	(Carrero *et al.*, 2006)
	Schistosoma mansoni	(Fallon *et al.*, 1998)
	Trypanosoma cruzi	(dos Santos *et al.*, 2005)
16α-bromoepiandrosterone (EpiBr or HE2000)	*Taenia crassiceps*	(Carrero *et al.*, 2010)
	Entamoeba histolytica	(Carrero *et al.*, 2010)
	AIDS	(Reading *et al.*, 2006)
	Feline immunodeficiency virus	(Pedersen *et al.*, 2003)
	Plasmodium falciparum *Plasmodium berghei*	(Freilich *et al.*, 2000)

Table 2. Therapeutic use of DHEA or an analogue (EpiBr) during several parasitic infections.

2. Concluding remarks

The evidence presented above illustrates the complexity and importance of neuroimmunoendocrine interactions during CC and provides clues to the many other possible mechanisms of parasite establishment, growth and reproduction in an immunocompetent host. Further, strong neuroimmunoendocrine interactions may have implications in the control of transmission and treatment of this parasitic disease in porcine and humans. In practical importance, the complexity of the cysticerci-host relationship suggests that all physiological factors (i.e., sex, age) should be taken into account in the design of vaccines and new drugs.

The differential response of cysticerci to sex steroids may also be involved in their ability to grow faster in the murine female or feminized male host. Host and parasite sex-associated biases may be combined to favor their evolution towards a mutually acceptable relationship. Moreover, the changes in behavior observed during CC, should not be regarded as simple biological curiosities but more as strong evidence of the plasticity of the host phenotype in response to infection by parasitic helminthes. Furthermore, by changing the reproductive, aggressive and dominant capacity of the host, parasites generate novel questions regarding to the evolution of host-parasite relationships in addition to only the prey/predator interaction.

Finally, we have documented here that a complex interactive network involving the immune, endocrine and nervous systems of the mouse, as well as the reproductive system of the cysticerci, is in control of the parasite load of each infected individual mouse. If such complex a management of the parasite loads, as that we shown here between mice and cysticerci, extends to other parasite diseases of mammals, as current research seems to indicate in a number of infections, their means of exploration, fuller understandings and forms of control must be reviewed and approached with designs matching in complexity and plasticity that of the infections.

Author details

Karen Nava-Castro
Facultad de Química, Departamento de Biología, Universidad Nacional Autónoma de México, México DF, México

Romel Hernández-Bello
Departamento de Microbiología, Facultad de Medicina, Universidad Autónoma de Nuevo León, Monterrey, NL, México, México

Lorena López-Griego, Jhonatan A. Hernández-Valdés,
Valeria López-Salazar, Nelly Tiempos-Guzmán and Jorge Morales-Montor
Departamento de Inmunología, Instituto de Investigaciones Biomédicas, Universidad Nacional Autónoma de México, México DF, México

Saé Muñiz-Hernández
Subdirección de Investigación Médica, Instituto Nacional de Cancerología, Secretaria de Salud, México

Acknowledgement

Financial support: Grant # 40072-Q from Consejo Nacional de Ciencia y Tecnología (CONACYT) de México, and Grant # IN-208103 from Programa de Apoyo a Proyectos de Investigación e Inovación Tecnológica (PAPIIT) from Dirección General de Asuntos del Personal Académico (DGAPA), U.N.A.M., both to J M-M. KNC received a postdoctoral fellowship from Dirección General de Asuntos del Personal Académico (DGAPA), U.N.A.M. and RHB received a postdoctoral fellowship from Instituto de Ciencia y Tecnología del Distrito Federal (ICyTDF).

3. References

Arteaga-Silva, M., Vargas-Villavicencio, J. A., Vigueras-Villasenor, R. M., Rodriguez-Dorantes, M. and Morales-Montor, J. (2009). Taenia crassiceps infection disrupts estrous cycle and reproductive behavior in BALB/c female mice. *Acta Trop,* 109,2,Feb,pp (141-145),1873-6254 (Electronic)

Baig, S., Damian, R. T., Morales-Montor, J., Olecki, P., Talhouk, J., Hashmey, R. and White, A. C., Jr. (2005). Characterization of excretory/secretory endopeptidase and metallo-aminopeptidases from Taenia crassiceps metacestodes. *J Parasitol,* 91,5,Oct,pp (983-987),0022-3395 (Print)

Besedovsky, H. O. and del Rey, A. (1996). Immune-neuro-endocrine interactions: facts and hypotheses. *Endocr Rev,* 17,1,Feb,pp (64-102),0163-769X (Print)

Besedovsky, H. O. and del Rey, A. (2000). The cytokine-HPA axis feed-back circuit. *Z Rheumatol,* 59 Suppl 2II/26-30),0340-1855 (Print)

Bojalil, R., Terrazas, L. I., Govezensky, T., Sciutto, E. and Larralde, C. (1993). Thymus-related cellular immune mechanisms in sex-associated resistance to experimental murine cysticercosis (Taenia crassiceps). *J Parasitol,* 79,3,Jun,pp (384-389),0022-3395 (Print)

Brehm, K., Wolf, M., Beland, H., Kroner, A. and Frosch, M. (2003). Analysis of differential gene expression in Echinococcus multilocularis larval stages by means of spliced leader differential display. *Int J Parasitol,* 33,11,Sep 30,pp (1145-1159),0020-7519 (Print)

Cardenas, G., Valdez, R., Saenz, B., Bottasso, O., Fragoso, G., Sciutto, E., Romano, M. C. and Fleury, A. (2012). Impact of Taenia solium neurocysticercosis upon endocrine status and its relation with immuno-inflammatory parameters. *Int J Parasitol,* 42,2,Feb,pp (171-176),1879-0135 (Electronic)

Carrero, J. C., Cervantes, C., Moreno-Mendoza, N., Saavedra, E., Morales-Montor, J. and Laclette, J. P. (2006). Dehydroepiandrosterone decreases while cortisol increases in vitro growth and viability of Entamoeba histolytica. *Microbes Infect,* 8,2,Feb,pp (323-331),1286-4579 (Print)

Carrero, J. C., Cervantes-Rebolledo, C., Vargas-Villavicencio, J. A., Hernandez-Bello, R., Dowding, C., Frincke, J., Reading, C. and Morales-Montor, J. (2010). Parasiticidal effect of 16alpha-bromoepiandrosterone (EpiBr) in amoebiasis and cysticercosis. *Microbes Infect,* 12,8-9,Aug,pp (677-682),1769-714X (Electronic)

Castellanos-Sanchez, V. O., Gomez-Conde, E., Rocha-Gracia, R. C., Pimentel, A., Aluja, A., Hernandez-Jauregui, P., Huerta, M. and Diaz-Orea, M. A. (2009). Chorionic gonadotropin hormone receptors on Taenia solium and Taenia crassiceps cysticerci in culture. *J Parasitol,* 95,6,Dec,pp (1287-1294),1937-2345 (Electronic)

Chikanza, I. C. and Grossman, A. B. (2000). Reciprocal interactions between the neuroendocrine and immune systems during inflammation. *Rheum Dis Clin North Am,* 26,4,Nov,pp (693-711),0889-857X (Print)

Crossgrove, K., Laudet, V. and Maina, C. V. (2002). Dirofilaria immitis encodes Di-nhr-7, a putative orthologue of the Drosophila ecdysone-regulated E78 gene. *Mol Biochem Parasitol,* 119,2,Feb,pp (169-177),0166-6851 (Print)

Crossgrove, K., Maina, C. V., Robinson-Rechavi, M. and Lochner, M. C. (2008). Orthologues of the Drosophila melanogaster E75 molting control gene in the filarial parasites Brugia malayi and Dirofilaria immitis. *Mol Biochem Parasitol,* 157,1,Jan,pp (92-97),0166-6851 (Print)

Damian, R. T. (1989). Molecular mimicry: parasite evasion and host defense. *Curr Top Microbiol Immunol,* 145101-115),0070-217X (Print)

dos Santos, C. D., Toldo, M. P. and do Prado Junior, J. C. (2005). Trypanosoma cruzi: the effects of dehydroepiandrosterone (DHEA) treatment during experimental infection. *Acta Trop,* 95,2,Aug,pp (109-115),0001-706X (Print)

Escobedo, G., Camacho-Arroyo, I., Nava-Luna, P., Olivos, A., Perez-Torres, A., Leon-Cabrera, S., Carrero, J. C. and Morales-Montor, J. (2011). Progesterone induces mucosal immunity in a rodent model of human taeniosis by Taenia solium. *International journal of biological sciences,* 7,9,1443-1456),1449-2288 (Electronic)

Escobedo, G., Larralde, C., Chavarria, A., Cerbon, M. A. and Morales-Montor, J. (2004). Molecular mechanisms involved in the differential effects of sex steroids on the reproduction and infectivity of Taenia crassiceps. *J Parasitol,* 90,6,Dec,pp (1235-1244),0022-3395 (Print)

Escobedo, G., Roberts, C. W., Carrero, J. C. and Morales-Montor, J. (2005). Parasite regulation by host hormones: an old mechanism of host exploitation? *Trends Parasitol,* 21,12,Dec,pp (588-593),1471-4922 (Print)

Escobedo, G., Romano, M. C. and Morales-Montor, J. (2009). Differential in vitro effects of insulin on *Taenia crassiceps* and *Taenia solium* cysticerci. *J Helminthol,* 83,4,Dec,pp (403-412),1475-2697 (Electronic)

Escobedo, G., Soldevila, G., Ortega-Pierres, G., Chavez-Rios, J. R., Nava, K., Fonseca-Linan, R., Lopez-Griego, L., Hallal-Calleros, C., Ostoa-Saloma, P. and Morales-Montor, J. (2010). A new MAP kinase protein involved in estradiol-stimulated reproduction of the helminth parasite Taenia crassiceps. *J Biomed Biotechnol,* 747121),1110-7251 (Electronic)

Fallon, P. G., Richardson, E. J., Jones, F. M. and Dunne, D. W. (1998). Dehydroepiandrosterone sulfate treatment of mice modulates infection with Schistosoma mansoni. *Clin Diagn Lab Immunol,* 5,2,Mar,pp (251-253),1071-412X (Print)

Ferone, D., Boschetti, M., Resmini, E., Giusti, M., Albanese, V., Goglia, U., Albertelli, M., Vera, L., Bianchi, F. and Minuto, F. (2006). Neuroendocrine-immune interactions: the role of cortistatin/somatostatin system. *Ann N Y Acad Sci,* 1069Jun,pp (129-144),0077-8923 (Print)

Forster, S., Gunthel, D., Kiss, F. and Brehm, K. (2011). Molecular characterisation of a serum-responsive, DAF-12-like nuclear hormone receptor of the fox-tapeworm Echinococcus multilocularis. *Journal of cellular biochemistry,* 112,6,Jun,pp (1630-1642),1097-4644 (Electronic)

Freebern, W. J., Osman, A., Niles, E. G., Christen, L. and LoVerde, P. T. (1999). Identification of a cDNA encoding a retinoid X receptor homologue from Schistosoma mansoni. Evidence for a role in female-specific gene expression. *The Journal of biological chemistry,* 274,8,Feb 19,pp (4577-4585),0021-9258 (Print)

Freilich, D., Ferris, S., Wallace, M., Leach, L., Kallen, A., Frincke, J., Ahlem, C., Hacker, M., Nelson, D. and Hebert, J. (2000). 16alpha-bromoepiandrosterone, a dehydroepiandrosterone (DHEA) analogue, inhibits Plasmodium falciparum and *Plasmodium berghei* growth. *Am J Trop Med Hyg,* 63,5-6,Nov-Dec,pp (280-283),0002-9637 (Print)

Gomez, Y., Valdez, R. A., Larralde, C. and Romano, M. C. (2000). Sex steroids and parasitism: Taenia crassiceps cisticercus metabolizes exogenous androstenedione to testosterone in vitro. *J Steroid Biochem Mol Biol,* 74,3,Oct,pp (143-147),0960-0760 (Print)

Gomez-Escobar, N., van den Biggelaar, A. and Maizels, R. (1997). A member of the TGF-beta receptor gene family in the parasitic nematode Brugia pahangi. *Gene,* 199,1-2,Oct 15,pp (101-109),0378-1119 (Print)

Gourbal, B. E., Lacroix, A. and Gabrion, C. (2002). Behavioural dominance and Taenia crassiceps parasitism in BALB/c male mice. *Parasitol Res,* 88,10,Oct,pp (912-917),0932-0113 (Print)

Gourbal, B. E., Righi, M., Petit, G. and Gabrion, C. (2001). Parasite-altered host behavior in the face of a predator: manipulation or not? *Parasitol Res,* 87,3,Mar,pp (186-192),0932-0113 (Print)

Guzman, C., Camacho-Arroyo, I., De Leon-Nava, M. A. and Morales-Montor, J. (2009). Neonatal exposure to estradiol induces resistance to helminth infection and changes in the expression of sex steroid hormone receptors in the brain and spleen in adult mice of both sexes. *Brain Behav Immun,* 23,5,Jul,pp (709-715),1090-2139 (Electronic)

Haddad, J. J., Saade, N. E. and Safieh-Garabedian, B. (2002). Cytokines and neuro-immune-endocrine interactions: a role for the hypothalamic-pituitary-adrenal revolving axis. *J Neuroimmunol,* 133,1-2,Dec,pp (1-19),0165-5728 (Print)

Hu, R., Wu, W., Niles, E. G. and Loverde, P. T. (2006). Isolation and characterization of Schistosoma mansoni constitutive androstane receptor. *Mol Biochem Parasitol,* 148,1,Jul,pp (31-43),0166-6851 (Print)

Huerta, L., Terrazas, L. I., Sciutto, E. and Larralde, C. (1992). Immunological mediation of gonadal effects on experimental murine cysticercosis caused by Taenia crassiceps metacestodes. *J Parasitol,* 78,3,Jun,pp (471-476),0022-3395 (Print)

Ibarra-Coronado, E. G., Escobedo, G., Nava-Castro, K., Jesus Ramses, C. R., Hernandez-Bello, R., Garcia-Varela, M., Ambrosio, J. R., Reynoso-Ducoing, O., Fonseca-Linan, R., Ortega-Pierres, G., Pavon, L., Hernandez, M. E. and Morales-Montor, J. (2011). A helminth cestode parasite express an estrogen-binding protein resembling a classic nuclear estrogen receptor. *Steroids,* 76,10-11,Sep-Oct,pp (1149-1159),1878-5867 (Electronic)

Jimenez, P., Valdez, R. A. and Romano, M. C. (2006). Metabolism of steroid hormones by *Taenia solium* and *Taenia crassiceps* cysticerci. *J Steroid Biochem Mol Biol,* 99,4-5,Jun,pp (203-208),0960-0760 (Print)

Khayath, N., Vicogne, J., Ahier, A., BenYounes, A., Konrad, C., Trolet, J., Viscogliosi, E., Brehm, K. and Dissous, C. (2007). Diversification of the insulin receptor family in the helminth parasite Schistosoma mansoni. *The FEBS journal,* 274,3,Feb,pp (659-676),1742-464X (Print)

Klein, S. L. (2000). Hormones and mating system affect sex and species differences in immune function among vertebrates. *Behav Processes,* 51,1-3,Oct 5,pp (149-166),1872-8308 (Electronic)

Konrad, C., Kroner, A., Spiliotis, M., Zavala-Gongora, R. and Brehm, K. (2003). Identification and molecular characterisation of a gene encoding a member of the insulin receptor family in Echinococcus multilocularis. *Int J Parasitol,* 33,3,Mar,pp (301-312),0020-7519 (Print)

Kurtis, J. D., Mtalib, R., Onyango, F. K. and Duffy, P. E. (2001). Human resistance to Plasmodium falciparum increases during puberty and is predicted by dehydroepiandrosterone sulfate levels. *Infect Immun,* 69,1,Jan,pp (123-128),0019-9567 (Print)

Laclette, J. P., Rodriguez, M., Landa, A., Arcos, L., de Alba, P., Mancilla, R. and Willms, K. (1989). The coexistence of Taenia solium cysticerci and the pig: role of the antigen B. *Acta Leiden,* 57,2,115-122),0065-1362 (Print)

Larralde, C., Laclette, J. P., Owen, C. S., Madrazo, I., Sandoval, M., Bojalil, R., Sciutto, E., Contreras, L., Arzate, J., Diaz, M. L. and et al. (1986). Reliable serology of Taenia solium cysticercosis with antigens from cyst vesicular fluid: ELISA and hemagglutination tests. *Am J Trop Med Hyg,* 35,5,Sep,pp (965-973),0002-9637 (Print)

Larralde, C., Sotelo, J., Montoya, R. M., Palencia, G., Padilla, A., Govezensky, T., Diaz, M. L. and Sciutto, E. (1990). Immunodiagnosis of human cysticercosis in cerebrospinal fluid. Antigens from murine Taenia crassiceps cysticerci effectively substitute those from porcine Taenia solium. *Arch Pathol Lab Med,* 114,9,Sep,pp (926-928),0003-9985 (Print)

Locksley, R. M. (1997). Exploitation of immune and other defence mechanisms by parasites: an overview. *Parasitology,* 115 SupplS5-7),0031-1820 (Print)

LoVerde, P. T., DeWald, J., Minchella, D. J., Bosshardt, S. C. and Damian, R. T. (1985). Evidence for host-induced selection in Schistosoma mansoni. *J Parasitol,* 71,3,Jun,pp (297-301),0022-3395 (Print)

Morales, J., Larralde, C., Arteaga, M., Govezensky, T., Romano, M. C. and Morali, G. (1996). Inhibition of sexual behavior in male mice infected with Taenia crassiceps cysticerci. *J Parasitol,* 82,5,Oct,pp (689-693),0022-3395 (Print)

Morales, J., Velasco, T., Tovar, V., Fragoso, G., Fleury, A., Beltran, C., Villalobos, N., Aluja, A., Rodarte, L. F., Sciutto, E. and Larralde, C. (2002). Castration and pregnancy of rural pigs significantly increase the prevalence of naturally acquired Taenia solium cysticercosis. *Vet Parasitol,* 108,1,Aug 30,pp (41-48),0304-4017 (Print)

Morales-Montor, J., Arrieta, I., Del Castillo, L. I., Rodriguez-Dorantes, M., Cerbon, M. A. and Larralde, C. (2004a). Remote sensing of intraperitoneal parasitism by the host's brain: regional changes of c-fos gene expression in the brain of feminized cysticercotic male mice. *Parasitology,* 128,Pt 3,Mar,pp (343-351),0031-1820 (Print)

Morales-Montor, J., Baig, S., Hallal-Calleros, C. and Damian, R. T. (2002a). Taenia crassiceps: androgen reconstitution of the host leads to protection during cysticercosis. *Exp Parasitol,* 100,4,Apr,pp (209-216),0014-4894 (Print)

Morales-Montor, J., Baig, S., Kabbani, A. and Damian, R. T. (2002b). Do interleukin-6 and macrophage-migration inhibitory factor play a role during sex-associated susceptibility in murine cysticercosis? *Parasitol Res,* 88,10,Oct,pp (901-904),0932-0113 (Print)

Morales-Montor, J., Baig, S., Mitchell, R., Deway, K., Hallal-Calleros, C. and Damian, R. T. (2001). Immunoendocrine interactions during chronic cysticercosis determine male mouse feminization: role of IL-6. *J Immunol,* 167,8,Oct 15,pp (4527-4533),0022-1767 (Print)

Morales-Montor, J., Chavarria, A., De Leon, M. A., Del Castillo, L. I., Escobedo, E. G., Sanchez, E. N., Vargas, J. A., Hernandez-Flores, M., Romo-Gonzalez, T. and Larralde, C. (2004b). Host gender in parasitic infections of mammals: an evaluation of the female host supremacy paradigm. *J Parasitol,* 90,3,Jun,pp (531-546),0022-3395 (Print)

Morales-Montor, J., Hallal-Calleros, C., Romano, M. C. and Damian, R. T. (2002c). Inhibition of p-450 aromatase prevents feminisation and induces protection during cysticercosis. *Int J Parasitol,* 32,11,Oct,pp (1379-1387),0020-7519 (Print)

Morales-Montor, J. and Larralde, C. (2005). The role of sex steroids in the complex physiology of the host-parasite relationship: the case of the larval cestode of Taenia crassiceps. *Parasitology,* 131,Pt 3,Sep,pp (287-294),0031-1820 (Print)

Morales-Montor, J., Rodriguez-Dorantes, M., Mendoza-Rodriguez, C. A., Camacho-Arroyo, I. and Cerbon, M. A. (1998). Differential expression of the estrogen-regulated proto-oncogenes c-fos, c-jun, and bcl-2 and of the tumor-suppressor p53 gene in the male mouse chronically infected with Taenia crassiceps cysticerci. *Parasitol Res,* 84,8,Aug,pp (616-622),0932-0113 (Print)

Pedersen, N. C., North, T. W., Rigg, R., Reading, C., Higgins, J., Leutenegger, C. and Henderson, G. L. (2003). 16alpha-Bromo-epiandrosterone therapy modulates experimental feline immunodeficiency virus viremia: initial enhancement leading to long-term suppression. *Vet Immunol Immunopathol,* 94,3-4,Aug 15,pp (133-148),0165-2427 (Print)

Pena, N., Morales, J., Morales-Montor, J., Vargas-Villavicencio, A., Fleury, A., Zarco, L., de Aluja, A. S., Larralde, C., Fragoso, G. and Sciutto, E. (2007). Impact of naturally acquired Taenia solium cysticercosis on the hormonal levels of free ranging boars. *Vet Parasitol,* 149,1-2,Oct 21,pp (134-137),0304-4017 (Print)

Rajan, B., Ramalingam, T. and Rajan, T. V. (2005). Critical role for IgM in host protection in experimental filarial infection. *J Immunol,* 175,3,Aug 1,pp (1827-1833),0022-1767 (Print)

Ramachandran, H., Skelly, P. J. and Shoemaker, C. B. (1996). The Schistosoma mansoni epidermal growth factor receptor homologue, SER, has tyrosine kinase activity and is localized in adult muscle. *Mol Biochem Parasitol,* 83,1,Dec 2,pp (1-10),0166-6851 (Print)

Rasmussen, K. R. and Healey, M. C. (1992). Dehydroepiandrosterone-induced reduction of Cryptosporidium parvum infections in aged Syrian golden hamsters. *J Parasitol,* 78,3,Jun,pp (554-557),0022-3395 (Print)

Reading, C., Dowding, C., Schramm, B., Garsd, A., Onizuka-Handa, N., Stickney, D. and Frincke, J. (2006). Improvement in immune parameters and human immunodeficiency virus-1 viral response in individuals treated with 16alpha-bromoepiandrosterone (HE2000). *Clinical microbiology and infection : the official publication of the European Society of Clinical Microbiology and Infectious Diseases,* 12,11,Nov,pp (1082-1088),1198-743X (Print)

Rivier, C. and Rivest, S. (1993). Mechanisms mediating the effects of cytokines on neuroendocrine functions in the rat. *Ciba Found Symp,* 172204-220; discussion 220-205),0300-5208 (Print)

Rodriguez-Dorantes, M., Cerbon, M. A., Larralde, C. and Morales-Montor, J. (2007). Modified progesterone receptor expression in the hypothalamus of cysticercotic male mice. *Acta Trop,* 103,2,Aug,pp (123-132),0001-706X (Print)

Sani, B. P., Vaid, A., Comley, J. C. and Montgomery, J. A. (1985). Novel retinoid-binding proteins from filarial parasites. *Biochem J,* 232,2,Dec 1,pp (577-583),0264-6021 (Print)

Sciutto, E., Fragoso, G., Trueba, L., Lemus, D., Montoya, R. M., Diaz, M. L., Govezensky, T., Lomeli, C., Tapia, G. and Larralde, C. (1990). Cysticercosis vaccine: cross protecting immunity with T. solium antigens against experimental murine T. crassiceps cysticercosis. *Parasite Immunol,* 12,6,Nov,pp (687-696),0141-9838 (Print)

Sciutto, E., Rosas, G., Hernandez, M., Morales, J., Cruz-Revilla, C., Toledo, A., Manoutcharian, K., Gevorkian, G., Blancas, A., Acero, G., Hernandez, B., Cervantes, J., Bobes, R. J., Goldbaum, F. A., Huerta, M., Diaz-Orea, A., Fleury, A., de Aluja, A. S., Cabrera-Ponce, J. L., Herrera-Estrella, L., Fragoso, G. and Larralde, C. (2007). Improvement of the synthetic tri-peptide vaccine (S3Pvac) against porcine Taenia solium cysticercosis in search of a more effective, inexpensive and manageable vaccine. *Vaccine,* 25,8,Feb 9,pp (1368-1378),0264-410X (Print)

Shea, C., Richer, J., Tzertzinis, G. and Maina, C. V. (2010). An EcR homolog from the filarial parasite, Dirofilaria immitis requires a ligand-activated partner for transactivation. *Mol Biochem Parasitol,* 171,2,Jun,pp (55-63),1872-9428 (Electronic)

Smith, J. K., Esch, G. W. and Kuhn, R. E. (1972). Growth and development of larval Taenia crassiceps (cestoda). I. Aneuploidy in the anomalous ORF strain. *Int J Parasitol,* 2,2,Jun,pp (261-263),0020-7519 (Print)

Spiliotis, M., Kroner, A. and Brehm, K. (2003). Identification, molecular characterization and expression of the gene encoding the epidermal growth factor receptor orthologue from the fox-tapeworm Echinococcus multilocularis. *Gene,* 323Dec 24,pp (57-65),0378-1119 (Print)

Terrazas, L. I., Bojalil, R., Govezensky, T. and Larralde, C. (1994). A role for 17-beta-estradiol in immunoendocrine regulation of murine cysticercosis (Taenia crassiceps). *J Parasitol,* 80,4,Aug,pp (563-568),0022-3395 (Print)

Terrazas, L. I., Bojalil, R., Govezensky, T. and Larralde, C. (1998). Shift from an early protective Th1-type immune response to a late permissive Th2-type response in murine cysticercosis (Taenia crassiceps). *J Parasitol,* 84,1,Feb,pp (74-81),0022-3395 (Print)

Terrazas, L. I., Cruz, M., Rodriguez-Sosa, M., Bojalil, R., Garcia-Tamayo, F. and Larralde, C. (1999). Th1-type cytokines improve resistance to murine cysticercosis caused by Taenia crassiceps. *Parasitol Res,* 85,2,Feb,pp (135-141),0932-0113 (Print)

Tzertzinis, G., Egana, A. L., Palli, S. R., Robinson-Rechavi, M., Gissendanner, C. R., Liu, C., Unnasch, T. R. and Maina, C. V. (2010). Molecular evidence for a functional ecdysone signaling system in Brugia malayi. *PLoS neglected tropical diseases,* 4,3,e625),1935-2735 (Electronic)

Unnasch, T. R., Bradley, J., Beauchamp, J., Tuan, R. and Kennedy, M. W. (1999). Characterization of a putative nuclear receptor from Onchocerca volvulus. *Mol Biochem Parasitol,* 104,2,Nov 30,pp (259-269),0166-6851 (Print)

Vargas-Villavicencio, J. A., Larralde, C., De Leon-Nava, M. A., Escobedo, G. and Morales-Montor, J. (2007). Tamoxifen treatment induces protection in murine cysticercosis. *J Parasitol,* 93,6,Dec,pp (1512-1517),0022-3395 (Print)

Vargas-Villavicencio, J. A., Larralde, C., De Leon-Nava, M. A. and Morales-Montor, J. (2005). Regulation of the immune response to cestode infection by progesterone is due to its metabolism to estradiol. *Microbes Infect,* 7,3,Mar,pp (485-493),1286-4579 (Print)

Vargas-Villavicencio, J. A., Larralde, C. and Morales-Montor, J. (2006). Gonadectomy and progesterone treatment induce protection in murine cysticercosis. *Parasite Immunol,* 28,12,Dec,pp (667-674),0141-9838 (Print)

Vargas-Villavicencio, J. A., Larralde, C. and Morales-Montor, J. (2008). Treatment with dehydroepiandrosterone in vivo and in vitro inhibits reproduction, growth and viability of Taenia crassiceps metacestodes. *Int J Parasitol,* 38,7,Jun,pp (775-781),0020-7519 (Print)

Wu, X., Zhao, B., Hong, Y., Li, X., Peng, J., Zhang, J., Wang, F., Shi, Y., Fu, Z. and Lin, J. (2012). Characterization of Schistosoma japonicum estrogen-related receptor beta like 1 and immunogenicity analysis of the recombinant protein. *Exp Parasitol,* 131,3,Jul,pp (383-392),1090-2449 (Electronic)

You, H., Zhang, W., Jones, M. K., Gobert, G. N., Mulvenna, J., Rees, G., Spanevello, M., Blair, D., Duke, M., Brehm, K. and McManus, D. P. (2010). Cloning and characterisation of Schistosoma japonicum insulin receptors. *PLoS One,* 5,3,e9868),1932-6203 (Electronic)

Chapter 3

The Burden of Cysticercosis

Rachana Bhattarai, Hélène Carabin and Christine Budke

Additional information is available at the end of the chapter

http://dx.doi.org/10.5772/51668

1. Introduction

Taenia solium cysticercosis is a major public health and agricultural problem in many developing countries. It is predominantly found and considered endemic in Latin American, Asian, and African countries where pigs are raised using traditional methods, veterinary meat inspection is insufficient, and sanitation is poor [1-3]. However, it is now increasingly being diagnosed in other regions such as the United States, Western Europe, and Canada due to an increasing flow of immigrants from endemic areas who may have taeniasis or cysticercosis [4-7]. The parasite not only impacts human health, but also pig farmers and their communities. In humans, the larvae of the parasite (metacestodes) may migrate to the brain resulting in neurocysticercosis (NCC). The natural history of NCC infection remains poorly understood, and the proportion of cases with lesions in their brains that will manifest at some point during the course of the infection remains unknown. According to a recent systematic review of the literature, among diagnosed NCC patients who sought care in clinics where imaging was available, epileptic seizures were by far the most common presenting symptom, followed by headaches, focal deficits, and cranial hypertension/hydrocephalus [8]. Depression has been reported to be very common among NCC patients, but it has not been determined if this is due to the presence of epilepsy or NCC itself [9]. Other manifestations of NCC include stroke and dementia, but those aspects have been very poorly described [10, 11]. The social consequences of NCC possibly include stigmatization, incapacitation, and decreased work productivity. Epilepsy has been shown, in several countries, to lead to social discrimination, and NCC-associated epilepsy is no different. In many endemic countries, the stigma associated with epilepsy may have a greater impact on patients' lives and families than the disease itself [12]. In addition, due to the reduction in quality of life and the psychological effects of the condition, work productivity might be further decreased.

In pigs, infection with the larval stages of the parasite results in the development of cysts primarily in the muscles, and less commonly in the tongue muscles, heart, diaphragm,

INTECH
open science | open minds

© 2013 Carabin et al., licensee InTech. This is a paper distributed under the terms of the Creative Commons Attribution License (http://creativecommons.org/licenses/by/3.0), which permits unrestricted use, distribution, and reproduction in any medium, provided the original work is properly cited.

brain, and other organ systems. The presence of these cysts can lead to partial or full condemnation of the carcass and economic losses in areas where meat is inspected. In some areas, pig traders look for the presence of cysts under the tongue before buying them, and will offer a lower price for animals affected. This parasite, therefore, can reduce the household income of farmers and whole communities that share the same environment. Porcine cysticercosis is most commonly associated with small holder farming practices and is often under-reported due to the absence of clinical signs in affected pigs and lack of meat inspection facilities and expertise in endemic countries.

Because cysticercosis impacts human and pig heath and results in economic losses, there is a need to evaluate the socioeconomic impact, or burden, of this condition on endemic communities. Both non-monetary and monetary methods can be employed. These estimates may then be compared among diseases to better target which diseases to control. Disease burden estimates can subsequently be used to compare alternative control strategies for cysticercosis, as well as other diseases affecting the population, through cost-utility and cost-benefit analyses. These analyses can guide stakeholders as to which diseases and control strategies should be prioritized to reduce the burden of diseases in the population.

2. Methods for evaluation of the burden of zoonotic infections

Taenia solium cysticercosis results in mortality, morbidity, and economic losses in affected human and animal populations. To evaluate the burden of cysticercosis, the monetary and non-monetary impacts of the disease on human health, agriculture, and society must be considered comprehensively. Measuring burden is challenging because it requires various types of data from valid studies conducted in humans and pig populations. Because of those challenges, it is recommended to focus the evaluation on a certain period and to one geographical area where high quality epidemiological and clinical studies have been conducted, preferably in both pigs and humans. The disadvantage of such an approach is that the data cannot be generalized to other areas. Some data are required for the estimation of both the non-monetary and the monetary burden of cysticercosis. In humans, these data include: the death rate of NCC (the number of deaths, if available, can also be used); the proportion of patients with NCC who seek care in clinics (and hospitals); the number (or incidence rate) of cases of NCC diagnosed after care has been sought; and the frequency and duration of each NCC manifestation. In pigs, the data required include the proportion of pigs that are inspected pre or post-mortem and the proportion of infected pigs diagnosed pre or post-mortem. Such data may be found in the published/unpublished literature and national or regional databases. When some aspects of the data are unavailable, opinion of local experts may be sought and uncertainty analyses can be run. In estimating the burden of NCC, there is the additional challenge that the internationally recognized definition of NCC requires the use of diagnostic imaging (computed tomography (CT) scan or magnetic resonance imaging (MRI)), autopsy or biopsy of skin nodules [13]. The absence of advanced diagnostic imaging facilities limits the evaluation of the burden of NCC in many areas of the world, and especially in the poorest regions where the disease is likely to be most prevalent.

Serological tests are designed to measure the exposure to, or current infection with, cysticercosis [14], but can show low specificity and sensitivity in the diagnosis of NCC, depending on the number and stages of lesions present in the brain [15].

3. Measuring the non-monetary burden of cysticercosis

Specific measures have been designed to estimate the non-monetary burden of human diseases [16, 17]. We will not discuss here measures of mortality and morbidity that can also be used in animals. The most informative measure of non-monetary burden is believed to be "utility", an economical concept which has been adapted to health economics, and measures the preference that people have for certain health status along a continuum [18].The greater the preference for a particular health state, the greater the "utility" associated with it. Several Health Adjusted Life Years (HALYs) metrics have been developed as indicators of "utility". HALYs are summary measures of population health that enable measures of mortality to be combined with measures of disability associated with each sequela (manifestation) of the disease of interest into one metric.

There are two types of HALYs that have been commonly used in estimating human burden of disease: Quality Adjusted Life Years (QALYs) and Disability Adjusted Life Years (DALYs). Even though QALYs and DALYs may be used to estimate utilities, they were developed to serve different purposes. Where DALYs are meant as an objective, population-based measure, QALYs are meant to be used as a subjective, individual-based measure of utility and health. In addition, these measures use opposite scales. The DALY is a negative concept, with one DALY being the equivalent of one year lived completely disabled (analogous to death) whereas the QALY is a positive concept, with one QALY being the equivalent of one year of healthy life [18]. Therefore, control strategies would aim to minimize DALYs and maximize QALYs.

3.1. Quality Adjusted Life Years (QALYs)

The ideal way of measuring quality of life is to attribute a utility, or a weighted preference for a certain health status, to each disease and its associated manifestations. In theory, the utility of health status is best measured with choice-based methods which include uncertainty, such as the standard gamble method. Other choice-based methods, without uncertainty, include paired person-trade-off and time-trade-off techniques [19]. Utility measures are based on the fact that Paretian welfare economics requires that each individual be the judge of his or her own welfare. However, in practice, these methods are difficult to implement because different people have different reactions when faced with uncertainty and choices, especially when these are theoretical. For example, in the standard gamble method, the patients are asked to find the probability "p" at which they would be unable to choose between remaining in their current state of health or dying immediately with a probability of p (and living healthy with a probability of $1-p$). Given the difficulty in implementing such measures, several groups of researchers have developed multi-attribute classification systems implemented in the form of scale-based questionnaires. Each answer to the scaled questions contributes a certain weight towards calculating utility. The utility weights are determined during studies where both the questionnaire and one of the choice-based methods are used, and then assumed to be generalizable to other contexts. Multi-attribute questionnaires are more commonly used than choice-based measures in QALYs studies. One advantage of multi-attribute questionnaires is that they may not only be used to estimate utility, but also to assess the perceptions of patients regarding different aspects of their health (i.e., mental, physical, social functioning, etc.).

When used at a population level, QALYs combine quantitative estimates of death, frequency and duration of disease with a qualitative assessment of how well (or not) patients can live with the disease. In other words, rather than just counting the number of people with the disease, QALYs try to "adjust" for how well people can live with the disease. Therefore, QALYs are a product of life expectancy and a measure of the quality of remaining life years, with weights placed on time spent in different health states. Most preferable state receives more weight. A year of perfect health is worth 1 and a year of less than perfect health is worth less than 1. Death is considered to be equivalent to 0. However, some health states may be considered worse than death and have negative values [19].

The multi-attribute measurement scales most commonly used in developing countries, where NCC is endemic, are the Euro-Qol (EQ-5D) and the Short Form-12 (SF-12) [20, 21]. These tools provide patient-based determination of quality of life and can be used to compare perceptions of physical, mental, and social health among patients with different diseases (or lack of disease), different stages of the same disease, or before and after treatment of the disease. The latter approach is often used in clinical trials where a drug, while very effective in treating the disease, may be linked to numerous side effects which could lead to worse quality of life than the disease itself.

The EQ-5D is a standardized measure of health status developed by the EuroQol Group. The EQ-5D questionnaire has 5 domains: mobility, self-care, usual activities, pain/discomfort, and anxiety/depression. For each domain, there are three levels of response: individuals are asked whether they have no problems, some problems, or severe problems. The answers to each domain are combined to generate a summary score, for a total of 125 possible combinations of answers, which indicates the overall utility. Table 1 provides an example of utility scores that can be allocated to different combinations of answers to the five EQ-5D questions [22].

The SF-12 is another tool developed by Quality Metric Inc. to assess the quality of life of an individual at a given time. It uses 12 questions to measure eight domains of functional health and well-being namely physical functioning, role physical, bodily pain, general health, vitality, social functioning, role emotional, and mental health (Table 2) [21]. Physical and mental component summary scores can be calculated by aggregating the eight domains [23].

Description	**Utility score**
No problems	1.000
No problems walking; no problems with self-care; some problems with performing usual activities; some pain or discomfort; not anxious or depressed	0.760
Some problems walking; some problems washing or dressing self; some problems with performing usual activities; moderate pain or discomfort; moderately anxious or depressed	0.5616
No problems walking; some problems washing or dressing self; unable to perform usual activities; some pain or discomfort; not anxious or depressed	0.329
Some problems walking; no problems with self-care; no problems with performing usual activities; moderate pain or discomfort; extremely anxious or depressed	0.222
Some problems walking; unable to wash or dress self; unable to perform usual activities; moderate pain or discomfort; moderately anxious or depressed	0.079
Confined to bed; unable to wash or dress self; unable to perform usual activities, extreme pain or discomfort; moderately anxious or depressed	-0.429

Table 1. Example of utility scores for the EQ-5D

Domain	**Description**
Physical functioning	Degree to which health limits everyday physical activities
Role physical	Degree to which physical problems interfere with usual daily activities such as work or school
Bodily pain	Degree of pain to the body
General health	Ratings of current health in general
Vitality	Ratings of energy level
Social functioning	Degree to which health interferes with social activities
Role emotional	Degree to which emotional problems interfere with usual daily activities such as school or work
Mental health	Degree to which health limits emotional well- being, including depression, anxiety and well being

Table 2. Description of the health domains used in the SF-12 v2 quality of life survey

Although QALYs are commonly used metrics in health economics, they also present some limitations. For example, adaptation of patients to certain symptoms may mask the impact of chronic disability. In addition, it is difficult to assign a single utility score to those diseases which cause a variety of clinical manifestations, such as NCC [24]. Another limitation is that scale-based measures can sometimes lead to "ceiling" or "flooring" effects where a majority of people consistently choose the "best" scenario or "worst" scenario. One important criticism of QALYs (which some view as an advantage), is that QALYs measures are subjective and not meant to be generalized to the society as a whole. QALYs associated with a disease in one country (or region) could not be used to estimate the burden in another region (or country). For example, having epilepsy in the United States would have very different social and role functioning values than in Sub-Saharan Africa. This difficulty in using QALYs for international comparison led a group of researchers to develop a completely different type of metric for measuring burden: the DALY.

3.2. Disability Adjusted Life Years (DALYs)

DALYs were first constructed for the Global Burden of Disease (GBD) Study in order to provide a comparable measure of output for interventions, program and sector evaluations, and planning [25]. The GBD Study was conducted to evaluate the non-monetary burden of a variety of infectious and non-infectious conditions, as well as risk factors, on pre-defined regions of the world. The latest comprehensive assessment of the burden of diseases is for the year 2004. However, DALY estimates from the 2010 GBD Study are expected to be released in late 2012 [26]. The DALY is a summary measure of population health that assesses the disability and early mortality associated with the condition of interest. DALYs measure the gap in years between age at death and gender-specific average life expectancy in Japan and combines it with time lived in states other than excellent health (disabled). They are obtained by summing years of life lost (YLL) from premature death and healthy years lost due to disability (YLD). The formulas used for the calculation of YLL and YLD are described below:

$$YLL = N * L \tag{1}$$

where N = number of deaths per age-sex group, L = remaining life expectancy at age of death

$$YLD = I * DW * D \tag{2}$$

where I = age and sex specific estimates of incidence, DW = disability weight, D = average duration of disability.

Disability weights are allocated according to the opinion of experts on how disabling a certain health status is perceived to be. Disability is placed on a uni-dimensional scale between 0 (perfect health) and 1 (death). In theory, utility is equal to 1-disability weight. Disability weights of clinical manifestations (referred to as indicator states) were determined for the original GBD Study by the person trade-off (PTO) method [27]. The PTO method is a way of estimating social preferences for different health states by asking people how many people affected by the health state of interest they would be willing to trade for extending the lives of 100 healthy people. This question is asked using two different formats. For the 2010 GBD Study, community assessment of selected sequelae using discrete choice methods, assessment by health professionals of all sequelae using ranking and visual analog scale methods, and multi-method studies among highly educated respondents were utilized rather than the PTO method [28]. Results from the new disability weights have not yet been published. Examples of disability weights used to calculate DALYs for the original GBD Study are provided in table 3.

Degree of morbidity	Disability weight
Healthy	0
Limited ability to perform at least one activity in one of the following areas: recreation, education, procreation or occupation	0.096
Limited ability to perform most activities in one of the following areas: recreation, education, procreation or occupation	0.220
Limited ability to perform most activities in two or more of the following areas: recreation, education, procreation or occupation	0.400
Limited ability to perform most activities in all of the following areas: recreation, education, procreation or occupation	0.600
Requires assistance with instrumental activities of daily living such as meal preparation, shopping or housework	0.810
Requires assistance with activities of daily living such as eating, personal hygiene or toilet use	0.920
Dead	1

Table 3. Examples of disability weights used to calculate DALYs [25]

Disability weights for NCC were not included in the original GBD study. However, in the 2010 GDB estimates, NCC will be included as causing an average of 29% of all epilepsy cases in endemic countries. This estimate is based on a meta-analysis of the percentage of NCC lesions present in the brain of people with epilepsy [29]. Disability weights of epilepsy will be used as there is no clinical difference between NCC-associated and other types of epilepsy. As better estimates of the distribution of manifestations among NCC patients become available, more sequelae will be added to DALYs estimates associated with NCC. The only two available estimates of DALYs associated with NCC used the disability weights associated with epilepsy (both studies) and migraine (1 study) [30, 31].

The original GBD Study calculations considered two additional parameters: 1) discounting future time and 2) age weighting [25]. Discounting future time is a common concept in economic and social policy. In burden of disease estimations, a discount rate is applied so that future healthy life has less value than the net value of life today [27]. In the context of DALYs, a disability occurring today is worth more than the same disability occurring in the future. The subject of discounting is complex and several papers have been published in favor and against its use in the context of DALYs and health outcomes [27, 32]. By including age weighting, the original GBD Study incorporated social preferences for the value of life lived during adulthood over life lived during childhood or later years. However, the newest version of the GBD Study (the GBD 2010 Study) will not include age weighting in the DALYs calculations. Therefore, the influence of age weighting will be eliminated.

The use of DALYs remains controversial, especially in measuring utilities. According to Anand (1997), DALYs understate the burden of disease of females relative to males since the standard expectation of life at birth in Japan is very similar in men and women [32]. DALYs also measure the burden of disease without considering cultural or socioeconomic differentiation of tested populations so that it underestimates the disease burden in developing countries [33]. DALYs also go against Paretian welfare economics where each individual is the best judge of his or her own welfare. By using utility weights measured by people that are unaffected by the disease of interest, this concept is not respected. Even with these controversies, the DALY remains a widely used summary measure of population health.

4. Measuring monetary burden

Estimates of the monetary burden of zoonotic diseases that impact both human and livestock health should include assessment of both animal health costs and human health costs. The overall estimated cost can be calculated using the following equation: [34]

$$\sum_{s=1}^{S}\sum_{a=1}^{A}\left[N_{a,s}\beta_{a,s}\left(\sum_{x=1}^{X}\pi_{x,a,s}C_{x,a,s}\right)\right] \tag{3}$$

This equation corresponds to the additive societal costs for all affected species (S) across all age groups (A). For the age-species-specific population of size ($N_{a,s}$), with the age-species-specific annual incidence ($\beta_{a,s}$), there is an age-species proportion ($\pi_{x,a,s,}$) of infected individuals with symptoms X. The treatment and consequences of each of these symptoms have a monetary burden of $C_{x,a,s}$. Ideally, the whole spectrum of symptoms and losses in humans and animals is included in the estimate [34].

4.1. Human health costs

Human health costs are classified into direct (health provider) and indirect (out-of-pocket) costs. Direct costs are costs associated with the diagnosis and treatment of patients. Commonly used diagnostic tests incorporated into direct costs include diagnostic imaging, sero-immunological and blood tests, and tests on cerebral spinal fluid (CSF). Diagnostic costs, for a neurological condition such as NCC, can be high since CT scans and MRI confirmatory tests are not readily available in developing countries and, if available, are often distantly located and expensive. Cost of treatment typically includes the cost of medicines, medical consultations, surgical charges, and hospital charges. In contrast to direct costs, indirect costs include costs of working days lost due to clinical manifestations or visits to hospitals, losses in productivity, buying over-the-counter drugs to relieve symptoms, costs of traditional treatment, and costs associated with transportation to and from medical treatment. Costs associated with the family members taking care of the patients would also need to be included.

4.2. Animal health costs

Animal health costs can be associated with partial or full condemnation of the carcass at slaughter or reduction in price of an infected carcass. The value of live animals can also be reduced when, in the case of *T. solium* cysticercosis, reduction in the price of pigs due to the presences of cysts can lower a farmer's household income. In addition, presence of *T. solium* in a country's pig population results in restrictions on the export of pork products.

4.3. Decision tree analysis

Decision trees are very helpful in organizing the information gathered on the distribution of manifestations and treatment seeking pattern in the study population. They can also be used to incorporate the probability of receiving different types of diagnoses and treatments. The tree usually starts with a "trunk" which is the disease of interest (in the case of NCC, this can be epilepsy). From this trunk, a probability (chance node) corresponding to the frequency of the disease is used to create the first two "branches" of the tree: the presence or absence of the disease in the study population. Additional branches are added each time a new probability is added. Each probability (node) may lead to more than two branches. The end of each branch corresponds to the probability that a patient has of following a certain treatment/diagnosis path, including the path of not seeking any medical care. The probability of each branch of a path can be multiplied by the costs corresponding to the options in this branch. An example, the use of decision tree analysis to estimate losses due cysticercosis in South Africa is shown in Figure 1 [35]. In this example, for the branch of people with epilepsy who have NCC but do not seek medical attention, we would multiply 1.33% by 36.7% by 70% to obtain the frequency of having NCC but not being treated (0.34%, as shown in Figure 1) [15, 36-41]. This percentage would be multiplied by the salary lost due to a reduction in productivity among people with epilepsy. Such trees can be developed for very complex treatment paths and for the impact of animal disease as well.

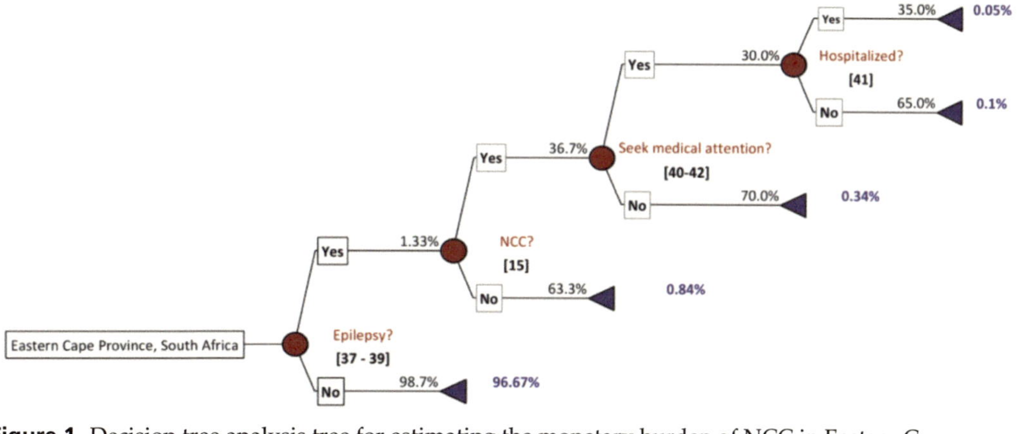

Figure 1. Decision tree analysis tree for estimating the monetary burden of NCC in Eastern Cape Province, South Africa. Circle is a chance node and triangle is an end node [35].

4.4. Uncertainty and sensitivity analysis

Common sources of epidemiological and economic data used in the assessment of disease burden include government and agency reports and values reported in the scientific literature. Values for neglected zoonotic diseases, such as *T. solium* cysticercosis, are often underreported or else the method of collection might be biased. In short, exact estimates of these parameters are difficult to identify. Therefore, in order to account for uncertainties, the distribution of these parameters should be selected carefully. So, instead of using an exact value for each probability and cost value, a distribution of values is used to reflect uncertainty. To include these distributions into the final estimate, sampling methods such as the Monte Carlo or Latin Hypercube are often applied. The final estimate will itself be a distribution reflecting the uncertainty of all included parameters. Uniform distribution can be applied to parameters for which we have very limited knowledge. For example, instead of assuming that 1.33% of the population has epilepsy in the Eastern Cape Province of South Africa, we could assume that the prevalence lies anywhere between 0.5% and 2.8%, with an average at 1.33% [35]. The sampling method would start by sampling one value (for example, 1%) from this distribution, provide and save the estimate of the cost of NCC using this value. Next, another value would be sampled from the distribution and lead to another estimated cost, which will also be saved. This process is usually repeated up to 10,000 times until a distribution of the overall costs is obtained. The Latin Hypercube and Monte Carlo sampling methods are simply efficient tools of sampling several uncertain parameters iteratively.

The sampling method described above will generate a database of 10,000 observations each associated with a different value for the uncertain parameters. We can then use linear regression using the estimated costs as the outcome and all of the uncertain parameters as "independent" variables to assess which parameters have the largest impacts on the estimated costs. The uncertain parameters with the largest impacts should be those that need to be better studied in the future because they have a strong influence on how much a disease costs a society. Sensitivity must be conducted with care to limit the values to those that are most likely and realistic. Including impossible values would lead to biased estimates and a false impression that they have an important impact on the overall cost estimate.

5. Review of morbidity and mortality associated with neurocysticercosis

There are only a few studies in the literature which report the distribution of manifestations among definitive or probable cases of NCC as defined by the Garcia and Del Brutto criteria (2005) [42]. The challenge in studying the natural history of NCC is that it is impossible to diagnose the presence of brain cysts without the use of imaging, and using radiation among a population without symptoms is unethical. Hence, the only information available is the distribution of manifestations among NCC patients that are already under care in facilities where imaging is available. This introduces a major selection bias which leads to likely overestimation of the frequency of more severe (and less stigmatizing) manifestations, or manifestations which are more likely to lead to a medical visit (and a referral to a clinic with imaging). In countries where epilepsy is stigmatized, people may be afraid to seek care which would lead to an underestimate of the distribution of epilepsy among people with

NCC. Similarly, people with cranial hypertension suffering from headaches may never seek medical attention. In contrast, people with hydrocephalus or stroke will most likely seek care.

In a systematic review of studies conducted in clinics or hospitals with imaging facilities, the distribution of presenting symptoms among diagnosed NCC patients was as follows: seizures/epilepsy were the most common (78.8%, 95% CI: 65.1% - 89.7%) followed by headaches (37.9%, 95% CI: 23.3% - 53.7%), focal deficits (16.0%, 95% CI: 9.7% - 23.6%), and signs of increased intracranial pressure (11.7%, 95%CI: 6.0% - 18.9%) [8]. These results, though consistent with what is usually believed for NCC, may be biased by what presenting symptoms the clinicians assessed at admission. This systematic review of the literature also revealed that NCC may contribute to an important percentage of stroke cases in endemic areas. Unfortunately, to our knowledge, there is only one case-control study which has been conducted on this topic [10]. If NCC is truly linked to strokes, this could lead to a very important burden in endemic regions.

The studies included in the systematic review described above were all clinical-based. There have also been several studies conducted in communities and small rural hospitals where, instead of sampling NCC cases, people with epilepsy received imaging for the diagnosis of NCC. When those studies were analyzed systematically, the percentage of people with epilepsy with lesions of NCC at imaging was 29% (95% CI: 23% - 36%) [29]. This finding is important as it suggests that nearly one third of all epilepsy cases living in endemic areas could possibly be prevented with appropriate control strategies. The measure of burden described above could help guide stakeholders as to which control strategy may lead to the best cost-utility or cost-benefit for their area.

Compared to other helminthic infections, the socioeconomic burden of cysticercosis tends to be higher because the condition not only causes severe clinical manifestations, but can also result in mortality. Although limited data exist on NCC-related mortality, a study conducted in the United States and a study conducted in Brazil reported age-adjusted annual mortality rates of 0.06 (95% CI: 0.05 - 0.07) and 1.68 (95% CI: 1.58 - 1.78) deaths per million population, respectively [4, 43]. Additional studies from the U.S. states of California and Oregon reported crude mortality rates of 0.33 (95% CI: 0.27 - 0.38) and 0.29 (95% CI: 0.11 - 0.64) deaths per million population, respectively [44, 45].

6. The monetary and non-monetary burden of neurocysticercosis

Very few studies have been conducted to evaluate the burden of NCC. At present, two studies have been carried out in Africa evaluating the burden of cysticercosis/NCC. A study in West Cameroon revealed that 1.0% of the total population had NCC-associated epilepsy (based on serological results) and 5.6% of the pig population had cysticercosis [31]. Average number of DALYs lost due to NCC was 9.0 per 1,000 person-years and the monetary burden per case of NCC-associated epilepsy was 194 Euro in 2009. The total annual costs due to *T. solium* cysticercosis in West Cameroon were estimated at 10,255,202 Euro (95% CR

6,889,048–14,754,044), of which 4.7% were due to losses in pig husbandry and 95.3% to direct and indirect losses caused by human cysticercosis. This estimate only accounted for the disease burden due to NCC-associated epilepsy and used serology for the diagnosis of NCC.

Similarly, another study conducted in the Eastern Cape Province of South Africa estimated that the monetary burden of NCC-associated epilepsy in 2004 varied from US$632 to US$844 per case, indicating high financial losses associated with this condition [35]. The total number of estimated NCC-associated epilepsy cases was 34,662 (95% CI: 17,167 – 50,068) and among them, expert opinion and a review of the literature suggested that 70% of cases of epilepsy did not seek medical attention. Annual losses to the agricultural sector were estimated at US$5.0 million (95% CI: 2.4 – 8.1), with the overall monetary burden estimated at US$34.2 million (95% CI: 12.8 – 70.0) using the mean wage approach, US$20.1 million (95% CI: 9.6 – 35.3) using generalist replacement costs, and US$18.6 million (95% CI: 9.0 – 32.3) using the traditional opportunity costs approach.

A study conducted in Mexico showed that 0.25 DALY was lost per 1,000 person-years due to NCC-associated epilepsy and severe headaches, with NCC associated epilepsy responsible for 90% of this value [30]. According to 2004 GBD estimates, 1.7 DALYs per 1,000 person-years were estimated to be lost due to epilepsy in Mexico, with approximately the same number of DALYs lost due to migraine. This indicates that almost 15% of DALYs lost due to epilepsy were associated with NCC. This study used only epilepsy and severe chronic headaches as clinical manifestations due to lack of frequency data and disability weights for other known clinical manifestations associated with NCC. Therefore, like the African studies, the total estimated number of DALYs lost was most likely underestimated.

Three studies have been conducted to evaluate the quality of life of NCC patients. A study conducted at two tertiary neurology referral hospitals in Mexico City, Mexico indicated that NCC outpatients had significantly lower scores for each of the SF-12's eight domains of health compared to an age-sex-hospital-day matched control group [46]. Similarly, a study conducted in Peru showed that patients with parenchymal NCC had decreased quality of life compared with healthy neighborhood controls and controls with epilepsy as measured by the short-form 36 (SF-36) quality of life survey [47]. In addition, a study conducted in Brazil showed the presence of depression had a significant impact on the quality of life of patients with NCC as measured by a direct subjective quantification scale and the Functional Assessment of Cancer Therapy Quality of Life Measurement System (FACT-HN version IV) [48].

7. Suggested methods to improve the burden assessment of neurocysticercosis

While there are currently numerous ways in which to evaluate disease burden, each method has its pros and cons. Table 4 provides an overview of the established measures of disease burden currently available with which to evaluate the non-monetary or monetary burden of

T. solium cysticercosis. While non-monetary burden metrics, such as the DALY, are most often used by international agencies, these metrics are not capable of capturing the burden of disease associated with animal infection. Therefore, in order to fairly compare the burden of cysticercosis with that of non-zoonotic diseases, studies need to be conducted to evaluate how cysticercosis in pigs affects individuals in endemic regions in terms of income/livelihood losses and social impact. This information can then be used to develop questions to incorporate into a QALY scale or else be added to DALYs to capture this burden.

Measure of burden	**Items**	**Availability / quality of data**	
		Humans	***Animals***
QALYs	Cause specific death rates	Quality highly variable between countries	Not applicable
	Life expectancy	Largely available	
	Disease-specific incidence rates	Notifiable / registry disease data Quality / completeness highly variable	
	Time evolution of disease states	Knowledge of natural history of disease needed	
	Quality of life measure at various disease states	Special studies Place / time specific	
DALYs	Cause specific death rates	Quality highly variable between countries	Not applicable
	Disease-specific incidence rates	Notifiable / registry disease data Quality / completeness highly variable	
	Distribution of sequelae associated with disease in treatment free individuals	Knowledge of natural history of disease needed	
	Duration of each sequelae in treatment free individuals	Knowledge of natural history of each sequelae needed	
	Distribution of sequelae associated with disease among people under treatment	Special studies required	
	Duration of each sequelae under treatment	Special studies required	

Measure of burden	Items	Availability / quality of data	
		Humans	*Animals*
	Disability weights for each sequela (treated / non treated)	Available from GBD initiative Not all sequelae have been attributed disability weights	
Monetary burden	Cause-specific death rates	Quality highly variable between countries	Rarely available except for notifiable diseases
	Disease-specific prevalence	National / special survey data Special survey data often overestimate the truth	Abattoir data where home slaughtering is rare Special survey data often overestimate the truth
	Distribution of sequelae associated with disease	Knowledge of natural history of disease needed	Knowledge of natural history of disease needed
	Frequency of care / treatments / diagnoses and productivity losses for each sequel	Special studies Expert opinion	Special studies Expert opinion
	Costs associated with care / treatments / productivity losses of each sequel	Country-level health / labor statistics Special surveys	Agricultural statistics Special surveys

Table 4. Comparison of using QALYs, DALYs and monetary estimates to evaluate the disease burden of cysticercosis/NCC and other neglected zoonotic diseases with a livestock component [17]

8. Conclusions

T. solium cysticercosis is believed to contribute to high levels of human morbidity and some mortality, as well as pig production losses. This parasitic disease tends to disproportionately affect areas of low socio-economic status and should be prioritized for preventive measures because the disease is, in essence, 100% preventable. However, in order to make *T. solium* cysticercosis/NCC a priority condition, efforts to obtain more accurate estimates of disease burden must be made. In particular, a better understanding of the distribution of manifestations among all NCC cases would be very helpful. In addition, studies on the impact of NCC on productivity are needed. Such estimates could be used to show policy makers the true socioeconomic impact of this disease in various regions of the world. One of the biggest limitations, for most of the measures of disease burden currently used for NCC/cysticercosis, is the lack of available high quality epidemiologic and/or financial data. Adherence to recommended guidelines for the diagnosis of cysticercosis in humans and pigs and declaring NCC a reportable disease would contribute greatly towards better burden estimates for this condition.

9. Nomenclature

Cysticercosis: Infection or disease of humans or animals caused by the larvae of *Taenia* spp. In this chapter, the term refers to infection of humans or pigs with *Taenia solium*.
Decision tree analysis: A method of organizing epidemiological data into infections and the frequency of their consequences.
Direct costs: Costs associated with the diagnosis and treatment of a medical condition, in addition to, costs associated with condemnation of all or part of an infected carcass.
Disability Adjusted Life Year (DALY): A measure of overall disease burden, expressed as the number of years lost due to ill-health, disability, or early death.
Disability weight: A score between 0 and 1 that is assigned to a condition depending on the degree of debilitation.
Euro-Qol (EQ-5D): A standardized instrument for use as a measure of health outcome.
Health Adjusted Life Year (HALY): An umbrella term for a family of measures of population health that includes, for example, Disability Adjusted Life Years (DALYs) and Quality Adjusted Life Year (QALYs).
Indirect costs: Costs associated with lost wages or decreased productivity arising indirectly from infection.
Neurocysticercosis (NCC): A neurological disease caused by invasion of the CNS by larvae of *Taenia solium*.
Quality Adjusted Life Year (QALY): A measure of disease burden, including both the quality and the quantity of life lived. It is used in assessing the value for money of a medical intervention. A year of full health is equivalent to 1 QALY, whereas, death corresponds to 0 QALYs.
Short-Form 12 (SF-12): A generic dual (i.e., mental and physical health) scale measure of quality of life.

Author details

Rachana Bhattarai and Christine M. Budke
Texas A&M University, College of Veterinary Medicine and Biomedical Sciences, College Station, Texas, USA

Hélène Carabin
Corresponding Author
University of Oklahoma Health Sciences Center, Department of Epidemiology and Biostatistics, Oklahoma City, Oklahoma, USA

10. References

[1] Rajshekhar V, Joshi DD, Doanh NQ, van De N, Xiaonong Z. *Taenia solium* taeniosis/cysticercosis in Asia: epidemiology, impact and issues. Acta Tropica 2003; 87(1) 53-60.

[2] Zoli A, Shey-Njila O, Assana E, Nguekam JP, Dorny P, Brandt J, Geerts S. Regional status, epidemiology and impact of *Taenia solium* cysticercosis in Western and Central Africa. Acta Tropica 2003; 87(1) 35-42.

[3] Flisser A, Sarti E, Lightowlers M, Schantz P. Neurocysticercosis: regional status, epidemiology, impact and control measures in the Americas. Acta Tropica 2003; 87(1) 43-51.

[4] Sorvillo FJ, DeGiorgio C, Waterman SH. Deaths from cysticercosis, United States. Emerging Infectious Diseases 2007; 13(2) 230-5.

[5] del la Garza Y, Graviss EA, Daver NG, Gambarin KJ, Shandera WX, Schantz PM, White AC Jr. Epidemiology of neurocysticercosis in Houston, Texas. American Journal of Tropical Medicine and Hygiene 2005; 73(4) 766-70.

[6] Del Brutto OH. A review of cases of human cysticercosis in Canada. Canadian Journal Neurological Sciences 2012; 39(3) 319-22.

[7] Del Brutto OH. Neurocysticercosis in Western Europe: a re-emerging disease? Acta Neurologica Belgica 2012; DOI: 10.1007/s13760-012-0068-3.

[8] Carabin H, Ndimubanzi PC, Budke CM, Nguyen H, Qian Y, Cowan LD, Stoner JA, Rainwater E, Dickey M. Clinical manifestations associated with neurocysticercosis: a systematic review. PLoS Neglected Tropical Diseases 2011; 5(5) e1152.

[9] Almeida SM, Gurjao SA. Frequency of depression among patients with neurocysticercosis. Arquios de Neuro-psiquiatria 2010; 68(1) 76-80.

[10] Alarcon F, Vanormelingen K, Moncayo J, Vinan I. Cerebral cysticercosis as a risk factor for stroke in young and middle-aged people. Stroke 1992; 23(11) 1563-5.

[11] Ciampi de Andrade D, Rodrigues CL, Abraham R, Castro LHM, Livramento JA, Machado LR, Leite CC, Carameli P. Cognitive impairment and dementia in neurocysticercosis. Neurology 2010; 74(16) 1288-1295.

[12] de Boer HM, Mula M, Sander JW. The global burden and stigma of epilepsy. Epilepsy & Behavior 2008; 12(4) 540-546.

[13] Del Brutto OH, Rajshekhar V, White AC Jr, Tsang VC, Nasht TE, Takayanagui OM, Schantz PM, Evans CA, Flisser A, Correa D, Botero D, Allan JC, Sarti E, Gonzalez AE, Gilman RH, Garcia HH. Proposed diagnostic criteria for neurocysticercosis. Neurology 2001; 57(2) 177-83.

[14] Praet N, Rodriguez-Hidalgo R, Speybroeck N, Ahounou S, Benitez-Oritz W, Berkvens D, Hul AV, Barrionuevo-Samaniego M, Saegerman C, Dorny P. Infection with versus exposure to Taenia solium: what do serological test results tell us? American Journal of Tropical Medicine and Hygiene 2010; 83(2) 413-5.

[15] Foyaca-Sibat H, Cowan LD, Carabin H, Targonska I, Anwary MA, Serrano-Ocana G, Krecek RC, Willingham AL. Accuracy of serological testing for the diagnosis of

prevalent neurocysticercosis in outpatients with epilepsy, Eastern Cape Province, South Africa. PLoS Neglected Tropical Diseases 2009; 3(12) e562.
[16] Carabin H, Budke CM, Cowan LD, Willingham AL, Torgerson PR. Methods for assessing the burden of parasitic zoonoses: echinococcosis and cysticercosis. Trends in Parasitology 2005; 21(7) 327-33.
[17] Budke CM, Carabin H, Togerson PR. Health impact assessment and burden of zoonotic diseases. In: Palmer SR.(ed.) Oxford textbook of zoonoses : biology, clinical practice, and public health control. Oxford u.a.: Oxford University Press: 2011. p30-37.
[18] Gold MR, Stevenson D, Fryback DG. HALYS and QALYS and DALYS, Oh My: similarities and differences in summary measures of population Health. Annual Review of Public Health 2002; 23: 115-34.
[19] Drummond MF. Methods for the economic evaluation of health care programmes. Oxford [u.a.]: Oxford Univ. Press: 2007.
[20] EQ-5D, EuroQol Group. http://www.euroqol.org/eq-5d.html (accessed 25 June 2012).
[21] Ware JE, Kosinski M, Turner-Bowker DM, Gandek B. How to Score Version 2 of the SF-12 Health Survey (With a Supplement Documenting Version 1). Lincoln, RI: QualityMetric Inc: 2002.
[22] Phillips C, Thompson G. What is a QALY? England: Hayward Medical Communications: 1998.
[23] Ware JE, Kosinski M, Turner-Bowker DM, Gandek B. Physical and Mental Health Summary Scales: A Manual for Users of Version 1. Lincoln, RI: QualityMetric Inc: 2002.
[24] Young T, Yang Y, Brazier JE, Tsuchiya A, Coyne K. The first stage of developing preference-based measures: constructing a health-state classification using Rasch analysis. Quality of Life Research, 2009; 18(2) 253-65.
[25] Murray CJ, Quantifying the burden of disease: the technical basis for disability-adjusted life years. Bulletin World Health Organization 1994; 72(3) 429-45.
[26] WHO GBD 2010.http://www.globalburden.org/. (accessed 25 June 2012).
[27] Murray CJ, Acharya AK, Understanding DALYs (disability-adjusted life years). Journal of Health Economics 1997; 16(6) 703-30.
[28] Global Burden of Diseases, Injuries and Risk Factors Study Operations Manual. Institute for Health Metrics and Evaluation http://www.globalburden.org/GBD_Study_Operations_Manual_Jan_20_2009.pdf (accessed 25 June 2012).
[29] Ndimubanzi PC, Carabin H, Budke CM, Nguyen H, Qian YJ, Rainwater E, Dickey M, Reynolds S, Stoner JA. A systematic review of the frequency of neurocyticercosis with a focus on people with epilepsy. PLoS Neglected Tropical Diseases 2010; 4(11) e870.
[30] Bhattarai R, Budke CM, Carabin H, Proano JV, Flores-Rivera J, Corona T, Ivanek R, Snowden KF, Flisser A. Estimating the non-monetary burden of neurocysticercosis in Mexico. PLoS Neglected Tropical Diseases 2012; 6(2) e1521.
[31] Praet N, Speybroeck N, Manzanedo R, Berkvens D, Nsame Nforninwe D, Zoli A, Quet F, Preux PM, Carabin H, Geerts S. The disease burden of Taenia solium cysticercosis in Cameroon. PLoS Neglected Tropical Diseases 2009; 3(3) e406.

[32] Anand S and Hanson K, Disability-adjusted life years: a critical review. Journal of Health Economics 1997; 16(6) 685-702.

[33] Reidpath DD, Allotey PA, Kouame A, Cummins RA. Measuring health in a vacuum: examining the disability weight of the DALY. Health Policy Plan 2003; 18(4) 351-6.

[34] Majorowski MM, Carabin H, Kilani M, Bensalah A. Echinococcosis in Tunisia: a cost analysis. Transactions of the Royal Society of Tropical Medicine and Hygiene 2005; 99(4) 268-78.

[35] Carabin H, Krecek RC, Cowan LD, Michael L, Foyaca-Sibat H, Nash T, Willingham AL. Estimation of the cost of Taenia solium cysticercosis in Eastern Cape Province, South Africa. Tropical Medicine & International Health 2006; 11(6) 906-16.

[36] Preux PM, Druet-Cabanac M. Epidemiology and aetiology of epilepsy in sub-Saharan Africa. Lancet Neurology 2005; 4(1) 21-31.

[37] Del Rio-Romero AH, Foyaca-Sibat H, Ibanez-Valdes L de F, Vega-Novoa E. Prevalence of epilepsy and general knowledge about neurocysticercosis at Nkalukeni village, South Africa. The Internet Journal of Neurology 2005; 3(2).

[38] Del Rio-Romero AH, Foyaca-Sibat H, Ibanez-Valdes L de F. Neuroepidemiology findings as contibutors for epilepsy due to Neurocysticercosis at Mngceleni Location, South Africa. The Internet Journal of Neurology 2008; 9(1).

[39] Coleman R, Loppy L, Walraven G. The treatment gap and primary health care for people with epilepsy in rural Gambia. Bulletin World Health Organization 2002; 80(5) 378-83.

[40] Pal DK, Das T, Sengupta S, Chaudhury G. Help-seeking patterns for children with epilepsy in rural India: implications for service delivery. Epilepsia 2002; 43(8) 904-11.

[41] Nsengiyumva G, Druet-Cabanac M, Ramanankandrasana B, Bouteille B, Nsizabira L, Preux PM. Cysticercosis as a major risk factor for epilepsy in Burundi, east Africa. Epilepsia 2003; 44(7) 950-5.

[42] Garcia HH, Del Brutto OH, Nash TE, White AC Jr, Tsang VC, Gilman RH. New concepts in the diagnosis and management of neurocysticercosis (*Taenia solium*). American Journal of Tropical Medicine and Hygeine 2005; 72(1) 3-9.

[43] Santo AH. Cysticercosis-related mortality in the State of Sao Paulo, Brazil, 1985-2004: a study using multiple causes of death. Cad Saude Publica 2007; 23(12) 2917-27.

[44] Sorvillo FJ, Portigal L, DeGiorgio C, Smith L, Waterman SH, Berlin GW, Ash LR. Cysticercosis-related deaths, California. Emerging Infectious Diseases 2004; 10(3) 465-9.

[45] Townes JM, Hoffmann CJ, Kohn MA. Neurocysticercosis in Oregon, 1995-2000. Emerging Infectious Diseases 2004; 10(3) 508-10.

[46] Bhattarai R, Budke CM, Carabin H, Proano JV, Flores-Rivera J, Corona T, Cowan LD, Ivanek R, Snowden KF, Flisser A. Quality of life in patients with neurocysticercosis in Mexico. American Journal of Tropical Medicine and Hygeine 2011; 84(5) 782-6.

[47] Wallin MT, Pretell EJ, Bustos JA, Caballero M, Alfaro M, Kane R, Wilken J, Sullivan C, Fratto T, Garcia HH. Cognitive changes and quality of life in neurocysticercosis: a longitudinal study. PLoS Neglected Tropical Diseases 2012; 6(1) e1493.

[48] de Almeida SM, Gurjao SA. Quality of life assessment in patients with neurocysticercosis. Journal of Community Health 2011; 36(4) 624-30.

Chapter 4

Agricultural Impact of Porcine Cyisticercosis in Africa: A Review

Helena A. Ngowi, Samson Mukaratirwa, Faustin P. Lekule, Ndichu Maingi, Charles Waiswa, Chummy Sikasunge, Sonia Afonso, Julienne Sumbu, Sylvia Ramiandrasoa, Mary Louise Penrith and Arve Lee Willingham

Additional information is available at the end of the chapter

http://dx.doi.org/10.5772/51196

1. Introduction

This chapter reviews the status of pig production and porcine cysticercosis caused by *Taenia solium* in Africa. First, it provides background information regarding pig production and porcine cysticercosis in the region. The chapter then reviews in some more details the current status of porcine cysticercosis in each of the countries based on available scientific literature. Furthermore, this chapter analyses extensively the economic impact of porcine cysticercosis, especially to the agricultural sector in Africa. Finally, the chapter provides conclusions and recommendations to guide future work in relation to porcine cysticercosis in the African continent. To simplify the reporting, the African continent has been divided into five regions based on the United Nations classification system. The regions are northern Africa, southern Africa, western Africa, central Africa, and eastern Africa.

2. Background

Porcine cysticercosis refers to as an infection of pigs with the larval form of *Taenia species*. *Taenia solium*, *T. saginata asiatica*, and *T. hydatigena* are the *Taenia species* that can infect pigs. While *T. saginata asiatica* is currently known to be limited to Asia, *T. solium* and *T. hydatigena* have a worldwide distribution. On the African continent, however, *T. solium* ('pork tapeworm') is the most important species of *Taenia* economically and for public health. The larval form of this parasite is capable of infecting humans leading to life-threatening neurological disorders, including epilepsy. In addition, *T. solium* cysticercosis in humans and pigs causes serious economic losses in affected countries because of condemnation of infected pigs and disability in neurocysticercotic patients. The human is the only natural definitive host of *T. solium*. An adult tapeworm is harboured in the small intestine of

INTECH
open science | open minds

© 2013 Ngowi et al., licensee InTech. This is a paper distributed under the terms of the Creative Commons Attribution License (http://creativecommons.org/licenses/by/3.0), which permits unrestricted use, distribution, and reproduction in any medium, provided the original work is properly cited.

humans, a condition referred to as taeniasis. *Taenia solium* taeniasis is acquired through ingestion of infective larvae of the parasite from infected meat. Raw or inadequately cooked pork provides the route for taeniasis transmission. On the other hand, the larval form of *T. solium*, cysticercosis, can infect both humans and pigs if the hosts ingest infective eggs of the parasite. The life cycle of *T. solium* is presented in Figure 1. Water and foodstuffs contaminated with faecal material from a human carrier of the adult tapeworm are the major sources of cysticercosis transmission. Several factors have been found to facilitate the occurrence of cysticercosis. These include open defaecation, poor personal hygiene, free ranging pigs, and lack of safe drinking water. These factors facilitate both human and animal host access to human faecal materials, which at times may contain *T. solium* eggs.

Although a number of animal species including dogs [1] can be infected with *T. solium* cysticercosis, domesticated pigs play the major role in the transmission cycle of the parasite because of their close proximity to humans, especially in rural areas, and the increasing popularity of pig keeping and pork consumption in many developing countries [2]. Therefore, most of the literature on *T. solium* has focused on the human-pig transmission cycle. This is also the focus in this chapter.

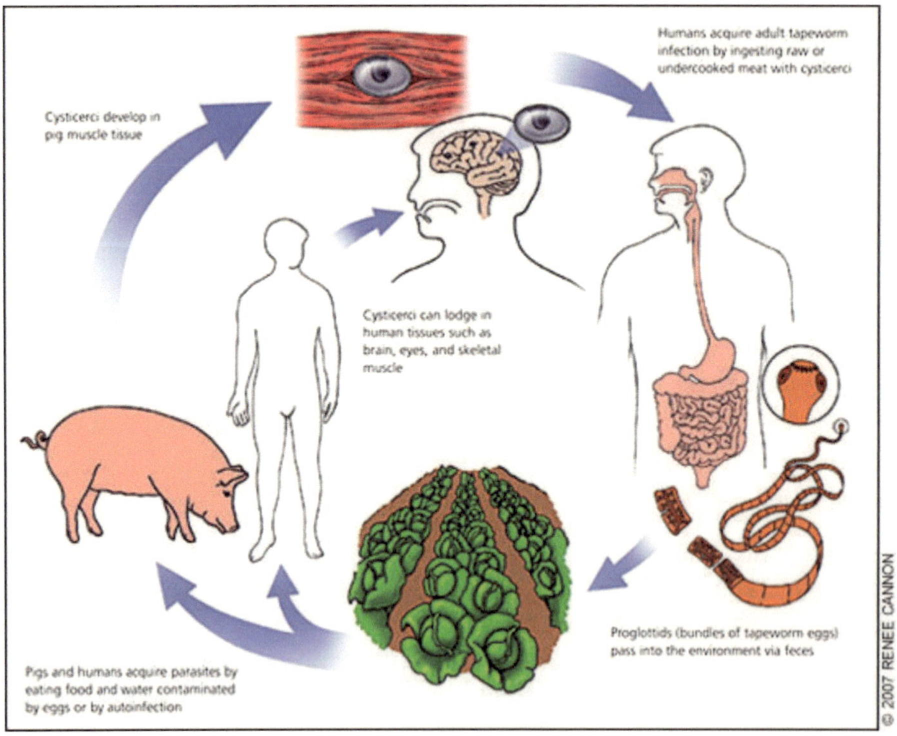

Source [3]

Figure 1. The life cycle of *Taenia solium*.

Taenia solium is prevalent in several countries of Africa, Asia and Latin America, providing the full life cycle of the parasite. Poverty has facilitated the parasite's endemicity by inhibiting adequate sanitation and good pig husbandry, which are primary in the control of *T. solium* transmission. The currently emergence and re-emergence of cysticercosis in some industrialised countries of the USA and Europe resulting from international migration have been limited to human-human transmission leading to human cysticercosis (including neurocysticercosis). However, because of improved sanitation and intensive pig rearing, porcine cysticercosis can rarely be (re)introduced in these countries, and hence, a full cycle of the parasite is virtually impossible. In such countries, the major impact of the parasite is related to human morbidity and associated economic losses.

In response to the WHO's effort to estimate the global burden of neurocysticercosis, four comprehensive studies have reported estimates of burdens of *T. solium* cysticercosis [4-7]. While three of the studies estimated the economic burden of cysticercosis, each focusing on a specific country [4,5,7], a global extensive systematic review of literature found that the frequency of neurocysticercosis in people with epilepsy was consistent across endemic countries. The pooled estimate was 29.0% (95%CI: 22.9%–35.5%) [6]. Knowledge on the proportion of epilepsy caused by neurocysticercosis is primary to enable estimation of the economic impact of neurocysticercosis in endemic countries. For the studies that have estimated the economic burden of cysticercosis in both human and pigs, the infected pigs have been found to contribute 4.7-26.9% of the overall costs of the infections [4,5]. The cost estimates in the pig industry have been entirely based on the prevalence of porcine cysticercosis and the economic loss of the pig's value due to the infection. Thus the observed variation between countries has been primarily due to the differences in porcine cysticercosis prevalence and reduced values of the infected pigs in the different country settings. A study in the Eastern Cape Province of South Africa also reported different values due to different data analytical methods [4]. Generally, the price of a finished pig was estimated to be reduced by 20-60% because of infection with cysticercosis [4,5].

While *T. solium* is progressively being recognized as an important parasite at the global level, to date scientists in several developing countries endemic for the parasite are struggling to bring the disease to the national attention. Failure of *T. solium* endemic countries to recognize the importance of the parasite is attributed partly to lack of knowledge by stakeholders on the presence, magnitude and impacts of the parasite. While understanding both the human health and agricultural impacts of the parasite is necessary in order to establish the overall societal burden of the parasite to countries, for endemic diseases such as cysticercosis, political decisions in most developing countries are often based on economic impacts of the diseases. This is because most long-term, persisting endemic diseases are difficult to quickly appreciate their impact, especially to non-professional policy makers. This is different from epidemic diseases, which draw significant attention when they occur, and hence, favourable measures are usually taken urgently to control such diseases. Political will is important for countries to allocate necessary resources to solve community related problems such as diseases. Specific knowledge on the contribution of the various sectors in the overall societal burden of *T. solium* is of particular importance to promote inter-sectoral collaboration towards control of the parasite [8].

In Africa, pig keeping is popular in many countries. However, there has been no study that has clearly described the pattern of pig production and the overall status of porcine cysticercosis on the continent. This is important in order to understand the importance of the pig enterprise in the region as well as the potential for porcine cysticercosis to constrain the industry. Africa is one of the regions where the full cycle of *T. solium* is occurring because of the favourable environmental conditions and poverty, which inhibit application of effective control measures for the parasite. Thus Africa provides a suitable ecology for *T. solium* endemicity. While information on human taeniasis and cysticercosis status in Africa is still scant, inhibiting a full appraisal of the parasite's burden to the affected countries, a number of scientific publications are presumed to be available with regard to the magnitude and impact of porcine cysticercosis to the agricultural sector in the affected African countries. The emergence of *T. solium* cysticercosis in eastern and southern Africa as a serious agricultural problem and public health risk was described earlier by the Cysticercosis Working Group in Eastern and Southern Africa (CWGESA) [2]. Other authors have described the taeniasis-cysticercosis complex in West and Central Africa [9]. These provide some of the evidence on the importance of cysticercosis caused by *T. solium* in Africa. Synthesizing the information on the burden of porcine cysticercosis to the agricultural sector in Africa would inform on the regional status and guide future efforts towards control and ultimately elimination of the parasite

3. Scope

In this chapter, we review the pig production and agricultural impact of porcine cysticercosis on the African continent based on available literature. Data on the pig population in Africa is based on the most current global pig population estimates [10]. For the prevalence of porcine cysticercosis, the most recent information is included, with a priority for prevalence estimated using antigen ELISA, where available, in order to reflect active infections. However, prevalence based on a less accurate diagnostic method is used if that is the only information available. Note that, the purpose of the review is to describe the current status of porcine cysticercosis in the African region rather than presenting all that has been done in the region with regard to porcine cysticercosis. For simplicity, the African continent is divided into five major regions as classified by the United Nations. That is northern Africa, southern Africa, western Africa, central Africa, and eastern Africa [Figure 2]. Only the 54 countries fully recognised by the United Nations are included. These consists of seven, five, 16, nine and 17 countries of the northern, southern, western, central and eastern Africa, respectively.

It is possible that porcine cysticercosis poses more economic losses than those only related to condemnation or reduced value of infected pigs. For example, studies have established possible reduced fertility of pigs naturally infected with cysticercosis, which would reduce the productive performance of the pigs [12]. Similar findings have been reported in human infected with neurocysticercosis [13]. In both the pig and human studies, cysticercosis was found to significantly reduce serum level of testosterone while increasing significantly the level of follicle stimulating hormones in males [12,13]. On the other hand, cysticercosis significantly reduced the level of progesterone in females [13]. These endocrinological changes are thought to exert significant inhibitory action in the reproduction function of the infected individuals. However, it has been observed that the effect is more intense in male than female hosts. Although the study of pigs included males only, there is strong evidence from laboratory trials, which suggests that the effect of the parasite in female pigs will most likely resemble that observed in female humans [12,13].

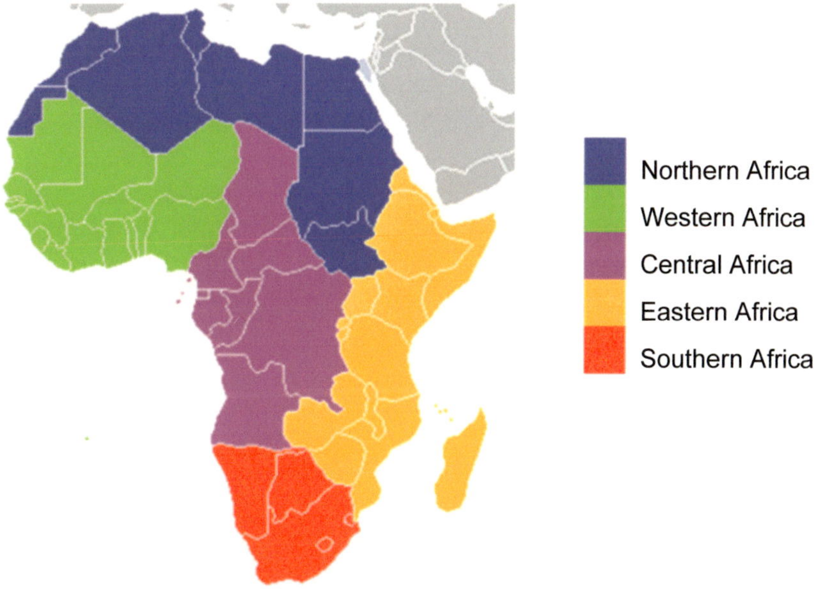

Source: [11]

Figure 2. Regions of Africa based on the United Nations system of classification.

Disability in persons infected with neurocysticercosis is another potential factor that is likely to contribute to further economic losses in the agricultural sector through reduced manpower, some of which would be used in pig production in the countries. This can be supported by studies in Eastern Cape Province of South Africa and Cameroon, which show that the majority of people in Africa are not employed in salaried jobs [4,5]. This significant proportion of the population is likely to engage in small-scale businesses, including pig farming. Those suffering from neurocysticercosis in this category of the population are likely to contribute significantly to agricultural losses in the pig industry.

Because of the current lack of information on the actual reduction of pigs' reproductivity as a result of cysticercosis and specific contribution of unemployed populations to pig production in endemic countries, the analysis of the agricultural impact of *T. solium* in this study is mostly based on the costs related to the partial or total condemnation of infected pigs. However, we observe possible gross underestimation of the impact.

4. Methodology

4.1. Study area and duration

This study was carried out between April and June, 2012 and included the 54 African countries that were fully recognised by the United Nations as of 2012 [14]

Collection of data on country pig populations and status of porcine cysticercosis

Pig population data for each of the 54 countries were downloaded from the FAO statistical database [10]. The most recent pig population estimates (those of 2010) were used. Thereafter, several Google searches were performed for each country name and key English phrases and words such as "porcine cysticercosis", *"Taenia solium"*, *"T. solium"*, and "cysticercosis" to gather scientific publications related to porcine cysticercosis in each country. When a relevant article was encountered, necessary information such as disease magnitude, sample size and diagnostic method was recorded as available. If more than one article was found to be relevant, a range of values was given and authors for all the articles used were cited. The most current literature was preferred.

Estimation of agricultural impact of porcine cysticercosis

This was the main focus of the study. Therefore, more attention was given to this aspect. A total of 200 articles were retrieved following several Google searches using the following four phrases in that order: (i) Burden-of Taenia-solium cysticercosis, (ii) Impact-of Taenia-solium, (iii) Economic-impact Taenia-solium, and (iv) Financial-impact Taenia-solium. For each search phrase, 50 first articles we retrieved from which the relevant ones were downloaded from their publishers for further analysis. This first screening was based on a quick assessment of information given in the abstracts. Following the first screening, a total of 18 articles were considered relevant and different from each other, and hence, were included. Out of the 18 articles, 10 were obtained from the first search, seven new articles from the second search, one form the third, and none new from the fourth search phrase. In the second screening, only those articles that included information for Africa were sub-selected from the 18 articles. Five were obtained at this sub-sampling stage. Finally, only those articles that included information on the economic burden of porcine cysticercosis in Africa were selected. Four articles met this criterion and were included for further analysis. The four articles were all peer-reviewed journal papers [4,5,16,17]. A flow diagram to illustrate the sampling procedure described above is given in Figure 3.

The information collected was recorded as reported by the author(s) of the article. If there was different information regarding the cost of porcine cysticercosis in a country, a range of values was given and data sources cited.

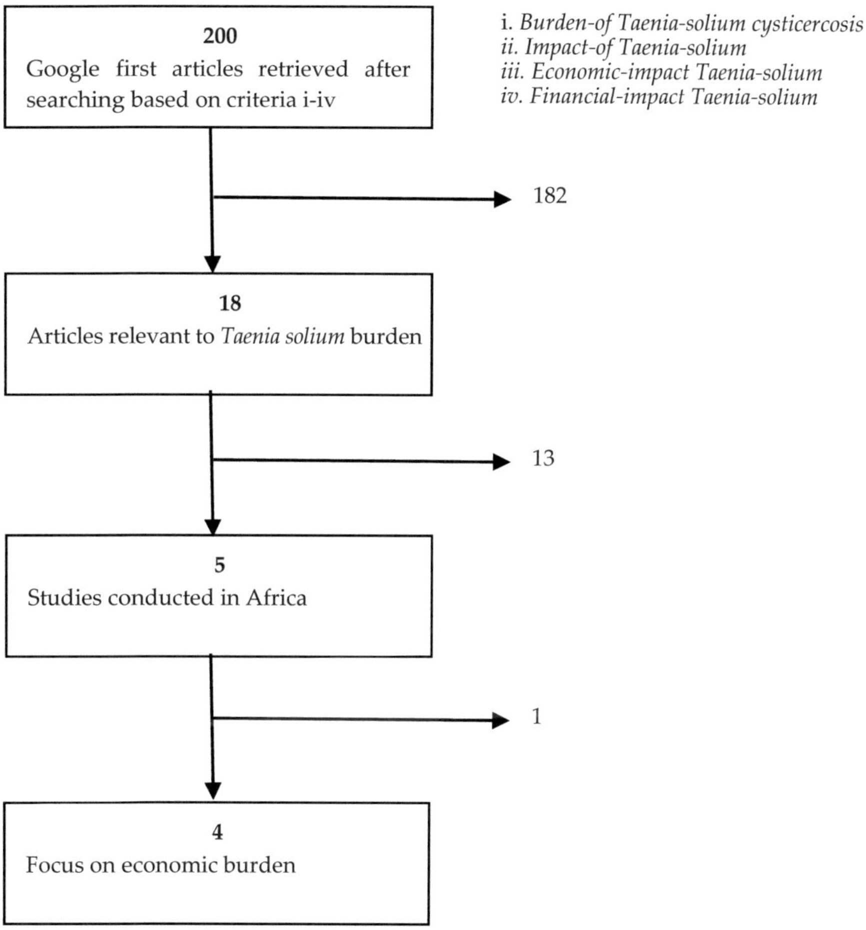

Figure 3. The flow diagram of the literature sampling procedure to analyse the economic impact of porcine cysticercosis in Africa.

5. Results

5.1. General results

The study area consisted of 54 countries. The total population of pigs estimated in the study area in 2010 amounted 29,606,438. This was approximately 3.1% of the world pig population estimate (N = 965,855,414) of 2010. Out of the Africa regional pig population, approximately 0.2% was reared in the northern countries, while 6.1%, 43.3%, 16,4%, and 34.0% were reared in the southern, western, central, and eastern Africa, respectively. Overall, 19 (35.2%) of the 54 study countries reported prevalence of cysticercosis in pigs. While no data were available in the northern region, the remaining regions provided prevalence data, with more reporting frequency observed in the eastern followed by central Africa.

Porcine cysticercosis in northern Africa

Countries of northern Africa comprise Algeria, Egypt, Libya, Morocco, Sudan, Southern Sudan, and Tunisia. Pig rearing in this region is minimal (Table 1). While there were no pigs reported for Libya, Sudan, and Southern Sudan, indicating possibly absence of or insignificant pig rearing in the countries, pig populations in the remaining four countries ranged from 5,700-38,000 in 2010, making an overall regional pig population of 58,200 pigs. The small number of pigs reared in the northern Africa region is likely to be due to drought and the fact that most of the inhabitants in the region are Muslims. Generally, there was no report available with regard to porcine cysticercosis in the northern Africa. While there is an indication of Egypt providing the most ancient known case of *T. solium* infection in humans, there was currently no information regarding prevalence of cysticercosis in pigs in that country. Pigs in Egypt are known to be kept mainly by Coptic Christians. Before, the 2009 suspected swine flu pandemic, which nevertheless did not prove true, pigs in the country have been very valuable in cleaning the city garbage by being fed on garbage traditionally collected from cities and urban centres [15]. Although this practice might have been reduced after the 2009 suspect swine flu pandemic, generally pigs in Egypt are at a greater risk of acquiring *T. solium* cysticercosis because of feeding on the garbage. The lack of reports on porcine cysticercosis in the country can be due to lack of research, which could also be enhanced by religious conflicts towards pig keeping in that country.

Country	Pig population 2010	Prevalence of PCC
Algeria	5,700	ND
Egypt	38,000	ND
Libya	-	ND
Morocco	8,500	ND
Sudan	-	ND
Southern Sudan	-	
Tunisia	6,000	ND
Total	**58,200**	

Table 1. Pig population estimates of North African countries in 2010 and the current status of porcine cysticercosis (PCC) caused by *Taenia solium*. ND indicates no data

Porcine cysticercosis in southern Africa

Table 2 presents the pig population estimates and status of porcine cysticercosis in southern Africa. South Africa is the only country in the region, which has reported prevalence of porcine cysticercosis. A number of studies have been conducted in several parts of the country for various periods of time. It is apparent that porcine cysticercosis is hyperendemic in some parts of the country. The possibility of the other countries in the region being free from porcine cysticercosis is yet to be scientifically proven. Such studies would be very valuable in guiding potential control measures for *T. solium* infections in South Africa by providing information on potential factors that may be encouraging the endemicity of the parasite in South Africa but not in the other countries if they prove to be free from the infections.

Country	Pig population 2010	Prevalence of PCC	Diagnostic method	Reference
Botswana	12,950	ND		
Lesotho	83,976	ND		
Namibia	65,000	ND		
South Africa	1,594,490	54.8 – 57	Ag-ELISA	[18]
Swaziland	50,000	ND		
Total	**1,806,416**			

Table 2. Pig population estimates of southern African countries in 2010 and the current status of porcine cysticercosis (PCC) caused by *Taenia solium*. ND indicates no data

Porcine cysticercosis in western Africa

Western Africa has the largest pig population in the region (Table 3). Six of the 16 countries of the region have reported presence of porcine cysticercosis. Burkina Faso seems to have high prevalence of porcine cysticercosis in some region, probably because of variations in pig management practices. Apart from Burkina Faso, Gambia and Senegal, data from the other countries are rather old. This suggests that research on porcine cysticercosis in these countries has been inactive for quite some time.

Country	Pig population 2010	Prevalence of PCC	Diagnostic method	Reference
Benin	354,000	ND		
Burkina Faso	1,920,200	0-39.6	Ag-ELISA	[16,19]
Cape Verde	238,600	ND		
Cote d'Ivoire	350,000	ND		
Gambia	28,500	4.8 (n = 371)	Ag-ELISA	[20]
Ghana	536,000	11.7		[16]
Guinea	95,180	ND		
Guinea Bissau	418,900	ND		
Liberia	265,300	ND		
Mali	75,015	ND		
Mauritania	-	ND		
Niger	40,000	ND		
Nigeria	7,471,730	15.3		[16]
Senegal	346,681	6.4-13.2 (n=1334)	Ag-ELISA	[20]
Sierra Leone	45,211	ND		
Togo	643,630	17		[16]
Total	**12,828,947**			

Table 3. Pig population estimates of West African countries in 2010 and the current status of porcine cysticercosis (PCC) caused by *Taenia solium*. ND indicates no data

Porcine cysticercosis in central Africa

Four out of the ten countries of central Africa have reported prevalence of porcine cysticercosis. Extensive studies have been conducted in Cameroon, ranging from epidemiological, intervention trials and disease burden analysis. Porcine cysticercosis prevalence in Cameroon seems to resemble that in the Democratic Republic of Congo. Central Africa also indicates high infection rates of porcine cysticercosis.

Country	Pig population 2010	Prevalence of PCC	Diagnostic method	Reference
Angola	791,000	0-6.8	Meat insp.	[16]
Cameroon	1,680,000	11-39.8	Ag-ELISA	[21]
Central Afr Rep	1,087,000	ND		
Chad	30,400	6.8-25.7	Tongue/Meat	[16]
Rep Congo	70,000	ND		
DR Congo	967,000	41.2 (n=153)	Ag-ELISA	[22]
Eq. Guinea	6,300	ND		
Gabon	215,000	ND		
Sao Tomé & Pr	2,620	ND		
Total	**4,849,320**			

Table 4. Pig population estimates of Central African countries in 2010 and the current status of porcine cysticercosis (PCC) caused by *Taenia solium*. ND indicates no data

Porcine cysticercosis in eastern Africa

The eastern Africa region consists of 17 countries and approximately 10 million pigs were reared in the region in 2010 (Table 5). The region includes ten out of 13 countries that belong to the CWGESA, an international non-governmental scientific organisation that was founded in 2002 with the overall objective of combating taeniasis/cysticercosis on a regional effort, considering that the disease has no border. As shown in the table below, a number of countries have reported prevalence of porcine cysticercosis, also suggesting high infection pressure in some countries. In Tanzania, an incidence rate of 69 per 100 pig-yeas was estimated in sentinel pigs based on antigen ELISA [23].

Economic impact of porcine cysticercosis in Africa

Quite a good amount of information regarding the monetary burden of porcine cysticercosis has been reported in the southern, western, central, and eastern Africa regions. Extensive and most recent studies are those conducted in South Africa and Cameroon [4,5]. These studies were also able to establish the disease burden in humans. Overall, the available information provides enough evidence of the agricultural impact of porcine cysticercosis in Africa, especially most of sub-Saharan Africa. Table 6 summarises the information on the monetary burden of porcine cysticercosis in Africa.

Country	Pig population 2010	Prevalence of PCC	Diagnostic method	Reference
Tanzania	495,000	30.7-32 (n=600)	Ag-ELISA	[24]
Kenya	347,400	4.0	Ag-ELISA	[25]
Uganda	2,300,000	8.6 (n=480)	Ag-ELISA	[26]
Rwanda	602,324	20		[16]
Burundi	244,791	2-39	Meat insp.	[16]
Djibouti	-	ND		
Eritrea	-	ND		
Ethiopia	29,000	ND		
Somalia	4,200	ND		
Mozambique	1,350,000	34.9 (n=661)	Ag-ELISA	[27]
Madagascar	1,380,250	ND		
Malawi	2,147,900	ND		
Zambia	500,000	8.2-23.3 (n=98-1691)	Ag-ELISA	[28, 29]
Zimbabwe	635,000	2.7-28.6	Meat insp.	[2]
Comoros	-	ND		
Mauritius	22,327	ND		
Seychelles	5,363	ND		
Total	**10,063,555**			

Table 5. Pig population estimates of East African countries in 2010 and the current status of porcine cysticercosis (PCC) caused by *Taenia solium*. ND indicates no data

Region	Country	Overall annual monetary losses	Losses due to PCC	Annual DALYs lost due to NCC	Reference
Northern Africa	-				
Southern Africa	S. Africa 04	US $18.6 - 34.2 M	US $5.0 M	ND	[4]
Western Africa	B/ Faso		€ 52,830		[16]
	Ghana		€ 594,945		[16]
	Nigeria		€ 17,442, 000		[16]
	Senegal		€ 57,600		[16]
	Togo		€ 2,167,500		[16]
Central Africa	Cameroon	€ 10,255,202	€ 478,844	€ 45,838.4	[5]
			€ 2,062,125		[16]
	Angola		€ 408,000		[16]
	Chad		€ 56,063		[16]
	D R Congo		€ 2,141,700		[16]
Eastern Africa	Burundi		€ 218,325		[16]
	Tanzania		*		[17]

* A community based health education intervention trial in Tanzania found out that over a period of 5 years, the health and pig management education intervention would have a significant financial benefit to a smallholder pig farmer receiving it [NPV: US $3507 (95% CI: 3421 to 3591); IRR: 370%].

Table 6. Monetary and non-monetary costs of *Taenia solium* cysticercosis in Africa

6. Conclusion

This extensive literature survey has established the agricultural impact of porcine cysticercosis in Africa. The results indicate a high disease burden and its economic impact to affected countries due to monetary losses in the agricultural sector, human health related costs and reduced manpower as a result of disabilities in neurocysticercotic patients. Most of the previous studies have focused on financial losses due to reduced value of infected pigs. This can grossly underestimate the burden of *T. solium* to the agricultural sector since disabilities in neurocysticercotic patients (including attached stigma) and possible reduced reproductive performance of infected pigs could add further to the impact of the parasite to the agricultural sector. Only two studies in the region have in addition analysed the cost of the parasite as a result of neurocysticercotic persons. These studies found that monetary losses due to pig condemnations account only approximately 5% of the overall cost of the disease [4,5]. In addition, the studies established significant Disability Adjusted Life Years (DALYs) lost by patients suffering from neurocysticercosis. Such opportunity costs are likely to exert additional burden of the parasite to the agricultural sector as a good number of rural communities are mostly engaged in agricultural activities, including pig farming. This study recommends urgent measures to control *T. solium* in endemic countries now that adequate epidemiological data are available in several countries. In addition, studies are needed to determine the impact of porcine cysticercosis to the fertility and eventually fecundity of infected pigs.

Author details

Helena A. Ngowi
Department of Veterinary Medicine and Public Health,
Sokoine University of Agriculture, Morogoro, Tanzania

Samson Mukaratirwa
School of Biological & Conservation Sciences,
University of KwaZulu-Natal, Durban, South Africa

Faustin P. Lekule
Department of Animal Science and Production,
Sokoine University of Agriculture, Morogoro, Tanzania

Ndichu Maingi
Department of Veterinary Pathology,
Microbiology & Parasitology,
University of Nairobi, Nairobi, Kenya

Charles Waiswa
Department of Veterinary Medicine,
Makerere University, Kampala, Uganda

Chummy Sikasunge
Department of Para-Clinical Studies,
University of Zambia, Lusaka, Zambia

Sonia Afonso
Faculty of Veterinary Medicine,
Eduardo Mondlane University,
Maputo, Mozambique

Julienne Sumbu
Department of Parasitology,
Central Veterinary Laboratory, Kinshasa,
Democratic Republic of Congo

Sylvia Ramiandrasoa
Division of Cysticercosis,
Ministry of Heath, Antananarivo, Madagascar

Mary Louise Penrith
Department of Veterinary Tropical Diseases,
Faculty of Veterinary Science,
University of Pretoria, Pretoria, South Africa

Arve Lee Willingham
WHO/FAO Collaborating Center for Research and Training on Emerging and Other Parasitic Zoonoses,
Danish Centre for Experimental Parasitology,
The Faculty of Life Sciences,
University of Copenhagen, Frederiksberg, Denmark
The Cysticercosis Working Group in Eastern and Southern Africa

Acknowledgement

Authors for the various studies and data sources used in the compilation of the information presented in this chapter are highly acknowledged.

7. References

[1] Ito A, Putra M. I, Subahar R, Sato M. O, Okamoto M, Sako Y, Nakao M, Yamasaki H, Nakaya K, Craig P. S, Margono S. S Dogs as alternative intermediate hosts of *Taenia solium* in Papua (Irian Jaya), Indonesia confirmed by highly specific ELISA and immunoblot using native and recombinant antigens and mitochondrial DNA analysis. Journal of Helminthology 2002; 76(4):311-314.

[2] Phiri I. K, Ngowi H, Afonso S, Matenga E, Boa M, Mukaratirwa S, Githigia S, Saimo M, Sikasunge C, Maingi N, Lubega G. W, Kassuku A, Michael L, Siziya S, Krecek R. C, Noormahomed E, Vilhena M, Dorny P, Willingham A. L 3rd The emergence of *Taenia solium* cysticercosis in Eastern and Southern Africa as a serious agricultural problem and public health risk. Acta Tropica 2003; 87(1) 13_23.

[3] Kraft R Cysticercosis an emerging parasitic disease. American Family Physician 2007; 76(1) 91-96.

[4] Carabin H, Krecek R. C, Cowan L. D, Michael L, Foyaca-Sibat H, Nash T, Willingham A. L Estimation of the monetary burden of Taenia solium cysticercosis in the Eastern Cape, South Africa. Tropical Medicine and International Health 2006; 11(6) 906–916.

[5] Praet N, Speybroeck N, Manzanedo R, Berkvens D, Nsame Nforninwe D, et al The Disease Burden of *Taenia solium* Cysticercosis in Cameroon. PLoS Neglected Tropical Diseases 2009; 3(3) e406. doi:10.1371/journal.pntd.0000406.

[6] Ndimubanzi P. C, Carabin H, Budke C. M, Nguyen H, Qian Y-J, et al A Systematic Review of the Frequency of Neurocyticercosis with a Focus on People with Epilepsy. PLoS Neglected Tropical Diseases 2010; 4(11) e870. doi:10.1371/journal.pntd.0000870.

[7] Bhattarai R, Budke C. M, Carabin H, Proan˜o J. V, Flores-Rivera J, et al Estimating the Non-Monetary Burden of Neurocysticercosis in Mexico. PLoS Neglected Tropical Diseases 2012; 6(2) e1521. doi:10.1371/journal.pntd.0001521.

[8] Zinsstag J, Schelling E, Wyss K, Bechir M Potential of cooperation between human and animal health to strengthen health systems. Lancet 2005; 366(9503) 2142.

[9] Geerts S, Zoli A, Nguekam J. P, Brandt J, Dorny P The taeniasis-cysticercosis complex in West and Central Africa Cameroon. Southeast Asian Journal of Tropical Medicine and Public Health 2004; 35 (suppl 1) 262–265.

[10] Anonymous. FAOSTAT. http://faostat.fao.org/site/573/default.aspx#ancor (accessed12 June 2012]

[11] Anonymous. Regional map of Africa. http://goafrica.about.com/od/africatraveltips/ig/Maps-of-Africa/Regional-Map-of-Africa-.htm (accessed 5 June 2012).

[12] Peña N, Morales J, Morales-Montor J, Vargas-Villavicencio A, Fleury A Impact of naturally acquired *Taenia solium* cysticercosis on the hormonal levels of free ranging boars. Veterinary Parasitology 200; (149(1-2) 134-137.

[13] Cárdenas G, Valdez R, Sáenz B, Bottasso O, Fragoso G, Sciutto E, Romano MC, Fleury A Impact of *Taenia solium* neurocysticercosis upon endocrine status and its relation with immuno-inflammatory parameters. International Journal of Parasitology 2012; 42(2)171-176.

[14] Anonymous. African countries. http://www.armoredpenguin.com/wordsearch/Data/best/africa/african.countries.01.html (accessed 13 June2012)

[15] Fahmi W, Sutton K Cairo's Contested Garbage: Sustainable Solid Waste Management and the Zabaleen's Right to the City. Sustainability 2010; 2 1765-1783; doi:10.3390/su2061765

[16] Zoli A, Shey-Njila O, Assana E, Nguekam J-P, Dorny P, Brandt J, Geerts S Regional status, epidemiology and impact of *Taenia solium* cysticercosis in Western and Central Africa. Acta Tropica 2003; 87(1) 35_42.

[17] Ngowi H. A, Mlangwa J. E. D, Carabin H, Mlozi M. R. S, Kassuku A. A, Kimera S. I, Willingham III A. L Financial effi ciency of health and pig management education intervention in controlling porcine cysticercosis in Mbulu District, northern Tanzania. Livestock Research for Rural Development. http://www.cipav.org.co/lrrd/lrrd19/5/ngow19062.htm (accessed 19 April 2012).

[18] Krecek R. C,, Mohammed H, Michael L. M, Schantz P. M, Ntanjana L, et al Risk Factors of Porcine Cysticercosis in the Eastern Cape Province, South Africa. PLoS ONE 2012; 7(5) e37718. doi:10.1371/journal.pone.0037718.

[19] Ganaba R, Praet N, Carabin H, Millogo A, Tamagda Z, Dorny P, Hounton A, Sow S, ,[7] Nitiéma P, Cowan L. D Factors Associated with the Prevalence of Circulating Antigens to Porcine Cysticercosis in Three Villages of Burkina Faso. PLoS Neglected Tropical Diseases 2011; 5(1): e927.

[20] Secka A, Marcotty T, Deken R. D, Mark E. V, Geerts S Porcine Cysticercosis and Risk Factors in The Gambia and Senegal. Journal of Parasitological Research 2010; 823892.

[21] Assana E, Amadou F, Thys E, Lightowlers M. W, Zoli A. P, Dony P, Geerts S Pig-farming systems and porcine cysticercosis in the north of Cameroon. Journal of Helminthology 2010; 84(4) 441–446.

[22] Praet N, Kanobana K, Kabwe C, Maketa V, Lukanu P, et al *Taenia solium* Cysticercosis in the Democratic Republic of Congo: How Does Pork Trade Affect the Transmission of the Parasite? PLoS Negl Trop Dis 2010; 4(9): e817. doi:10.1371/journal.pntd.0000817.

[23] Ngowi H. A, Carabin H, Kassuku A. A, Mlozi M. R. S, Mlangwa J. E. D, et al A health-education intervention trial to reduce porcine cysticercosis in Mbulu District, Tanzania. Preventive Veterinary Medicine 2008; 85: 52–67.

[24] Komba EVG. Prevalence of porcine cysticercosis in Mbozi and Mbeya rural districts, Tanzania. MSc Dissertaion. MSc Dissertation. Sokoine University of Agriculture; 2008.

[25] Kagira J. M, Maingi N, Kanyari P. W, Githigia S. M, Ng'ang'a J. C, Gachohi J. M Seroprevalence of Cysticercus cellulosae and associated risk factors in free-range pigs in Kenya. Journal of Helminthology 2010; 84(4):398-403.

[26] Waiswa C, Fèvre E. M, Nsadha Z, Sikasunge C. S, Willingham III A. L Porcine Cysticercosis in Southeast Uganda: Seroprevalence in Kamuli and Kaliro Districts. Journal of Parasitology Research 2009; doi:10.1155/2009/375493

[27] Pondja A, Neves L, Mlangwa J, Afonso S, Fafetine J, Willingham A. L 3rd, Thamsborg S. M, Johansen M. V Prevalence and risk factors of porcine cysticercosis in Angónia District, Mozambique. PLoS Neglected Tropical Diseases 2010; 4(2):e594.

[28] Phiri I. K, Dorny P, Gabriel S, Willingham A. L, Speybroeck N, Vercruysse J, The prevalence of porcine cysticercosis in Eastern and Southern Provinces of Zambia. Veterinary Parasitology 2002;108(1)31-39.

[29] Sikasunge C. S, Phiri I. K, Phiri A. M, Siziya S, Dorny P, Willingham A. L 3rd Prevalence of *Taenia solium* porcine cysticercosis in the Eastern, Southern and Western provinces of Zambia. Veterinary Journal 2008;176(2) 240-244.

Chapter 5

Control of *Taenia Solium* Transmission of Taeniosis and Cysticercosis in Endemic Countries: The Roles of Continental Networks of Specialists and of Local Health Authorities

Agnès Fleury, Edda Sciutto, Aline S. de Aluja, Carlos Larralde, Sonia Agudelo, Gisela Maria Garcia, Jaime Fandiño, Randy Guerra, Cáris Nunes, Samuel Carvalho de Aragão, Marcello Sato, Ronaldo Abraham, Arturo Carpio, Franklin Santillan, Maria Milagros Cortez A., Glenda Rojas, Elizabeth Ferrer, Cruz Manuel Aguilar, Juan Carlos Durán and R. Michael E. Parkhouse

Additional information is available at the end of the chapter

http://dx.doi.org/10.5772/51286

1. Introduction

Neurocysticercosis (NCC) is still an endemic disease in most of the countries of Asia, Africa and Latin America, despite the important progress made in the development of effective tools for its prevention, diagnosis and treatment. Although the infection disappeared in many European countries during the nineteenth century, in some Eastern European countries control was not achieved until the beginning of the twentieth century, mainly due to the improvement of their political, social and economic status. Alarming recent reports show the persistence of the endemia in Africa [1-3] **(Table 1)**, as well as in the Americas [25] **(Table 2)** and in Asia **(Table 3).** None of the endemic countries has been able to eradicate *Taenia solium´s* Taeniosis/Cysticercosis (T/C). Similarly, the frequency of human cases of NCC is increasing in some industrialized countries, such as the United States, Canada and Spain, due mostly to migrant workers, although some autochthonous cases have also occurred [92-97].

In this paper, we will try to understand the reasons behind such failures and propose strategies that can improve the control of the T/C.

2. Actual tools for diagnosis and treatment

It is clear that there are efficient tools for diagnosis and treatment, although investigations must surely go on and progress will be made.

INTECH
open science | open minds

© 2013 Fleury et al., licensee InTech. This is a paper distributed under the terms of the Creative Commons Attribution License (http://creativecommons.org/licenses/by/3.0), which permits unrestricted use, distribution, and reproduction in any medium, provided the original work is properly cited.

Country	Reference	Type of study	Subject included	Diagnosis based on	Seroprevalence Cysticercosis	Prevalence NCC
Burkina Faso	[4]	Population-based	763	Ag-ELISA	10,3%; 1.4%; 0%	
	[5]	Population-based	734	Ag-ELISA	4.5%	
Burundi	[6]	Case-control	324 PWE 648 controls	Ab-ELISA	59.6 % PWE 31,5% controls	
	[7]	PWE	250	Ab-ELISA	61%	
	[8]	Case-control	303 PWE 606 Controls	Ab/Ag - ELISA	Ab 58,7% ; Ag 38,3 PWE Ab 31, 4% Ag 20 % controls	
	[9, 10]	Population-based	168	Ab-ELISA	1,2%	
	[11]	Population-based	500	EITB	25,8%	
Cameroon	[12]	Population-based	137 Butchers 198 Controls	Ag-ELISA	Butchers 3,6% Controls: 4,5%	
	[13]	Population-based	504 PWE	Ab/Ag ELISA	1,2% Ag 44,6% Ab	
	[14]	Population-based	4993	Ag-ELISA CT scan	0,4% 1,0 % 3,0%	59.1% of sero+
	[15]	Population-based	93 PWE 81Controls	Ab-ELISA	18,3% PWE 14,8% Controls	
Democratic Republic of Congo	[16]	Population-based	943	Ag-ELISA	21.6%	
Madagascar	[17]	Population-based	4375	Ab-ELISA EITB	7-21%	
	[18]	US Peace Corps	73	EITB	8,2%	
Mozambique	[19]	Urban children	269	Abs	20,8%	
Senegal	[20]	Population-based	403	Ag-ELISA EITB CT scan	11,9%	23,3% of sero+
South Africa	[21]	PWE (Hospital)	92	CT scan		37%
Tanzania	[22, 23]	Hospital-based	212 PWE	CT scan		16.5%
Zambia	[24]	Population-based	708	Ag-ELISA	5,8%	

Table 1. Prevalence (sero prevalence) of human neurocysticercosis in Africa.
Only 2002-2012 articles were considered.

Improvement of neuroimaging techniques permits a sensitive and accurate diagnosis of NCC in the great majority of cases, the problem being its limited accessibility to the principal rural population. Immunodiagnosis based on serum antibody detection is an efficient marker of contact with the parasite, permitting the identification of endemic areas in which control and preventive measures must be intensified. Detection of parasite antigens in serum and cerebrospinal fluid permits a confident diagnosis of severe neurocysticercosis forms, allowing opportune and adequate treatment and reducing the morbidity [98]. Regarding NCC treatment, two cestocidal drugs (Praziquantel and

Albendazole) have been used for at least 30 years. Although different studies evaluating their efficacy have shown that these drugs are not efficient in all patients, they also revealed that they eliminate the parasites and diminish the symptomatology significantly more than placebo [99-101]. As a consequence, investigation in this area must continue.

Country	Reference	Type of study	Subject included	Diagnosis based on	Seroprevalence Cysticercosis (%)	Prevalence NCC
Bolivia	[26]	Population-based	10124 (124 PWE)	EITB CT-scan		27.4% PWE
Brazil	[27]	Blood donors	1133	Ab-ELISA	5.6	
	[28]	Population-based	694	EITB	1.6	
	[29]	Hospital-based	36379	CT-scan		0.20%
	[30]	Population-based	110 PWE	EITB, Ag-ELISA	8.2 (EITB) 3.6 (ELISA)	
	[31]	Hospital-based	5 105 259	Admission		0.01%
	[32]	Population-based	354	Ab-ELISA, EITB	11.3	
	[33]	Population-based	84	Ab-ELISA	5.9	
	[34]	Population-based	Deaths Sao Paulo state	Death certificate		0.55/1000,000**
	[35]	Hospital-based	1501	Autopsies		4.80**
	[36]	Hospital-based	1009	CT-scan		9.02
	[37]	Hospital- based	6500	Autopsies		0.80
Colombia	[38]	Hospital based	Psychiatric patients with neurological signs (98) Primary psychiatric patients (153) Controls (246)	EITB	Group 1: 5.1 Group 2: 2.6 Group 3: 2	
	[39]	Population-based	399	Ab- ELISA	52.9	
	[40]	Patients with neurological symptoms	1890 sera 989 CSF 52 sera + CSF	Ab-ELISA CTscan/MRI	14.9	82.2
	[41]	Population-based	157	Ab-ELISA	28.7	
	[42]	Pig-breeders	46	EITB	8,7	
	[43]	Population-based	665	Ab-ELISA	28.4	
	[44]	PWE	111	Ab- ELISA	17,1	
	[45]	PWE	223	Ab-ELISA	35,9	
	[46]	Population-based	29360	Ab-ELISA	8.55	
Ecuador	[47]	Population-based	4306	Ag-ELISA	4.99	
	[48]	Population-based	2415 (24 PWE)	CT scan		33% PWE

Country	Reference	Type of study	Subject included	Diagnosis based on	Seroprevalence Cysticercosis (%)	Prevalence NCC
	[49]	Population-based	800	Ag-ELISA, EITB	2.25	
	[50]	Hospital-based	194 PWE (late-onset)	CT scan/MRI		19.6*
Haiti	[51]	Medical visits	216	EITB	2.8	
Honduras	[52]	Population-based	6473 (151 PWE)	EITB CT scan		37 (PWE)
	[53]	Population-based	5609 (33 PWE)	EITB CT scan		13.9 (PWE)
Mexico	[54]	Population-based	154	CT scan		9.1
	[55]	Population-based	649	CT scan		9.1
	[56]	Psychiatric patients	105	Ab-ELISA EITB	7.6 (ELISA) 0.9 (EITB)	
	[57]	PWE (late-onset)	455	CT scan		21.1
	[58]	All NC patients diagnosed at INNN in 2004	4706	CT scan/ MRI		2.5
Nicaragua	[59]	PWE	88	Ab-ELISA EITB	8.0 (ELISA) 14.8 (EITB)	
Peru	[60]	Population-based	2583	EITB	13.9	
	[61]	Population-based	316	EITB	21	
	[62]	Population-based	903	EITB (825) CTscan (150)	24.2	27.3
	[63]	Housemaids	1178	EITB CT-scan	14.6	50 (of sero+)
	[64]	Population-based	803	EITB CT-scan	24.4	3
	[65]	Population-based	817 (8 PWE)	EITB CT-scan		50 (PWE)
	[66]	Population-based	368	Ab-ELISA, EITB	3.3	
Venezuela	[67]	Population-based	68	Ag/Ab ELISA	Ag: 64.7, Ab: 79	
	[68]	Population-based (3)	1254	Ag/Ab ELISA	Ag: 9.1; 6.1; 5.7 Ab: 36.5;36.5; 4	
	[69]	Hospital-based	158 psychiatric patients 127 controls	EITB	Patients:18.3 Controls:1.6	

EITB: Electro immune transfer blot; PWE: people with epilepsy. Ag: Circulating antigens of *T. solium* metacestodes, Ab: Antibodies anti-cysticercal. * Only patients diagnosed between 2000 and 2009 were included. ** Cases of cysticercosis in general were reported

Table 2. Prevalence (sero prevalence) of human neurocysticercosis in Latin America. Only 2002-2012 articles were considered.

Country	Reference	Type of Study	Subject included	Diagnosis Based on	seroprevalence	Prevalence NCC
China	[70]	Population-based	202	Ab-ELISA	2.97%.	
India	[71]	Population-based	72	CT-scan		26%
	[72]	Hospital study	1026 PWE	CT-scan		34.6%
	[73]	Population-based	1063	EITB	15.9%	
	[74]	Population-based	450	Ab-ELISA	22.4%	
	[75]	Population-based	595	CT-scan		15.1%
	[76]	Population-based	141 PWE	CT-scan		24.8%
	[77]	Population-based	1064 (sera)	Ab / Ag-ELISA CT-scan	15.9% (Ac) / 4.5% (Ag)	
	[78]	Neurological patients	103	Ac-ELISA	33 (32%)	
	[79]	Population-based	1442 controls 91 suspected cases of NCC 100 healthy students	Indirect haemaggluti nation (IHA)	6.1% controls 21.97% suspected cases 0% healthy students	
	[80]	Blood donors	216	Ab-ELISA / Ag-Co-agglutination	14 (6.48 %)	
Indonésia	[81]	Population-based (1539 people)	1120 cases of burns, 293 PWE (Papua) / 74 PWE, 746 controls (Bali)	Ab-ELISA	67% PWE, 65% SCN (Papua) 13.5% PWE 12.5% controls (Bali)	
	[82]	Population-based	17 PWE 32 SCN 47 control	Ab-ELISA	70.6% PWE 62.5% SCN 25.5% control	
	[83]	Population-based	96	Ab-ELISA	45.8%	
	[84]	Population-based	311	Ab-ELISA	0.3%	
Korea	[85]	Population-based	74,448	Ab-ELISA	8.3% (1993) 2.2% (2006)	
Malasya	[86]	Population-based	135	Ab-ELISA	2.2%.	
Nepal	[87]	Hospital study	300 PWE	MRI		47%
Philippines	[88]	Population-based	497	Ab-ELISA	24.6%	
Thailand	[89]	Population-based	159	Ab-ELISA	5.70%	
Viet Nam	[90]	Population-based	210	Ag-ELISA	5.7%	
	[91]	Population-based	707 (303 mountain, 175 coast 229 urban)	Ag-ELISA, CT scan	5.3% (mountain) 0.6% (coast) 0% (urban)	
PWE: people with epilepsy / SCN: subcutaneous nodules						

Table 3. Prevalence (seroprevalence) of human neurocysticercosis in Asia only 2002-2012 articles were considered.

Regarding porcine cysticercosis, diagnosis based on tongue inspection has been conventionally used, but does not detect all affected pigs. Serology permits, although not with ideal sensibility and specificity, identification of the areas where the life-cycle of the parasite persists. Echography (ultrasound) has recently been introduced as a sensitive (95%) and specific (97%) method of diagnosis (Kappa coefficient of 90%) [102]. Treatment of cysticercotic pigs with oxfendazole has shown a good efficiency [103].

Diagnosis of the adult form of *T. solium* is perhaps the topic where more efforts must be made. Although a species-specific coproantigen ELISA was developed, reaching very good performance [104], further studies are required to evaluate it in field conditions. And this is not so easy, as prevalence of taeniosis seems to be much lower than that of cysticercosis, a fact understandable as one tapeworm carrier can infect hundreds of people and thousands of pigs. Treatment of taeniosis with niclosamide or praziquantel has shown to be very efficient [105].

In conclusion, although efforts must continue in some areas, today we have tools that allow the detection of endemic areas and the effective diagnosis and treatment of patients in most circumstances. This situation, adding to the existence of specific tools for prevention (vaccine), allows the design of extensive and effective preventive and control programs.

3. Strategies to eradicate the disease

Cysticercosis is considered a neglected "tools-ready disease" according to WHO [106] and as a potentially eradicable disease since 1993 [107].This is feasible because there are no animal reservoirs besides humans and pigs, the only source of *T. solium* infection for pigs being humans (the definitive host), interrupting the parasite´s life cycle seems an easy task by intervention strategies acting upon different stages of the parasite´s development.

Different strategies have been proposed and tested, generally experimental and at small scale, to eradicate the (T/C) complex, the most notable being:

1. Massive cestocidal treatment to humans in order to reduce the number of tapeworm carriers [108-110].
2. Health education programs aiming to promote the understanding of the mechanisms of transmission of the parasite and to improve hygienic behavior, pig-management and sanitary conditions which fosters transmission [111-113].
3. Treatment of infected pigs [103, 114-116].
4. Vaccination of rural pigs: different vaccines have been tested in field conditions and have demonstrated their efficacy in preventing swine cysticercosis [117-120].
5. Combinations of different strategies: pig vaccination and treatment [121], massive human cestocidal treatment associated with pig vaccination and treatment [122,123].

Almost all these strategies have shown some degree of efficacy, this fact contrasting with the persistence of the parasite in all the endemic countries in the 1950's. It should be noted that, to our knowledge, programs promoting letrinization of rural communities and construction of pig housing have not been tested (probably due to economic and logistic costs) although it seems to be a very efficient strategy for many parasitic and infectious disease transmitted by faeces.

4. What must be done?

This is a truly kafkian situation: we are in the presence of a parasite that causes a potentially severe human disease, as well as important economic losses; paradoxically, it is clear that the disease is potentially eradicable and, in fact, scientists and health authorities know how to eradicate it and have strategies to reach this goal. Despite all these resources, and their demonstrated effectiveness, the signs of a decrease of the transmission rate in the endemic countries are inconclusive or doubtful and, worse yet, in some non-endemic countries, an increase in the number of neurocysticercosis cases is occurring.

Faced with this perspective, it becomes evident that we will not attain the eradication of *T. solium* without:

4.1. The intervention of the national and international health authorities in control programs

International initiatives have been concerned with the problem of cysticercosis for many years and several meetings were organised, the most important being: WHO Technical Consultation (Geneva, 1983), Pan American Health Organization (PAHO) Informal Consultation on Taeniasis/Cysticercosis (Porto Allegre, 1990), International Task Force for Disease Eradication (ITFDE, Atlanta, 1993), PAHO/WHO Informal Consultation on the Taeniasis/Cysticercosis Complex (Brasilia, 1995), North Atlantic Treaty Organization (NATO) Seminar on Emergent Helminth Zoonoses, (Pozna, 2000), Fifty-Fifth World Health Assembly, (Geneva, 2002), ITFDE II (Atlanta, 2003), WHO Expert Consultation on Foodborne Trematode Infections (Ventiane, 2009). In most of them, strategies for prevention and control of T/C were analyzed and recommendations were made. Since 2008, the WHO has included T/C in its Global Plan to combat Neglected Tropical diseases [124].

Regarding national health authorities, not much has been done. In very few countries, specific norms have been recommended. Such is the case of Latin America where only Mexico has an official norm for the vigilance, the prevention and the control of T/C in the first level of attention which was published in 1994 (modified in 2004) [125]. The Mexican norm includes the implementation of education and information programs, the identification and treatment of tapeworm carriers, the referral of subjects with suspected of NCC to a second level of attention, the confiscation of infected pigs, and the obligation to notify the diagnosed cases of NCC, taeniosis and swine cysticercosis to the corresponding authorities. The effort must be applauded, and has surely contributed to the awareness of the general population and of the medical personnel about the problem. Unfortunately, still, 15 years after its promulgation, cases of swine and human cysticercosis are still being diagnosed and not notified in Mexico. Probably, this is due to the fact that this norm did not reach the rural zones where the life-cycle of *T. solium* is still active and notification is not equally honored by all professionals (or because there are no health facilities in these areas).

It is important to promote the confiscation of infected pigs, but who is going to pay the owners, and who will go to the endemic communities (for example >2500 municipalities in Mexico) and make the diagnosis in more than six million rural pigs that get renewed every year? Clearly, pig owners must be included in a control program, for the obvious reason that they are the most interested in not having infected pigs.

It is highly relevant to promote the notification of infected individuals, but who will make this notification? Hospitals with an efficient epidemiologic department are scarce and medical doctors in public institutions are generally over loaded by the clinical workload. The comparison of the official statistics and the statistics published from only one hospital center can demonstrate the problem: in 2004, in the Instituto Nacional de Neurología y Neurocirugía, located in Mexico City, an institution that treats only patients lacking social security, 120 new cases of NCC were diagnosed [58], while in the official statistics, in this same year, approximately 400 new NCC cases were reported throughout Mexico [126]. It is very improbable that a sole institution accounts for a quarter of all the Mexican NCC cases, and probably this is due to a significant under-reporting of cases. Faced with this undesirable practice, what actions can the governments take? It is probably necessary: 1) to maintain a continuing health education program available to the population and the medical personnel, insisting on their obligation to notify the cases and promoting the establishment of epidemiological departments and surveillance system in all the hospitals, 2) to actively lobby for the implementation of a National Control Program that could be started as a priority in the areas from where most cases are referred. In relation to this point, the critical question is, who can organize a preventive program? The scientists probably not, as the logistics of such programs require an established structure supported by a recognized local authority. Since 2009, in Mexico, an extensive pilot control program is under way, in certain areas of the poorest states, based on health and sanitary education and associated with vaccination of pigs. Local authorities are part of the efforts, helping with the identification of the endemic areas, by furnishing sera collected from the pigs, and by funding the program. The results so far are encouraging. People in the remote areas accept suggestions for improvement in their pig raising methods and for their personal hygiene, including the indispensable installation of latrines [127]. What has become clear is that programs must be of long duration, at least 5 years. It is of little use to visit communities, give talks, vaccinate pigs and leave. People in theses "forgotten" areas need long-lasting help, advice and supervision. Therefore, without the active participation of the governments, failure of any control program is predictable because scientists cannot apply it at large enough scales and sufficient time. Finally, the presence of cysticercosis is an objective indicator of unacceptable conditions in a rural community, and their improvement will not only contribute to the eradication of cysticercosis, but will also bring collateral benefits, such as the control of other soil transmitted diseases and increased public awareness of respect for adequate simple public health measures.

4.2. Implementation of regional networks

As *T. solium* does not respect frontiers, it is necessary to organize multidisciplinary regional networks of specialists that must be the interlocutors of the local government and international organizations, and that must participate in the decision of where the preventive measures must be applied, and what type of measures are the most adequate regarding the individual characteristics of the country affected. Such efforts are currently established:

- In Asia, the Regional Network for Asian Schistosomiasis and other important zoonoses (RNAS+) was created in 2006 (extension of the RNA created in 2000) and since this date has published several papers and has maintained discussions on preventive measures to be applied to effectively combat zoonoses.
- In Africa: the Cysticercosis Working Group in Eastern and Southern Africa (CWGESA) was established in 2002 to promote communication, collaboration and coordination of integrated research and control activities to combat cysticercosis.
- In Europe, The European Cysticercosis Working Group, inaugurated in 2008 and receiving organizational support from the World Health Organization (WHO)/Food and Agricultural Organization of the United Nations (FAO) Collaborating Centre for Parasitic Zoonoses in Denmark and the University of Edinburgh, Scotland, and aimed at finding ways to achieve a more effective, concerted approach to combat cysticercosis in Europe, as well as in the main cysticercosis-endemic areas of Africa, Asia, and Latin America [128].
- In Latin America, since 1987, the Cysticercosis Working Group in Peru has made several epidemiological, diagnostic and control studies in this country [129] and recently a new Ibero-Latinamerican network was created to promote the investigation and the implementation of preventive measures in the entire continent.

At the moment, although some objectives have been reached, their scope is still limited. To improve the situation, it is necessary: 1) to expand exchanges between the different networks; 2) to open ways of communication between these networks and the national and international authorities.

In conclusion, to reach the control of *T.solium* infections it is very important to open new ways of communication between the scientists, grouped in networks, and with the international and the national health authorities. Agreements must be made in which the role and responsibilities of each of them are clearly defined. If one of these conditions fails, we are afraid that in 50 years, today's T/C epidemiological situation will persist.

Author details

Agnès Fleury*
For the Ibero Latinamerican Cysticercosis Network
Peripheral Unit of the Institute of Biomedical Research in the National Neurology Institute,
National Autonomous University of Mexico, Mexico DF

* Corresponding Author

Edda Sciutto and Carlos Larralde
Immunology Department, Institute of Biomedical Research, National Autonomous University of Mexico, Mexico DF

Aline S. de Aluja
Department of Pathology, School of Veterinary Medicine and Zootecnies, National Autonomous University of Mexico, Mexico DF

Sonia Agudelo and Maria Garcia Gisela
Department of Parasitology, Academic Corporation for the Study of Tropical Pathologies, School of Medicine, Antioquia University, Medellin, Colombia

Jaime Fandiño and Randy Guerra
Latin America Research Center in Epilepsy, Cartagena, Colombia

Cáris Nunes and Samuel Carvalho de Aragão
School of Veterinary Medicine, University Estadual Paulista Julio de Mesquita Filho, Brazil

Marcello Sato
University Federal Do Tocantins, Brazil

Ronaldo Abraham
Medicine Department, Taubaté University, Brazil

Arturo Carpio
University of Cuenca, Ecuador

Franklin Santillan
Santa Ana Clinic, Cuenca, Ecuador

Maria Milagros Cortez A., Glenda Rojas and Elizabeth Ferrer
Biomedical Research Institute "Dr. Francisco J. Triana Alonso", Faculty of Health Sciences, University of Carabobo, Maracay, Venezuela

Cruz Manuel Aguilar
Tropical Diseases Research Center, University of Carabobo, San Carlos, Cjedes state, Venezuela

Juan Carlos Durán
Higher University of San Andrés, La Paz, Bolivia

Teresa Garate
Carlos III Institute of Health, National Center of Microbiology, Majadahonda, Madrid, Spain

R. Michael E. Parkhouse
Instituto Gulbenkian de Ciencias, Oeiras, Portugal

Acknowledgement

The authors acknowledge the CYTED program (Ibero-American Programme for Science, Technology and Development) that has founded partially the network.

5. References

[1] Pondja A, Neves L, Mlangwa J, Afonso S, Fafetine J, Willingham AL 3rd, Thamsborg SM, Johansen MV. Prevalence and risk factors of porcine cysticercosis in Angónia District, Mozambique. PLoSNegl Trop Dis. 2010;4(2):e594

[2] Assana E, Amadou F, Thys E, Lightowlers MW, Zoli AP, Dorny P, Geerts S. Pig-farming systems and porcine cysticercosis in the north of Cameroon. J Helminthol. 2010;84(4):441-6.

[3] Praet N, Kanobana K, Kabwe C, Maketa V, Lukanu P, Lutumba P, Polman K, Matondo P, Speybroeck N, Dorny P, Sumbu J. *Taenia solium* cysticercosis in the Democratic Republic of Congo: how does pork trade affect the transmission of the parasite? PLoS Negl Trop Dis. 2010;4(9).

[4] Carabin H, Millogo A, Praet N, Hounton S, Tarnagda Z, Ganaba R, Dorny P, Nitiéma P, Cowan LD. Evaluation du Fardeau Economique de la Cysticercose Au Burkina Faso (EFECAB)- Seroprevalence to the antigens of *Taenia solium* cysticercosis among residents of three villages in Burkina Faso: a cross-sectional study. PLoS Negl Trop Dis. 2009;3(11):e555.

[5] Nitiéma P, Carabin H, Hounton S, Praet N, Cowan LD, Ganaba R, Kompaoré C, Tarnagda Z, Dorny P, Millogo A. Prevalence case-control study of epilepsy in three Burkina Faso villages. Acta Neurol Scand. 2012 Jan 31. doi: 10.1111/j.1600-0404.2011.01639.x.

[6] Nsengiyumva G, Druet-Cabanac M, Ramanankandrasana B, Bouteille B, Nsizabira L, Preux PM. Cysticercosis as a major risk factor for epilepsy in Burundi, east Africa. Epilepsia. 2003;44(7):950-5.

[7] Diagana M, Nsengiyumva G, Tuillas M, Druet-Cabanac M, Bouteille B, Preux PM, Tapie P. Electroencephalograms (EEG) in 250 patients with epilepsy in a cysticercosis endemic area in Burundi. Neurophysiol Clin. 2005;35(1):1-10.

[8] Prado-Jean A, Kanobana K, Druet-Cabanac M, Nsengyiumva G, Dorny P, Preux PM, Geerts S. Combined use of an antigen and antibody detection enzyme-linked immunosorbent assay for cysticercosis as tools in an epidemiological study of epilepsy in Burundi. Trop Med Int Health. 2007;12(7):895-901.

[9] Nkouawa A, Sako Y, Itoh S, Kouojip-Mabou A, Nganou CN, Saijo Y, Knapp J, Yamasaki H, Nakao M, Nakaya K, Moyou-Somo R, Ito A. Serologica studies of neurologic helminthic infections in rural areas of southwest cameroon: toxocariasis, cysticercosis and paragonimiasis. PLoS Negl Trop Dis. 2010;4(7):e732.

[10] Nkouawa A, Sako Y, Moyou-Somo R, Ito A. Serological and molecular tools to detect neurologic parasitic zoonoses in rural Cameroon. Southeast Asian J Trop Med Public Health. 2011;42(6):1365-74.

[11] O'Neal SE, Townes JM, Wilkins PP, Noh JC, Lee D, Rodriguez S, Garcia HH, Stauffer WM. Seroprevalence of antibodies against *Taenia solium* cysticerci among refugees resettled in United States. Emerg Infect Dis. 2012;18(3):431-8.

[12] Vondou L, Zoli AP, Nguekam, Pouedet S, Assana E, Kamga Tokam AC, Dorny P, Brandt J, Geerts S. *Taenia solium* taeniasis/cysticercosis in the Menoua division (West Cameroon). Parasite. 2002;9(3):271-4.
[13] Zoli AP, Nguekam, Shey-Njila O, Nsame Nforninwe D, Speybroeck N, Ito A, Sato MO, Dorny P, Brandt J, Geerts S. Neurocysticercosis and epilepsy in Cameroon. Trans R Soc Trop Med Hyg. 2003;97(6):683-6.
[14] Nguekam JP, Zoli AP, Zogo PO, Kamga AC, Speybroeck N, Dorny P, Brandt J, Losson B, Geerts S. A seroepidemiological study of human cysticercosis in West Cameroon. Trop Med Int Health. 2003;8(2):144-9.
[15] Dongmo L, Druet-Cabanac M, Moyou SR, Zebaze DR, Njamnshi AK, Sini V, Mapoure N, Echouffo TJ, Djeumen WC, Ndumbe PM. Cysticercosis and epilepsy: a case-control study in Mbam Valley, Cameroon. Bull Soc Pathol Exot. 2004;97(2):105-8.
[16] Kanobana K, Praet N, Kabwe C, Dorny P, Lukanu P, Madinga J, Mitashi P, Verwijs M, Lutumba P, Polman K. High prevalence of *Taenia solium* cysticercosis in a village community of Bas-Congo, Democratic Republic of Congo. Int J Parasitol. 2011;41(10):1015-8.
[17] Andriantsimahavandy A, Ravaoalimalala VE, Rajaonarison P, Ravoniarimbinina P, Rakotondrazaka M, Raharilaza N, Rakotoarivelo D, Ratsitorahina M, Rabarijaona LP, Ramarokoto CE, Leutscher P, Migliani R. The current epidemiological situation of cysticercosis in Madagascar. Arch Inst Pasteur Madagascar. 2003;69(1-2):46-51.
[18] Leutscher P, Andriantsimahavandy A. Cysticercosis in Peace Corps volunteers in Madagascar. N Engl J Med. 2004;350(3):311-2.
[19] Noormahomed EV, Pividal JG, Azzouz S, Mascaró C, Delgado-Rodríguez M, Osuna A. Seroprevalence of anti-cysticercus antibodies among the children living in the urban environs of Maputo, Mozambique. Ann Trop Med Parasitol. 2003;97(1):31-5.
[20] Secka A, Grimm F, Marcotty T, Geysen D, Niang AM, Ngale V, Boutche L, Van Marck E, Geerts S. Old focus of cysticercosis in a senegalese village revisited after half a century. Acta Trop. 2011;119(2-3):199-202.
[21] Foyaca-Sibat H, Cowan LD, Carabin H, Targonska I, Anwary MA, Serrano-Ocaña G, Krecek RC, Willingham AL 3rd. Accuracy of serological testing for the diagnosis of prevalent neurocysticercosis in outpatients with epilepsy, Eastern Cape Province, South Africa. PLoS Negl Trop Dis. 2009;3(12):e562.
[22] Winkler AS, Blocher J, Auer H, Gotwald T, Matuja W, Schmutzhard E. Epilepsy and neurocysticercosis in rural Tanzania-An imaging study. Epilepsia. 2009;50(5):987-93.
[23] Blocher J, Schmutzhard E, Wilkins PP, Gupton PN, Schaffert M, Auer H, Gotwald T, Matuja W, Winkler AS. A cross-sectional study of people with epilepsy and neurocysticercosis in Tanzania: clinical characteristics and diagnostic approaches. PLoS Negl Trop Dis. 2011;5(6):e1185.
[24] Mwape KE, Phiri IK, Praet N, Muma JB, Zulu G, Van den Bossche P, de Deken R, Speybroeck N, Dorny P, Gabriël S. *Taenia solium* Infections in a rural area of Eastern Zambia-A community based study. PLoS Negl Trop Dis. 2012; 6(3): e1594.

[25] Morales J, Martínez JJ, Rosetti M, Fleury A, Maza V, Hernandez M, Villalobos N, Fragoso G, de Aluja AS, Larralde C, Sciutto E. Spatial distribution of *Taenia solium* porcine cysticercosis within a rural area of Mexico. PLoS Negl Trop Dis. 2008;2(9):e284.

[26] Nicoletti A, Bartoloni A, Sofia V, Bartalesi F, Chavez JR, Osinaga R, Paradisi F, Dumas JL, Tsang VC, Reggio A, Hall AJ. Epilepsy and neurocysticercosis in rural Bolivia: a population-based survey. Epilepsia. 2005;46(7):1127-32.

[27] Silveira-Lacerda Ede P, Machado ER, Arantes SC, Costa-Cruz JM. Anti-*Taenia solium* metacestodes antibodies in serum from blood donors from four cities of Triângulo Mineiro area, Minas Gerais, Brazil, 1995. Rev Inst Med Trop Sao Paulo. 2002;44(4):229-31.

[28] Gomes I, Veiga M, Embirucu EK, Rabelo R, Mota B, Meza-Lucas A, Tapia-Romero R, Carrillo-Becerril BL, Alcantara-Anguiano I, Correa D, Melo A. Taeniasis and cysticercosis prevalence in a small village from Northeastern Brazil. Arq Neuropsiquiatr. 2002;60(2-A):219-23.

[29] Mendes EC, da Silva SS, Fonseca EA, de Souza HR, de Carvalho RW. Human neurocysticercosis in Baixada Fluminense, Rio de Janeiro State, Brazil. Arq Neuropsiquiatr. 2005;63(4):1058-62.

[30] Freitas FI, Meza-Lucas A, Lima CB, Costa W, Melo A. Cysticercosis research in epileptic patients dwelling in towns of the western Cariri in the State of Paraíba, Brazil. Arq Neuropsiquiatr. 2005;63(3A):656-60.

[31] Façanha MC. Cysticercosis' admissions in public health hospitals: Ceará State distribuition. Rev Soc Bras Med Trop. 2006;39(5):484-7.

[32] Oliveira HB, Rodrigues RM, Barcelos IS, Silva LP, Costa-Cruz JM. Anti-*Taenia solium* metacestode IgG antibodies in serum samples from inhabitants of a central-western region of Brazil. Rev Inst Med Trop Sao Paulo. 2006;48(1):49-52.

[33] Prestes-Carneiro LE, Freitas Sde B, Zago SC, Miguel NA, Primo OB, Iha AH, Espíndola NM, Vaz AJ. Taeniosis-cysticercosis complex in individuals of a peasants' settlement (Teodoro Sampaio, Pontal of Paranapanema, SP, Brazil). Mem Inst Oswaldo Cruz. 2006 ;101(1):15-20.

[34] Santo AH. Cysticercosis-related mortality in the State of São Paulo, Brazil, 1985-2004: a study using multiple causes of death. Cad Saude Publica. 2007;23(12):2917-27.

[35] Faleiros AC, Lino-Junior R, Lima V, Cavellani C, Corrêa RR, Llaguno M, Reis M, Teixeira V. Epidemiological analysis of patients coinfected with Chagas disease and cysticercosis. Biomedica. 2009;29(1):127-32.

[36] Grazziotin AL, Fontalvo MC, Santos MB, Monego F, Grazziotin AL, Kolinski VH, Bordignon RH, Biondo AW, Antoniuk A. Epidemiologic pattern of patients with neurocysticercosis diagnosed by computed tomography in Curitiba, Brazil. Arq Neuropsiquiatr. 2010;68(2):269-72.

[37] de Almeida SM, Torres LF. Neurocysticercosis--retrospective study of autopsy reports, a 17-year experience. J Community Health. 2011;36(5):698-702.

[38] Sanzón F, Osorio AM, Morales JP, Isaza R, Cardona E, Moncayo LC, Villota GE, Zapata OT, Palacio CA, Arbeláez MP, Restrepo BI. Serological screening for cysticercosis in mentally altered individuals. Trop Med Int Health. 2002;7(6):532-8

[39] Torres F, Vásquez R, Gonzales F, Vergara D, Alvarado E, Giraldo J, Medina G, Zamora T. Cisticercosis en el departamento de Cauca. Revista de la Asociación Colombiana de Ciencias Biológicas. Ibagué (Colombia). 2004; 16(2).

[40] Montero Y, Rojas R. Estudio retrospectivo de la seroprevalencia de neurocisticercosis en Colombia. Dentro del Periodo de enero de 1995 a diciembre de 2005. Programa de Vigilancia por el Laboratorio. Instituto Nacional de Salud. Tesis de pregrado Bacteriología Pontifica Universidad Javeriana. Colombia. 2005

[41] Caldera O, Acuña E, Guzman E, Giraldo J, Yanine H. Prevalencia de anticuerpos frente a las fracciones polipeptídicas 53 y 92 kDa del metacéstodo de *Taenia solium* en habitantes del corregimiento Sabanas de Pedro, Sucre. Biomédica. 2005; 25(1): 188.

[42] Agudelo-Flórez P, Restrepo B, Palacio G. Knowledge and practices concerning taeniasis-cysticercosis in Colombian pig-breeders. Rev. salud pública. Colombia. 2009;11 (2): 191-199.

[43] Vásquez L, Agudelo-Florez P, Giraldo J, Vergara D , Samper D, Nieto-S D, Ramos O, Bonilla L, Campo V. Prevalencia de cisticercosis humana en el área rural de mercaderes, cauca. Revista de la Asociación Colombiana de Ciencias Biológicas. 2010;22(1): 68

[44] Vergara J, Ortega M, Vásquez L, Casas J, Giraldo J. Cisticercosis humana en pacientes con diagnóstico de epilepsia en un centro de salud de Popayán, Cauca Introducción. Biomédica 2011. 31(3):83.

[45] Giraldo J, Franco C, Vásquez L. Detección de anticuerpos anti-cisticerco en pacientes que asistieron a consulta médica durante el período 2009-2010 a la Liga contra la Epilepsia, Capítulo Cauca. Biomédica. 2011;31(3):159.

[46] Flórez A, Pastrán S, Vargas N, Enríquez Y, Peña A, Benavides A, Villarreal A, Rincón C, Garzón I, Muñoz L, Guasmayan L, Valencia C, Parra S, Hernández N. Seroprevalencia de la cisticercosis en 23 departamentos de Colombia, 2010. Biomédica. 2011; 31(3): 29-32.

[47] Rodríguez-Hidalgo R, Benítez-Ortiz W, Dorny P, Geerts S, Geysen D, Ron-Román J, Proaño-Pérez F, Chávez-Larrea MA, Barrionuevo-Samaniego M, Celi-Erazo M, Vizcaíno-Ordóñez L, Brandt J. Taeniosis-cysticercosis in man and animals in the Sierra of Northern Ecuador. Vet Parasitol. 2003;118(1-2):51-60.

[48] Del Brutto OH, Santibáñez R, Idrovo L, Rodrìguez S, Díaz-Calderón E, Navas C, Gilman RH, Cuesta F, Mosquera A, Gonzalez AE, Tsang VC, García HH. Epilepsy and neurocysticercosis in Atahualpa: a door-to-door survey in rural coastal Ecuador. Epilepsia. 2005;46(4):583-7.

[49] Rodriguez-Hidalgo R, Benitez-Ortiz W, Praet N, Saa LR, Vercruysse J, Brandt J, Dorny P. Taeniasis-cysticercosis in Southern Ecuador: assessment of infection status using multiple laboratory diagnostic tools. Mem Inst Oswaldo Cruz. 2006;101(7):779-82.

[50] Del Brutto OH, Del Brutto VJ. Reduced percentage of neurocysticercosis cases among patients with late-onset epilepsy in the new millennium. Clin Neurol Neurosurg. 2012 Apr 11.

[51] Raccurt CP, Agnamey P, Boncy J, Henrys JH, Totet A. Seroprevalence of human *Taenia solium* cysticercosis in Haiti. J Helminthol. 2009;83(2):113-6.

[52] Medina MT, Durón RM, Martínez L, Osorio JR, Estrada AL, Zúniga C, Cartagena D, Collins JS, Holden KR. Prevalence, incidence, and etiology of epilepsies in rural Honduras: the Salamá Study. Epilepsia. 2005;46(1):124-31.

[53] Medina MT, Aguilar-Estrada RL, Alvarez A, Durón RM, Martínez L, Dubón S, Estrada AL, Zúniga C, Cartagena D, Thompson A, Ramirez E, Banegas L, Osorio JR, Delgado-Escueta AV, Collins JS, Holden KR. Reduction in rate of epilepsy from neurocysticercosis by community interventions: the Salamá, Honduras study. Epilepsia. 2011;52(6):1177-85.

[54] Fleury A, Gómez T, Alvarez I, Meza D, Huerta M, Chavarria A . High prevalence of calcified silent neurocysticercosis in a rural village of Mexico. Neuroepidemiology 2003;22:139-145.

[55] Fleury A, Morales J, Bobes RJ, Dumas M, Yánez O, Piña J, . An Epidemiological study of familial neurocysticercosis in an endemic Mexican community. Trans R Soc Trop Med Hyg 2006;100: 551-558.

[56] Alvarado-Esquivel C, Arreola-Valenzuela MA, Rodríguez-Briones A, Alanís-Quiñones OP, Estrada-Martínez S, Luevanos-Becerra C, . Seroprevalence of selected viral, bacterial and parasitic infections among inpatients of a public psychiatric hospital of Mexico. Rev Inst Med Trop Sao Paulo 2008;50:161-164.

[57] Suástegui R, Gutiérrez J, Ramos R, Bouchan S, Navarrete H, Ruiz J, . Clinical characteristics of the late-onset epilepsy in Mexico to the beginning of the new millennium: 455 cases. Rev Invest Clin 2009;61:354-363.

[58] Fleury A, Moreno García J, Valdez Aguerrebere P, de SayveDurán M, Becerril Rodríguez P, Larralde C, Sciutto E. Neurocysticercosis, a persisting health problem in Mexico. PLoS Negl Trop Dis. 2010;4(8):e805.

[59] Bucardo F, Meza-Lucas A, Espinoza F, García-Jerónimo RC, García-Rodea R, Correa D. The seroprevalence of *Taenia solium* cysticercosis among epileptic patients in León, Nicaragua, as evaluated by ELISA and western blotting. Ann Trop Med Parasitol. 2005 Jan;99(1):41-5.

[60] García HH, Gilman RH, Gonzalez AE, Verastegui M, Rodriguez S, Gavidia C, Tsang VC, Falcon N, Lescano AG, Moulton LH, Bernal T, Tovar M; Cysticercosis Working Group in Perú. Hyperendemic human and porcine *Taenia solium* infection in Perú. Am J Trop Med Hyg. 2003;68(3):268-75.

[61] Moro PL, Lopera L, Bonifacio N, Gilman RH, Silva B, Verastegui M, Gonzales A, Garcia HH, Cabrera L; Cysticercosis Working Group in Peru. *Taenia solium* infection in a rural community in the Peruvian Andes. Ann Trop Med Parasitol. 2003;97(4):373-9.

[62] Montano SM, Villaran MV, Ylquimiche L, Figueroa JJ, Rodriguez S, Bautista CT, Gonzalez AE, Tsang VC, Gilman RH, Garcia HH; Cysticercosis Working Group in Peru. Neurocysticercosis: association between seizures, serology, and brain CT in rural Peru. Neurology. 2005;65(2):229-33.

[63] Huisa BN, Menacho LA, Rodriguez S, Bustos JA, Gilman RH, Tsang VC, Gonzalez AE, García HH; Cysticercosis Working Group in Perú. Taeniasis and cysticercosis in housemaids working in affluent neighborhoods in Lima, Peru. Am J Trop Med Hyg. 2005;73(3):496-500.

[64] Lescano AG, Garcia HH, Gilman RH, Gavidia CM, Tsang VC, Rodriguez S, Moulton LH, Villaran MV, Montano SM, Gonzalez AE; Cysticercosis Working Group in Peru. *Taenia solium* cysticercosis hotspots surrounding tapeworm carriers: clustering on human seroprevalence but not on seizures. PLoS Negl Trop Dis. 2009;3(1):e371.

[65] Villarán MV, Montano SM, Gonzalvez G, Moyano LM, Chero JC, Rodriguez S, Gonzalez AE, Pan W, Tsang VC, Gilman RH, Garcia HH; Cysticercosis Working Group in Peru. Epilepsy and neurocysticercosis: an incidence study in a Peruvian rural population. Neuroepidemiology. 2009;33(1):25-31.

[66] Cordero A, Miranda E, Segovia G, Cantoral V, Huarcaya I. Taeniosis prevalence and human cysticercosis seroprevalence in Pampa Cangallo, Ayacucho, Peru 2008. Rev Peru Med Exp Salud Publica. 2010;27(4):562-8.

[67] Ferrer E, Cortez MM, Perez H, De la Rosa M, de Noya BA, D'Avila I, Harrison LJ, Foster-Cuevas M, Parkhouse RM, Cabrera A. Serological evidence for recent exposure to *Taenia solium* in Venezuelan Amerindians. Am J Trop Med Hyg. 2002;66(2):170-4.

[68] Ferrer E, Cabrera Z, Rojas G, Lares M, Vera A, de Noya BA, Fernandez I, Romero HU, Harrison LJ, Parkhouse RM, Cortez MM. Evidence for high seroprevalence of *Taenia solium* cysticercosis in individuals from three rural communities in Venezuela. Trans R Soc Trop Med Hyg. 2003;97(5):522-6.

[69] Meza NW, Rossi NE, Galeazzi TN, Sánchez NM, Colmenares FI, Medina OD, Uzcategui NL, Alfonzo N, Arango C, Urdaneta H. Cysticercosis in chronic psychiatric inpatients from a Venezuelan community. Am J Trop Med Hyg. 2005;73(3):504-9.

[70] Chung JY, Eom KS, Yang Y, Li X, Feng Z, Rim HJ, Cho SY, Kong Y. A seroepidemiological survey of *Taenia solium* cysticercosis in Nabo, Guangxi Zhuang Autonomous Region, China. Korean J Parasitol. 2005;43(4):135-9.

[71] Prasad KN, Chawla S, Jain D, Pandey CM, Pal L, Pradhan S, Gupta RK. Human and porcine *Taenia solium* infection in rural north India. Trans R Soc Trop Med Hyg. 2002;96(5):515-6.

[72] Singh G, Singh P, Singh I, Rani A, Kaushal S, Avasthi G. Epidemiologic classification of seizures associated with neurocysticercosis: observations from a sample of seizure disorders in neurologic care in India. Acta Neurol Scand. 2006;113(4):233-40.

[73] Prabhakaran V, Raghava MV, Rajshekhar V, Muliyil J, Oommen A. Seroprevalence of *Taenia solium* antibodies in Vellore district, south India. Trans R Soc Trop Med Hyg. 2008;102(3):246-50.

[74] Vora SH, Motghare DD, Ferreira AM, Kulkarni MS, Vaz FS. Prevalence of human cysticercosis and taeniasis in rural Goa, India. J Commun Dis. 2008;40(2):147-50.

[75] Prasad KN, Verma A, Srivastava S, Gupta RK, Pandey CM, Paliwal VK. An epidemiological study of asymptomatic neurocysticercosis in a pig farming community in northern India. Trans R Soc Trop Med Hyg. 2011;105(9):531-6.

[76] Goel D, Dhanai JS, Agarwal A, Mehlotra V, Saxena V. Neurocysticercosis and its impact on crude prevalence rate of epilepsy in an Indian community. Neurol India. 2011;59(1):37-40.

[77] Jayaraman T, Prabhakaran V, Babu P, Raghava MV, Rajshekhar V, Dorny P, Muliyil J, Oommen A. Relative seroprevalence of cysticercus antigens and antibodies and

antibodies to Taenia ova in a population sample in south India suggests immunity against neurocysticercosis. Trans R Soc Trop Med Hyg. 2011;105(3):153-9.

[78] Kumar A, Khan SA, Khan S, Das S, Anurag, Negi KS. A study of neurocysticercosis in the foothills of the Himalayas. Int J Infect Dis. 2006;10(1):79-82.

[79] Parija SC, Sahu PS. A serological study of human cysticercosis in Pondicherry, South India. J Commun Dis. 2003;35(4):283-9.

[80] Parija SC, Balamurungan N, Sahu PS, Subbaiah SP. Cysticercus antibodies and antigens in serum from blood donors from Pondicherry, India. Rev Inst Med Trop Sao Paulo. 2005;47(4):227-30.

[81] Margono SS, Subahar R, Hamid A, Wandra T, Sudewi SS, Sutisna P, Ito A. Cysticercosis in Indonesia: epidemiological aspects. Southeast Asian J Trop Med Public Health. 2001;32 Suppl 2:79-84.

[82] Wandra T, Ito A, Yamasaki H, Suroso T, Margono SS. *Taenia solium* Cysticercosis, Irian Jaya, Indonesia. Emerg Infect Dis. 2003;9(7):884-5.

[83] Suroso T, Margono SS, Wandra T, Ito A. Challenges for control of taeniasis/cysticercosis in Indonesia. Parasitol Int. 2006;55 Suppl:S161-5.

[84] Wandra T, Sutisna P, Dharmawan NS, Margono SS, Sudewi R, Suroso T, Craig PS, Ito A. High prevalence of *Taenia saginata* taeniasis and status of *Taenia solium* cysticercosis in Bali, Indonesia, 2002-2004. Trans R Soc Trop Med Hyg. 2006;100(4):346-53.

[85] Lee MK, Hong SJ, Kim HR. Seroprevalence of tissue invading parasitic infections diagnosed by ELISA in Korea. J Korean Med Sci. 2010;25(9):1272-6.

[86] Noor Azian MY, Hakim SL, Sumiati A, Norhafizah M. Seroprevalence of cysticercosis in a rural village of Ranau, Sabah, Malaysia. Southeast Asian J Trop Med Public Health. 2006;37(1):58-61.

[87] Rajbhandari KC. Epilepsy in Nepal. Can J Neurol Sci. 2004;31(2):257-60.

[88] Xu JM, Acosta LP, Hou M, Manalo DL, Jiz M, Jarilla B, Pablo AO, Ovleda RM, Langdon G, McGarveyST,Kurtis JD, Friedman JF, Wu HW. Seroprevalence of cysticercosis in children and young adults living in a helminth endemic community in leyte, the Philippines. J Trop Med. 2010;2010:603174

[89] Anantaphruti MT, Okamoto M, Yoonuan T, Saguankiat S, Kusolsuk T, Sato M, Sato MO, Sako Y, Waikagul J, Ito A. Molecular and serological survey on taeniasis and cysticercosis in Kanchanaburi Province, Thailand. Parasitol Int. 2010;59(3):326-30.

[90] Erhart A, Dorny P, Van De N, Vien HV, Thach DC, Toan ND, Cong le D, Geerts S, Speybroeck N, Berkvens D, Brandt J. Taenia solium cysticercosis in a village in northern Viet Nam: seroprevalence study using an ELISA for detecting circulating antigen. Trans R Soc Trop Med Hyg. 2002;96(3):270-2.

[91] Somers R, Dorny P, Nguyen VK, Dang TC, Goddeeris B, Craig PS, Vercruysse J. Taenia solium taeniasis and cysticercosis in three communities in north Vietnam. Trop Med Int Health. 2006;11(1):65-72.

[92] Esquivel A, Diaz-Otero F, Gimenez-Roldan S. Growing frequency of neurocysticercosis in Madrid (Spain).Neurologia. 2005;20(3):116-20.

[93] O'Neal S, Noh J, Wilkins P, Keene W, Lambert W, Anderson J, Compton Luman J, Townes J. *Taenia solium* Tapeworm Infection, Oregon, 2006-2009. Emerg Infect Dis. 2011;17(6):1030-6.

[94] Sorvillo F, Wilkins P, Shafir S, Eberhard M. Public health implications of cysticercosis acquired in the United States. Emerg Infect Dis. 2011;17(1):1-6.

[95] Del Brutto OH. Neurocysticercosis among international travelers to disease-endemic areas. J Travel Med. 2012a;19(2):112-7.

[96] Del Brutto OH. Neurocysticercosis in Western Europe: a re-emerging disease? Acta Neurol Belg. 2012b, Apr 18.

[97] Del Brutto OH. A review of cases of human cysticercosis in Canada. Can J Neurol Sci. 2012c;39(3):319-22.

[98] Fleury A, Hernández M, Avila M, Cárdenas G, Bobes RJ, Huerta M, Fragoso G, Uribe-Campero L, Harrison LJ, Parkhouse RM, Sciutto E. Detection of HP10 antigen in serum for diagnosis and follow-up of subarachnoidal and intraventricular human neurocysticercosis. J Neurol Neurosurg Psychiatry. 2007;78(9):970-4.

[99] Garcia HH, Pretell EJ, Gilman RH, Martinez SM, Moulton LH, Del Brutto OH, Herrera G, Evans CA, Gonzalez AE; Cysticercosis Working Group in Peru. A trial of antiparasitic treatment to reduce the rate of seizures due to cerebral cysticercosis. N Engl J Med. 2004;350 (3):249–58.

[100] Del Brutto O, Roos K, Coffey C, Garcia HH. Meta-analysis: Cysticidal drugs for neurocysticercosis: albendazole and praziquantel. Ann Intern Med. 2006;145(1):43-51.

[101] Carpio A, Kelvin EA, Bagiella E, Leslie D, Leon P, Andrews H, Hauser WA; Ecuadorian Neurocysticercosis Group. The effects of albendazole treatment on neurocysticercosis: a randomized controlled trial. J Neurol Neurosurg Psychiatry. 2008; 79(9):1050-5.

[102] Herrera-García SC, de Aluja AS, Méndez Aguilar RE. El uso de la ultrasonografía para el diagnóstico de la cisticercosis porcina. Vet Mex. 2007;38(1):125-133.

[103] Pondja A, Neves L, Mlangwa J, Afonso S, Fafetine J, Willingham AL 3rd, Thamsborg SM, Johansen MV. Use of oxfendazole to control porcine cysticercosis in a high-endemic area of mozambique. PLoS Negl Trop Dis. 2012;6(5):e1651.

[104] Guezala MC, Rodriguez S, Zamora H, Garcia HH, Gonzalez AE, Tembo A, Allan JC, Craig PS. Development of a species-specific coproantigen ELISA for human *Taenia solium* taeniasis. Am J Trop Med Hyg. 2009;81(3):433-7.

[105] Pawlowski ZS. Role of chemotherapy of taeniasis in prevention of neurocysticercosis. Parasitol Int. 2006; 55 Suppl:S105-9.

[106] WHO, "Global Plan to Combat Neglected Tropical Diseases 2008-2015. World Health Organization 2007.

[107] Recommendations of the International Task Force for Disease Eradication. MMWR Recomm Rep. 1993;42:1–38.

[108] Cruz M, Davis A, Dixon H, Pawlowski ZS, Proano J. Operational studies on the control of *Taenia solium* taeniasis/cysticercosis in Ecuador. Bull World Health Organ. 1989;67(4):401-7.

[109] Allan JC, Velasquez-Tohom M, Fletes C, Torres-Alvarez R, Lopez-Virula G, Yurrita P, Soto de Alfaro H, Rivera A, Garcia-Noval J. Mass chemotherapy for intestinal *Taenia solium* infection: effect on prevalence in humans and pigs. Trans R Soc Trop Med Hyg. 1997;91(5):595-8.

[110] Sarti E, Schantz PM, Avila G, Ambrosio J, Medina-Santillán R, Flisser A. Mass treatment against human taeniasis for the control of cysticercosis: a population-based intervention study. Trans R Soc Trop Med Hyg. 2000;94(1):85-9.

[111] Keilbach NM, de Aluja AS, Sarti GE. Programme to control Taeniasis-cysticercosis (*T.solium*): Experiences in a Mexican village. Acta Leidensia, 1989;57(2): 181-9.

[112] Sarti E, Flisser A, Schantz PM, Gleizer M, Loya M, Plancarte A, Avila G, Allan J, Craig P, Bronfman M, Wijeyaratne P. Development and evaluation of a health education intervention against *Taenia solium* in a rural community in Mexico. Am J Trop Med Hyg. 1997;56(2):127-32.

[113] Ngowi HA, Carabin H, Kassuku AA, MloziMR,Mlangwa JE, Willingham AL 3rd.A health-education intervention trial to reduce porcine cysticercosis in Mbulu District, Tanzania. Prev Vet Med. 2008;85(1-2):52-67.

[114] Gonzales AE, Garcia HH, Gilman RH, Gavidia CM, Tsang VC, Bernal T, Falcon N, Romero M, Lopez-Urbina MT. Effective, single-dose treatment or porcine cysticercosis with oxfendazole. Am J Trop Med Hyg. 1996;54(4):391-4.

[115] Gonzalez AE, Gavidia C, Falcon N, Bernal T, Verastegui M, Garcia HH, Gilman RH, Tsang VC; Cysticercosis Working Group in Peru. Protection of pigs with cysticercosis from further infections after treatment with oxfendazole. Am J Trop Med Hyg. 2001;65(1):15-8

[116] Sikasunge CS, Johansen MV, Willingham AL 3rd, Leifsson PS, Phiri IK. *Taenia solium* porcine cysticercosis: viability of cysticerci and persistency of antibodies and cysticercal antigens after treatment with oxfendazole. Vet Parasitol. 2008;158(1-2):57-66.

[117] Molinari JL, Rodríguez D, Tato P, Soto R, Arechavaleta F, Solano S. Field trial for reducing porcine *Taenia solium* cysticercosis in Mexico by systematic vaccination of pigs. Vet Parasitol. 1997;69(1-2):55-63.

[118] Huerta M, de Aluja AS, Fragoso G, Toledo A, Villalobos N, Hernández M, Gevorkian G, Acero G, Díaz A, Alvarez I, Avila R, Beltrán C, Garcia G, Martinez JJ, Larralde C, Sciutto E. Synthetic peptide vaccine against *Taenia solium* pig cysticercosis: successful vaccination in a controlled field trial in rural Mexico. Vaccine. 2001;20(1-2):262-6.

[119] Sciutto E, Rosas G, Hernández M, Morales J, Cruz-Revilla C, Toledo A, Manoutcharian K, Gevorkian G, Blancas A, Acero G, Hernández B, Cervantes J, Bobes RJ, Goldbaum FA, Huerta M, Diaz-Orea A, Fleury A, de Aluja AS, Cabrera-Ponce JL, Herrera-Estrella L, Fragoso G, Larralde C. Improvement of the synthetic tri-peptide vaccine (S3Pvac) against porcine *Taenia solium* cysticercosis in search of a more effective, inexpensive and manageable vaccine. Vaccine. 2007;25(8):1368-78.

[120] Morales J, Martínez JJ, Manoutcharian K, Hernández M, Fleury A, Gevorkian G, Acero G, Blancas A, Toledo A, Cervantes J, Maza V, Quet F, Bonnabau H, de Aluja AS, Fragoso G, Larralde C, Sciutto E. Inexpensive anti-cysticercosis vaccine: S3Pvac

expressed in heat inactivated M13 filamentous phage proves effective against naturally acquired *Taenia solium* porcine cysticercosis. Vaccine. 2008;26(23):2899-905.

[121] Assana E, Kyngdon CT, Gauci CG, Geerts S, Dorny P, De Deken R, Anderson GA, Zoli AP, Lightowlers MW. Elimination of *Taenia solium* transmission to pigs in a field trial of the TSOL18 vaccine in Cameroon. Int J Parasitol. 2010;40(5):515-9.

[122] Garcia HH, Gonzalez AE, Gilman RH, Moulton LH, Verastegui M, Rodriguez S, Gavidia C, Tsang VC; Cysticercosis Working Group in Peru. Combined human and porcine mass chemotherapy for the control of *Taenia solium*. Am J Trop Med Hyg. 2006;74(5):850-5.

[123] Garcia HH, Gonzalez AE, Rodriguez S, Gonzalvez G, Llanos-Zavalaga F, Tsang VC, Gilman RH; Grupo de Trabajo en Cisticercosis en Perú. Epidemiology and control of cysticercosis in Peru. Rev Peru Med Exp Salud Publica. 2010;27(4):592-7.

[124] Prichard RK, Basáñez MG, Boatin BA, McCarthy JS, García HH, Yang GJ, Sripa B, Lustigman S. A research agenda for helminth diseases of humans: intervention for control and elimination. PLoS Negl Trop Dis. 2012;6(4):e1549.

[125] Mexican Health Secretary. Modificación a la Norma Oficial Mexicana NOM-021-SSA2-1994, para la prevención y control del complejo taeniosis/cisticercosis en el primer nivel de atención médica. Diario Oficial de la Federación, 2004. http://www.salud.gob.mx/unidades/cdi/nom/m021ssa294.html. (accessed 12 June 2012)

[126] Flisser A, Correa D. Neurocysticercosis may no longer be a public health problem in Mexico. PLoS Negl Trop Dis 2010;4: e831

[127] de Aluja A, Morales Soto J, Sciutto E. A Programme to Control Taeniosis-Cysticercosis (*Taenia solium*) in Mexico, Current Topics in Tropical Medicine, Dr. Alfonso Rodriguez-Morales (Ed.), ISBN: 978-953-51-0274-8, InTech, 2012. Available from: http://www.intechopen.com/books/current-topics-in-tropical-medicine/a-program-to-control-taeniosis-cysticercosis-taenia-solium-in-mexico

[128] Willingham AL 3rd, Harrison LJ, Fèvre EM, Parkhouse ME; Cysticercosis Working Group in Europe. Inaugural meeting of the Cysticercosis Working Group in Europe. Emerg Infect Dis. 2008;14(12):e2.

[129] Garcia HH, Gonzalez AE, Rodriguez S, Gonzalvez G, Llanos-Zavalaga F, Tsang VC, Gilman RH; Grupo de Trabajo en Cisticercosis en Perú. Epidemiology and control of cysticercosis in Peru. Rev Peru Med Exp Salud Publica. 2010;27(4):592-7.

Chapter 6

Orbital Cisticercosis. A Challenger for Neurologists, Ophthalmologists, Neuro-Opthalmologists, and General Practitioners

Humberto Foyaca Sibat, María Carolina Salazar Campos
and Lourdes de Fátima Ibañez Valdés

Additional information is available at the end of the chapter

http://dx.doi.org/10.5772/52515

1. Introduction

Cysticercosis is a disease closely related to poverty in general and in particular with a poor personal hygiene and food, socio-cultural factors, environmental, education for health in the community, and also very closely related to the hygienic and sanitary conditions of each region. This is a preventable and an eradicable disease [1] that currently affects more than 50 million people in the entire world, of which 400 thousand live in Latin America [2] is internationally accepted that the onset of epilepsy, intracranial hypertension or headache of unknown cause in a person originating, visitor or in contact with another person from an area where *T solium* is endemic suggests considering the diagnosis of NCC. The patient affected by the NCC can remain asymptomatic for several months or years, and its diagnosis can be confirmed by accident when a CT scan is carried out in search of another diagnosis. [3,4] According to WHO figures confirmed by Roman and collaborators [5] around 50 thousand people die each year as a result of the NCC and the epilepsy secondary to the NCC (ESNCC).

Taenia solium produces two different diseases: taeniasis (Te) and/or cysticercosis (CC). When the parasite is an adult expels its mature proglotides and eggs with the stool to the environment; the subsequent ingestion of these eggs of pork cause porcine cysticercosis (PCC). When a person swallows raw pork meat or not well cooked and infected with cysticerci (CT) then develops a new adult parasite. The human then becomes an accidental intermediate host. These oncosphere (primary larvae) penetrate the intestinal mucosa and enter the circulatory system. The Hematogenous spread of neural, muscular, and ocular tissues occurs. Within these tissues, the oncosphere develop into secondary larvae (i.e., the cysticerci).

INTECH
open science | open minds

© 2013 Foyaca Sibat et al., licensee InTech. This is a paper distributed under the terms of the Creative Commons Attribution License (http://creativecommons.org/licenses/by/3.0), which permits unrestricted use, distribution, and reproduction in any medium, provided the original work is properly cited.

When man eats the eggs of *T. solium* acquires CC which can be found in any tissue including heart, liver, lungs, pancreas, spleen, kidneys, and peritoneal cavity among others. (See Chapter 3) [6-32] As has been mentioned, the location of Ct (larval stage) in the CNS and the eye (considering the retina as an extension of the CNS) is called NCC and is considered the neurological disease more important of parasitic origin in man and the main cause of epilepsy late onset. [33] In the brain NCC is located mainly at the level of gray substance cortical or at the level of the union between the gray and white matter because it is the best blood supplied area. [34] The CC is considered is a serious problem for public health in several developing countries where social conditions, economic and cultural levels favor the maintenance of this zoonotic disease and it is seen as a growing community problem in those developed countries with a high rate of immigrants from endemic areas. WHO includes the NCC between neglected diseases or forgotten that cause a significant impact on the economy in several regions of the world. It affects 4% of the population in endemic areas [35,36] where the personal and food hygiene habits and sometimes the religious tendencies determine the incidence and prevalence of the disease, for example: Islamism. Islam was not the first religion to prohibit the consumption of pork, before that Judaism made it perhaps less severe restrictions; however some cases have been reported in the Jewish community in New York. [37]

Due to globalization a growing number of uncontrolled migrants from endemic areas of Latin America came to the USA every day therefore a significantly increasing number of cases of NCC are gradually diagnosed in the country, especially in the southwest, including Texas and California. [4, 6-8,33, 37, 38-41] It suffices to mention that a total of 1494 patients with NCC were confirmed between 1980 and 2004 of which 66% suffered from epilepsy, 16% had an obstructive hydrocephalus and 15% headache due to intraparenchymal NCC [IpNCC] (91%), intraventricular (6 %) or subarachnoid (2 %) either because travelled to endemic areas, were of Hispanic origin or had any contact with carriers of the parasite. [42] In Latin America has been described the existence of the NCC in 18 countries with an estimated 350,000 patients infected by the complex TE/CC. In 2008, Pawlowski [43] stipulated that in the world would have 2.5 million owning approximate mind of disabled people of *Taenia solium,* at least 20 million with CC, which causes on average 50.000 deaths a year. In his recent book, Hotez [2] reported that in the United States were confirmed between one and two thousand cases of NCC each year and considering the growing Latino population could have more than 41,000 Hispanics suffer from NCC in that country. [2,43,44] Neurocysticercosis is also virtually endemic in certain countries in Europe such as Romania, Poland and even Portugal. In Spain the growing strength of the migration of individuals coming from endemic areas has conditioned an increase in the frequency of this entity. [45]

Other less frequent locations of *T solium* in the CNS include: intra ventricular (Iv), subarachnoid (Sa), medullary (Me), intraocular (Io) and intraspinal (Ip). Some authors report a list of frequencies for these locations and some combinations among of them such as: IpNCC (55.23 %), IvNCC (15,69 %) %), SaNCC (11.63 %), MeNCC (3.4 %), IoNCC (0.58 %), IpNCC (0.09 %) and the frequency of different combinations in the following manner:

Iv-Ip (6.98 %), Sa-Ip (3.49 %) and Sa-Iv (2.32 %) reported by Amaral et al. [46] In a hospital-based study conducted in Mexico is reported a rate of up to 8.6 cases of NCC per 100 hospitalized, and in the series of necrosis of up to 2 453 per 100 000 inhabitants and pointed out that 43.3 % of the cases were asymptomatic [35, 47] and 80% were autopsy findings. [48] Official statistics report an annual average of 500 cases of CC, with a national rate raw 0.6 per 100,000 inhabitants. [49-51] this report does not include the cases that were not attended by professional health personnel or that were not included in the study for other reasons, and does not include the extra-parenchymal presentations or even other modalities of CC. In Brazil, the prevalence in autopsies varies from 0.12 to 9% and in a series of clinical cases it varies from 0.03 to 7.5 %; in studies sero-epidemiological of 0.6 to 5.2 %. [52] In Colombia there is not much information on the CC, only some work in the departments of Antioquia and Santander that reported 1 to 2% of affectation to the population and 2% in Ecuador. [53, 54] On the other hand it has been estimated that 50 million people are infected by *T solium* in the world, of which 350 thousand live in Latin America [55] especially in those countries that do not have an adequate health infrastructure and proper health education program. [56] The main risk factors associated with the CC are the presence of peoples infected by *T solium* in the community with inadequate primary health care system, without proper health education and personal and food hygiene and without a sustainable supply of safe and clean water and where free-range pigs are able to ingest contaminated human feces [57-62] and the use of infected feces as an agricultural fertilizer. [63] The NCC has become a public health problem in different countries in Africa, Asia and Latin America [56, 64-68]

The orbits are two bony cavities occupied by the eyes and associated muscles, nerves, blood vessels, fat, and much of the lacrimal apparatus. Each orbit is shaped like a pear or a four-sided pyramid, with its apex situated posteriorly and its base anteriorly. The orbit is related to its superior side to the anterior cranial fossa and usually to the frontal sinus, laterally to the temporal fossa in (anterior) and to the middle cranial fossa (posterior), on its inferior side of the maxillary sinus, and medially to the ethmoid bone and the anterior extent of the sphenoid sinus.

Orbital cysticercosis is caused by the infestation of the larval form of the pork tapeworm Taenia solium in the orbital cavity affecting the eyeball (ocular cysticercosis) or the extra ocular structures found within the orbital cavity such as: extra ocular muscles, nerves, ganglions, and fatty tissue. Orbital cysticercosis may cause significant visual loss, especially if the cyst is located intraocularly or is compressing the optic nerve. [70]

Ocular cysticercosis may be extraocular (in the sub-conjunctival or orbital tissues) or intraocular (in the vitreous, sub-retinal space, or anterior chamber). [70-72] Ocular manifestations of cysticercosis vary from asymptomatic to painful blind eye and may be associated with neurological symptoms such as headache, fits, diplopia, and restriction of the ocular movements, nystagmus and papilloedema.

According to some authors the most common location of the Ocular CC is the sub retinal region (35 %), followed by the vitreous cysticercosis (22 %), conjunctival cysticercosis (22 %), and anterior segment cysticercosis. (5 %) [73] While involvement of other regions (e.g., extraocular muscles, optic nerve) are relatively less common. [70]

Sub retinal cysticercosis (SrCC), vitreous cysticercosis (VCC) and anterior segment cysticercosis (AsCC) are more common in India. While either eye may be affected, bilateral involvement is rare [74] and multiple cysts may develop in the same eye. [75] Ocular manifestations may be devastating as the cysticercus enlarges. The cysticercus may lead to blindness in 3-5 years. [76] Decreased vision, pain, and recurrent redness of the involved eye are common symptoms of intraocular cysticercosis. [70]

Some authors consider that intraocular cysticercosis is predominant in the Western countries, whereas extraocular is more common in the Indian population attributed to geographic and environmental factors. [77, 79] However, other affirm that intraocular involvement is more common in India compared with Western countries. [78,] and involvement of conjunctiva is most commonly reported in India [80-99], whereas involvement of posterior segment of the eye is most commonly seen in Western countries. [100-109] compared with conjunctival region but it also can be seen in India. [110-112]

Orbital cysticercosis should be suspected in patients who have lived in an endemic area and who develop uveitis, leucocoria or Neuro-Ophthalmological signs, also in the presence of sub conjunctival cysts or lids nodules. Cysts deep within the orbit are best treated conservatively with a 4-week regimen of oral albendazole (15 mg/kg/d) in conjunction with oral steroids (1.5 mg/kg/d) in a tapering dose over a 1-month period. Treatment may increase inflammation as the cyst involutes, leading to worsening clinical status. Thus, concomitant administration of corticosteroids is recommended to avert an inflammatory response. [113,114]

In 2010, Rath et al., Studied 93 patients presenting orbital cysticercosis with mean age of 13 years and they concluded that orbital cysticercosis is a common clinical condition in the developing world which typically affects young individuals and has a wide spectrum of clinical manifestations; B-scan ultrasonography and computed tomography scan are useful in confirming the diagnosis and despite resolution of cysticercosis with medical management, a significant proportion of patients may have residual functional deficits. [77, 115,116]

1.1. Is orbital metastasis another challenger for differential diagnosis?

It may be, therefore our readership should remember that renal cell carcinoma (RCC) is a tumor of middle-aged men that metastasizes to the lung, liver, and bone. When this tumor spreads to the orbit, the orbital metastasis is likely to be the first indication of the cancer and up to 1993 only a few cases were reported. [117] In 1994, Schmidt et al [118] reported a 69 years-old-male patient with similar condition. Konya et al [119] reported two cases: a 44 and 59-years-old- male patients with proptosis and a tongue tumor due to RCC. Another patient was: 39-year-old black man with sickle cell trait, presented with a rapidly progressive painful proptosis of the left eye due to metastasis from renal medullary carcinoma. [120]

Most of patient reported at that time were from non-endemic areas for cysticercosis, this information was very important in the diagnostic process but at the present moment cysticercosis can be found in almost all countries. The next report came from India. It was a 69-year-old male who presented with pulsatile proptosis owing to metastasis of an asymptomatic renal cell carcinoma [121] this case was an example of the great challenger. In 2007, another three patients: two males of 67 and 58 years old males and a 23-years-old-female from India presenting iris mass, orbital metastasis were reported. [122] At this time, a total of 71 patients was reported in the international medical literature. This report suggested that patients presenting with atypical orbital or ocular masses, the possibility of renal cell carcinoma metastasis should be considered, especially if there is a history of previous renal disorder. Incisional biopsy with histopathological evaluation may be an important means to diagnose this condition and facilitate appropriate therapy. Other author reported similar findings. [123-126] Based on this review of the medical literature we can conclude that differential diagnosis between orbital metastasis and orbital cysticercosis it is not difficult considering that only three patients presenting proptosis of the eyes as the first clinical manifestation of RCC have been reported to the medical literature. [125]

Patients with hepatic cell carcinoma presenting primary symptoms of metastatic disease are rare and the retro-orbital mass as the initial manifestation of disease is also very uncommon as well. [127] Nevertheless, this an uncommon pathological disorder can also affect intracranial structures mainly in elderly patients or presenting as rapid onset of proptosis and visual loss (only three patients reported), or painful proptosis as the most common clinical sign of hepatocellular carcinoma metastatic to the orbit (ten patients reported). [128-132] In conclusion, hepatocellular carcinoma is a rare source of metastasis to the orbit, and only 14 histopathologically proven cases have been reported in the international medical literature. Proptosis is the most common presenting feature in the reviewed reports and a majority of patients have occult primary tumors at presentation and the diagnosis of the orbital mass is based on histopathology. [131]

The age of the patients, clinical features of the orbital lesion, presence of other metastatic lesions, epidemiological features of cysticercosis, CT scans, and ultrasonographic studies are elements that allow you to make a certain diagnosis.

In the previous chapter we reviewed some aspects on orbital cysticercosis according to their different locations within and outside of the eyeball without exceeding the limits of orbit, mainly those clinical features of the ocular cysticercosis associated with damage of other organs as part of the disseminated cysticercosis at the same time.

2. Vitreous cysticercosis and anterior chamber cysticercosis

2.1. Intraocular cysticercosis

It may be asymptomatic in the early stages. As the parasite grows, it causes a painless, progressive loss of vision related to the area of location.

Patients` complaints about an intermittent roundish, dark mobile mass (intravitreal location) or may experience visual field defects (sub retinal or CNS location).

Intraocular lesions caused by cysticercosis most commonly occur in the vitreous or subretinal space, but subchoroidal, sub hyaliod, and into the anterior chamber, also occur. [133-138] Lens involvement also can occur but it is extremely rare. (139)

A cyst in the anterior chamber can be manifested as an acute anterior uveitis, sometimes is so severe that is difficult to differentiate a cyst from a dislocated lens and always there is a cataract formation. The parasite can be seen moving freely into the cavity. (See figure 1)

When the parasite is freely mobile it may contribute to the absence of reaction in the anterior chamber. The portal of entry of the parasite into the anterior chamber has not been well documented although some author refers that the cyst may enter the anterior chamber either from the posterior ciliary arteries or from the angle. [154].

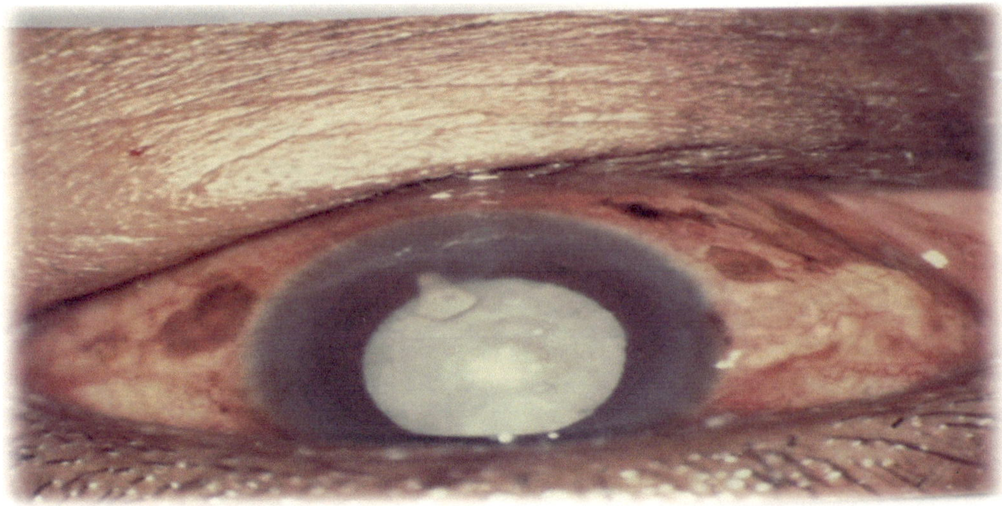

Figure 1. Anterior chamber cysticercosis with freely mobile cysticercus into the aqueous humor.

In the posterior segment, parasites gain access presumably through the posterior ciliary arteries. From this location, they usually pass through a rent in the retina into the vitreous. In rare cases the parasite may pass from the vitreous, through the pupil, into the anterior chamber. Infestation of the ocular adnexa is probably through the anterior ciliary arteries. [101-134,140]

The intraocular location of the cyst can cause retinal detachment, macular scarring, retinal vasculitis and vitritis [141] and usually affects young patients unilaterally. The cyst may be in either the vitreous cavity or the sub retinal space, and visual acuity at presentation is often poor. [142]

Most patients presenting intraocular cysticercosis can tolerate it well while the cysticercus is alive, however when the parasite dies, there is a marked inflammatory response to toxic products released from the cyst, and the patient presents a blind painful eye. [136,142.143]. Only a few cases about cysticercosis resulting in glaucoma due to pupillary block have been reported. [72]

2.2. Intravitreal cysticercosis

It can be recognized through clear media, the translucent cyst with a dense white spot formed by the invaginated scolex and the undulating movements are typical. We can see the scolex returning rapidly to the cyst when exposed to the ophthalmoscope or slit lamp light. [144,145] The frequency of different location of intraocular cysticercosis can be seen in the figure below.

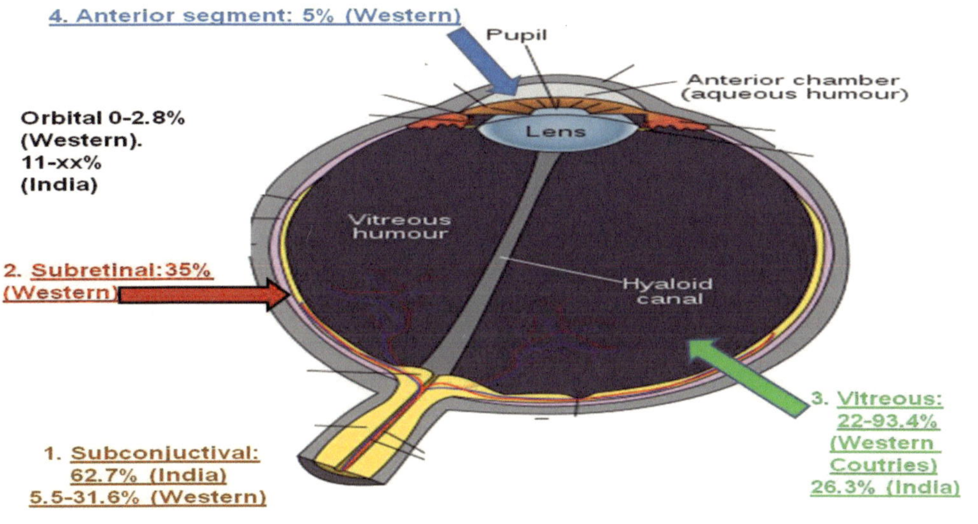

Figure 2. Frequency of intraocular cysticercosis in Western countries and India

After migration into the vitreous, a chorioretinal scar may develop in this area.

Laboratory tests:

Diagnostic paracentesis of the anterior chamber cysticercosis can show more than 50% of leukocytes in the aqueous humor with eosinophils . ELISA IgG serology test for cysticercosis and Western blot contribute to confirm the diagnosis although some cross reaction can be found in patients presenting Diphyllobothriosis, Taeniasis, Cysticercosis, Echinococcosis (Hydatidosis), Coenuriosis or Sparganosis.

Stool samples:

May not show any proglottids or eggs of T. solium.

Blood tests:

Are of limited value in diagnosing intraocular cysticercosis. FBC, serum chemistries and ESR may all be normal; eosinophilia is uncommon.

EITB (enzyme-linked immuno-electro transfer blot assay) has been shown to have greater than 98% sensitivity and specificity in patients with systemic disease, and can be completed with the determination of circulating antibody and antigen in the aqueous humor.
In ocular cysticercosis, serologic tests are helpful if positive, but false-negative tests may be reported, and their negativity does not rule out the disease. [143,146]

Imagenology

Fluorescein Angiography is useful in delineating the sub-retinal cyst located in the periphery of the retina. Plain X-rays of soft tissue or skull often reveal calcified cysticerci. The enhanced CT scan is valuable for identifying and following the evolution of orbital cysticercosis, which may appear as solid, cystic or calcified nodules.

MRI provides detailed images of living and degenerating cysticerci. [141]

Ultrasonography is an effective and economical alternative to MRI and CT for the detection of the intra-ocular cysticerci. It is a real time, dynamic examination, also allows direct visualization of the movements of the parasite when it is intraocular. U/S is effective for the detection of the cysts in the orbit and muscles too.

A cysticercus cyst with the scolex attached to the inner wall composes the "hanging drop sign." This sign was seen in cases studied using simultaneous A-and B-scan ultrasonography. This appearance was consistent and reproducible, regardless of whether the cyst was intraocular or extraocular in location. Serial B-scan ocular ultrasonography or CT scans of the orbit helps to follow the resolution of the cyst, which is recognized by the disappearance of the scolex. [15]

Optical Coherence Tomography (OCT) exam is seen as hyporeflective area due to the presence of fluid in the cyst cavity. Sometimes the height of the cyst obscured the visualization of the scolex. In children, intraocular cysticercosis can simulate retinoblastoma mainly in the inflammatory response.

Therapeutic aspects

Medical treatment for intraocular cysticercosis is not advisable while that Albendazole or Praziquantel (PZQ), in conjunction with corticosteroids can be used for extraocular presentations with very good results.

Surgical treatment is used to remove the cysts from the adnexa, anterior and posterior segment. Removal of the cyst is mandatory to remove the source of the toxins causing inflammation and early removal has been advocated by many authors. [144,147] Reviews of treated cases suggest that early removal of the organism is associated with preservation of visual function. [137] If possible, ocular cysts should be removed before systemic treatment is undertaken to prevent damage from the dying process of the parasite. Freely mobile live cysticercus in the anterior chamber associated to NCC in patients complete asymptomatic has been reported in the medical literature. [148] or may be attached by inflammatory membranes to surrounding structures, such as the cornea, lens capsule, or iris. [149] In general these cysts are around 2x2 mm in size, grayish-white in color and are freely mobile (See figure 2), changing its shape by protruding and retracting its scolex from and into the cyst cavity; sometimes the parasite is not neither attached to the iris, cornea or other intra-ocular anatomical structure and usually there are not an associated conjunctival or ciliary congestion and not abnormalities of the retina, macula vitreous or optic disc with preservation of the visual acuity but it can be associated with iridocyclitis [150-152] and secondary glaucoma [153] and as a rule the parasite is attached to the iris and only occasionally to the corneal endothelium or lens capsule.

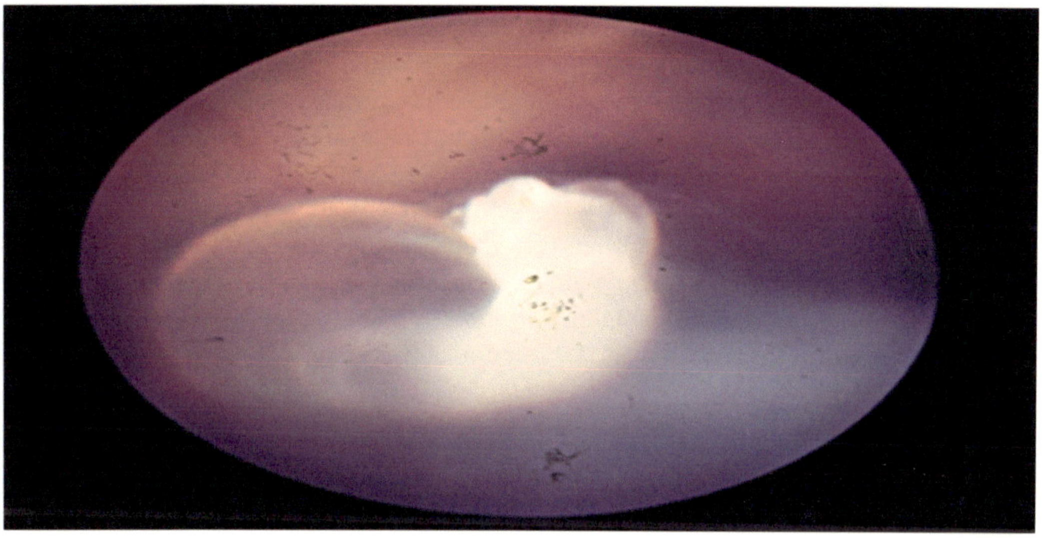

Figure 3. Intravitreous cysticercus moving freely

2.3. Ocular cysticercosis in South Africa

Some author reported a frequency of ocular involvement in cysticercosis around 13 to 46% [155,156] and its associated intraocular inflammation may also cause cataract formation [154] and iris atrophy. We found some differences and similarities compared with South African's patients that we will comment below.

Most of studies done in India and Western countries confirmed that orbital cysticercosis with ocular involvement is an uncommon pathological process that may cause severe damage of the eyes and an important involvement of the visual acuity. [80-84, 93, 142, 150, 156-158] The pathogenesis of ocular injury due to an intense inflammatory reaction secondary to intravitreous cysticercosis has been documented throughout an experimental animal model for intravitreous cysticercosis using New Zealand rabbits and Taenia crassiceps cysticerci since 1996. [159]

In 1964, Proctor [160] estimated a 1% incidence in South Africa of infestation by tapeworm cysts in 7 597 autopsies. Pammenter and Rossouw in 1984, [161] reported the results of serological tests in 79 patients with systemic cysticercosis in South Africa, from this study they confirmed that in isolated ocular cysticercosis serological tests are usually negative:

45,5% ELISA positive, the indirect haemagglutination test 33,3% positive, and the fluorescent antibody test 48,9% positive. Almost always these tests were positive in cases of systemic cysticercosis in our region. This experience was confirmed also by other. [162, 164].

In 1987, Welsh et al [106] studied thirteen cases of ocular cysticercosis at King Edward VIII Hospital over an 8-year period from 1976 to 1984. All patients came from rural areas, a reflection on the low standards of hygiene. At that time, adolescent females ingested tapeworm eggs for slimming purposes, but none of this report was under that category. From their review of the medical literature they found that up to 1952, 1 216 cases of ocular cysticercosis were reported and when studied their patients most of them were occasional and came to South Africa from India. Of the 13 patients with ocular cysts nine were found in the vitreous, three in the anterior chamber and one under the conjunctiva of the eye. The majority of patients were female and all were Zulus living in areas of KwaZulu Natal, most of them complained of loss of vision for an average of 3 months. The only exception was one patient with the sub-conjunctival cyst who had waited 2 years before seeking treatment, since the lump had not affected his vision. Today all types of cysticercosis in KwaZulu Natal practically disappeared and patients with cysticercosis can be seen only at the former Transkei or another province but emigrated from this region (currently region C and D) of the Eastern Cape Province which does not mean that cysticercosis is going to disappear in the next decade how we explained in the previous chapter.

All patients from Welsh' series [107] presenting vitreous cysticercosis complained of severe loss of vision, and there was always a marked vitreoretinal reaction and the patients with cysts in the anterior chamber showed severe anterior chamber reactions with anterior uveitis. The vision was reduced in all patients to where hand movements could not be seen or to perception of light being absent or to complete blindness, except for the patient with the subconjunctival cyst . In this series of patients because of the severity of the lesions, surgical removal, although partly successful, did not improve vision and the distribution of the cysts in the various structures of the eye was similar to cases reported in the literature. We would like to highlight that around 70's and 80's years several cases presenting bilateral involvement of the eyes and/or multifocal intra-ocular cysts were most commonly seen. [74,104,107,164,165]

Medical treatment for intraocular cysticercosis is not recommended based on South African's experiences with praziquantel (isquinoline pyrazine) [106] and another report from the same period of time. [166] Surgical removal is strongly recommended as the best treatment because complications associated with the cyst were minimal. Removal of vitreous cysts by pars plana vitrectomy is the method of choice. [110,167]

Removal of a cyst from the anterior chamber is relatively simple excepting cases pre-existing vitreoretinal-uveal reaction. [110, 168] The treatment of anterior chamber cysticercosis is essentially surgical. The different modalities used to remove the cyst include paracentesis, extraction with capsule forceps, cryo-extraction, diathermia, and viscoexpression. [78, 110,136, 168, 169]

In individuals with uveitis, the perioperative corticosteroid administration is recommended. Although surgical excision of orbital cysts was considered the ideal treatment modality, deep orbital dissection and difficulty in completely excising the cyst because of the surrounding inflammatory response, increase the chances of postoperative complications (e.g., decreased vision, diplopia). [110, 169]

Destruction of the larvae in situ of photocoagulation [170] cryotherapy, and diathermy has been attempted with some success. However, as intraocular cysticercosis may lead to severe inflammation following larval death, early surgical removal of the cyst is the treatment of choice. [137]

In years the 70s and 80s systemic cysticercosis was very common in rural areas of South Africa but ocular cysticercosis was not associated with any other systemic features and CT suggested that some patients with ocular cysticercosis had neurocysticercosis as well, although none was reported with accompanying systemic physical signs or symptoms. All patients had severe reactions to the cyst, whereas in the majority of reported cases there was a little ocular reaction. [107]

The treatment of anterior chamber cysticercosis is essentially surgical. The different modalities used to remove the cyst include paracentesis, extraction with capsule forceps, cryo-extraction, erysiphake extraction, and viscoexpression. [15,78] Viscoexpression allows removal of an intact cyst through a small limbal incision. In the treatment of intraocular cysticercosis, the most common surgical approach is removal through the pars plana route following vitrectomy. [168] Sub retinal cyst anterior to the equator may be removed trans-sclerally, whereas sub retinal cysts posterior to the equator and intravitreal cysts are best removed trans-vitreally. [137] Ideally, the cyst should be removed in toto. Complete surgical removal of the intact cyst results in good functional recovery in eyes with intraocular cysticercosis. [110, 136,137, 167]

3. Subretinal cysticercosis and optic nerve neurocysticercosis

3.1. Subretinal cysticercosis

The macular region is the site of choice for the subretinal cysticercus to lodge, maybe because of the high vascularization of this area but it can be seen in another subretinal area as well. In early stages, subretinal cysticercosis can appear as an acute central retinitis with retinal edema and subretinal exudates. The subretinal organism eventually develops into a cyst and the parasite and its movements can be recognized through the thin muscular layers. The observation of the cyst is more difficult when it is located in the periphery of the retina because scleral depression has to be used and the movements of the parasite cannot be observed clearly. (See figure 4 and 5)

Reportedly 35% of the cysts are in the subretinal space, 22% in the vitreous, 22% in the subconjunctival space, 5% in the anterior segment and 1% in the orbit. Among the intraocular cysts, 60% are found intravitreally and 40% are subretinal. [137,153]

When the parasite dies, an intraocular inflammation develops. Signs of acute anterior uveitis are present and severe opacification of the vitreous is observed. There are reports of dead and degenerating cysticerci causing a severe inflammatory reaction and ultimately loss of the eye. The cysts are known to release toxic products that cause severe inflammation mimicking endophthalmitis and even intraocular tumor. [171] The differential diagnosis with other parasitic infections and tumors has to be done. [144, 172, 173]

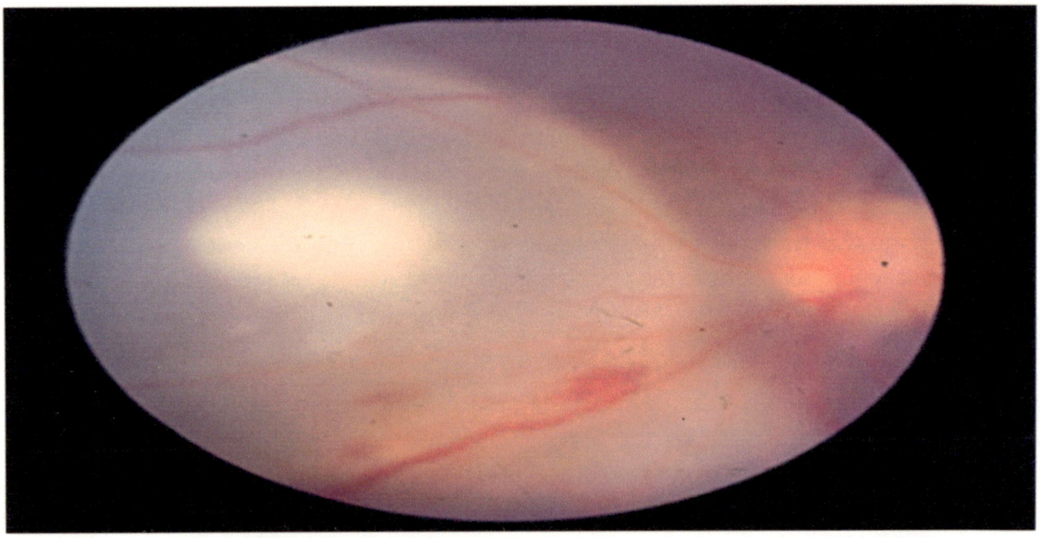

Figure 4. Shows subretinal cysticercosis seen by fundoscopy.

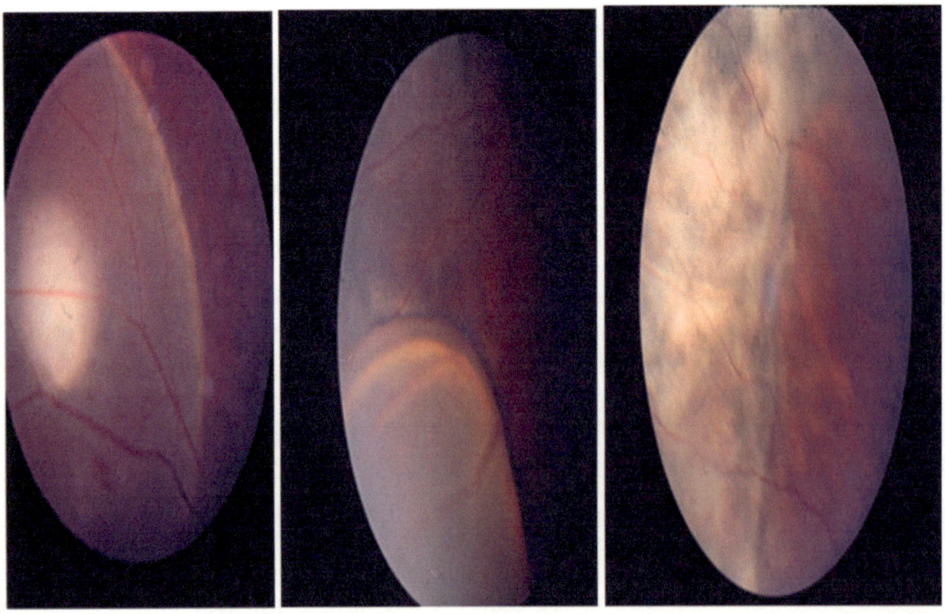

Figure 5. Another view of subretinal cysticercosis seen by fundoscopy (left & center) and picture of the fundus after surgical treatment on the right.

Seems to be that the viable cysts can evoke less inflammatory response, [170] while the degenerating cyst rapidly increases in size due to osmotic regulation and causes compression of the surrounding tissues and release of antigens into the surrounding tissue inducing inflammatory response. [106, 156,170, 173]

After the pars plana vitrectomy approach for removal of intravitreal cysts has developed, the prognosis of these eyes has improved. Another technique in conjunction with endolaser, diathermy, cryocoagulation, photocoagulation, and internal tamponade according to the retinal damage had been advocated for the treatment of cysticercosis. However, these methods will give rise to severe intraocular inflammation due to the toxins released from the dead larval tissues.

[137, 172, 174, 175] If the cyst is ruptured, care should be taken to remove all of the residual debris to prevent severe postoperative inflammation. Without treatment for intraocular parasites, the eyes go to the blindness in a short period of time.

Some report confirmed that the cyst usually presents in the sub-retinal space or vitreous cavity, where it can be observed ophthalmoscopically. The site of entry into the eye is most probably the choroidal vasculature from here the parasite can shift its location from sub-retinal space into the vitreous through a retinal break which could seal spontaneously, this passage incites inflammation, leaving behind a chorioretinal scar or even moves from anterior to posterior chamber and vice versa. [106,176-1978]

At this point, is good to remember what we explained before about cysts moving freely in the posterior chamber: apart from uveitis cysticercus may also lead to retinal hemorrhages, proliferative vitreoretinopathy, retinal detachment, disc edema, cyclitic membrane formation, and phthisis. [177,178]

In places where specialized retinal services are not available, external approach for the removal of sub retinal cyst is used. One of us (MCSC) has been used this surgical technique in places where other surgical approaches cannot be applied.

3.2. Approach to subretinal cyst removal using a conventional surgery technique

The conventional serial approach is a well-established surgical procedure for the treatment of subretinal cysts. This technique was the only one performed for many years to remove intraocular cysticercus (See figure 6) until advanced modern and easy methods were developed as the pars plana vitrectomy and internal tamponades.

The conventional method is more time consuming but it can be done in places where other facilities are not available.

Number one priority is localizing the cyst by indirect ophthalmoscopy at the pre-operatory stage and then to proceed as follows:

1. To retract the lids using a wire lid retractor or sutures.
2. To perform a limbal peritomy by grasping the conjunctiva and Tenon`s capsule at the level of the limbus with a toothed forceps and with a conjunctival scissors. The

extension varies according to the size of the cyst. Radial relaxing incisions is made through the conjunctiva and Tenon`s capsule in oblique meridians to prevent tearing of the conjunctiva during the surgery and avoid further complications as a symblepharon formation.

3. Scleral exposure has taken care to avoid damage of the vortex veins.
4. Isolated two or three rectus muscles according to the place the surgeon is going to do the scleral incision. Here is important to highlight do not cut the muscle belly to avoid bleeding. Using a muscle hook passed underside and 4-0 silk suture is passed around the muscle to do the fixation.

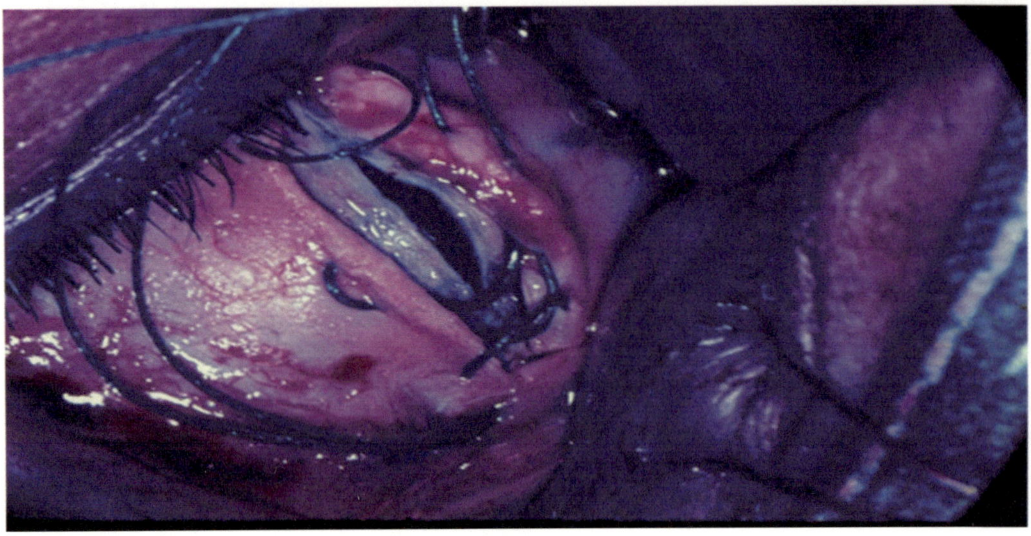

Figure 6. External approach to subretinal cysticercosis.

5. Localization of the subretinal cyst is done again with the indirect ophthalmoscope and the assistant help to mark the limits on the sclera where the incision will be made. These marks can be done with the use of the diathermy or with a surgical pen.
6. The Scleral incision has to be made at right angles to the surface of the sclera to maintain a uniform depth of the undermining. The incision should extend more than two thirds of the scleral thickness to have a floor for the placement of the diathermy treatment to avoid bleeding trans operators
7. 4-0 or 5-0 polyester sutures with spatulated needle to close the scleral flap are used. The sutures are placed 2mm apart in a radial fashion and approximately 1.5 mm from the edge of the scleral flap. Two or three mattress sutures are placed in each quadrant. If the incision is bigger than a single quadrant with 2 sutures in each one is enough. The sutures cannot be placed under the muscles.
8. The scleral lamina is perforated and the cyst is expressed out through a choroidal incision.
9. Sometimes more diathermy is necessary
10. Scleral sutures are closed, suture of the muscles release and closure of the Tenon`s and the conjunctiva with Vicryl is done.

11. In case the cyst burst during the extraction a thorough irrigation has to be done.

Subretinal cyst anterior to the equator may be removed trans sclerally, whereas subretinal cysts posterior to the equator and intravitreal cysts are best removed transvitreally. [112]

Under conventional surgical procedures by sclerotomy exactly over the subretinal *cyst* localized by scleral depression under indirect ophthalmoscopy, other authors also obtained successful surgical removal of subretinal cysticerci including patients with an associated exudative retina detachment with extensive gliosis, fixed folds, focal retinitis, and multiple subretinal precipitates specially near to the cyst but fatal results in patients presenting multifocal intraocular cysticercosis and severe NCC (even in the non-pork eaters) is obtained. [178]

In the treatment of intraocular cysticercosis, the most common surgical approach is removal through the pars plana route following vitrectomy. Ideally, the cyst should be removed in toto. Complete surgical removal of the intact cyst results in good functional recovery in eyes with intraocular cysticercosis. [29] Systemic corticosteroids are used before and after surgical removal of the cysticercus.

Patnaik and Kalsi [178] also reported a progressive pre-retinal gliosis with the passage of time with the evagination of the scolex against the retina, the latter is perforated, often in more than one point. They comment that the cyst through one of these perforations can escape into the vitreous cavity and the detached retina continues to shrink with increasing gliosis and vitreous becomes progressively hazy which becomes totally impenetrable with massive exudation then the parasite cannot be located. It may be presumed that the sudden advent of massive inflammation is associated with rupture of the cyst or death of the parasite. The eye is lost with massive inflammation. Even the successful removal of the subretinal cyst if not conducted early enough may not prevent the progressive deterioration of the retina and vitreous probably because of continued inflammation. The same results were reported by others. [178-182]

3.3. Optic nerve neurocysticercosis

The cysticercosis does not affect the spinal nerves or cranial nerves.

The optic (second cranial) nerve is the nerve of sight, and it extends from the eye to the optic chiasm. Developmentally, it may be considered as a tract between the retina (a derivative of the brain) and the brain. The nerve fibers, which arise in the retina, converge on the optic disc, pierce the layers of the eye, and receive myelin sheaths. The optic nerve, itself, is surrounded by meningeal sheaths continuous with those of the brain, and also by the subarachnoid space. As is known the optic nerve originates from the axonal extensions of the ganglion cells of the retina which is an extension of the central nervous system. Therefore this type of presentation of cysticercosis should be grouped within the category of Neurocysticercosis. (NCC)

Although other zoonotic parasites (Trematode) have been found in the layers of the retina at longitudinal position [183] the size and shape of cysticercus exceed the thickness of the retina so that its location is below it, and in close relation to the vascular layer of which is nourished. For certain reasons when the larva is leaving the subretinal region only has the option to do so toward the vitreous cavity because the resistance given by the sclera to be crossed.

The NCC of the optic nerve is extremely uncommon and until today no more than 10 patients have been well documented. [184-200]

As we discussed in the previous chapter orbital cysticercosis as a presentation of disseminating cysticercosis has not been reported in the medical literature excepting one anecdotal case [194]. The first well documented patient presenting optic nerve cysticercosis was from India (1991). Other authors [185] reported a 15-years-old female with progressive deterioration of her visual acuity of seven months duration. Her CT scan revealed a right retrobulbar optic nerve thickened with small area of low attenuation in the thickened portion of the optic nerve. A diagnosis of optic nerve glioma or granulomas was considered and a right frontal craniotomy and extradural frontal orbitomy was performed, they found an intense fibrosis and or deeper incision a sago grain like cyst was identified and excised. Histopathology revealed it to be a cysticercosis. Postoperatively the patient's vision full was completely recovered but there was an oculomotor nerve paresis. Similar patient was not described previously. Five years later, Bousquest et al [186] reported a first case of intraoptic neurocysticercosis in a 12-year-old boy living on Reunion Island (France). They also initially considered a diagnosis of optic nerve tumor and later computerized tomography scans and surgical aspects confirmed a diagnosis of retrobulbar optic nerve cysticercosis recommending a conservative removal using en bloc orbitotomy because of good functional and aesthetic results. Despite a first case was reported before we would like to highlight that Bousquest [186] was the first to use the correct terminology for cysticercosis involving the optic nerve such as: Intraoptic neurocysticercosis.

Other anecdotic report about the occurrence of optic neuritis following oral albendazol therapy for orbital cysticercosis was done in 1998 [187] but this one served to highlight the importance of adding a steroid medication to Albendazole in the treatment of all cases of orbital cysticercosis mainly when cysts are in close proximity to the optic nerve. They confirmed a full visual recovery after resolution of optic neuritis after four weeks treatment with Prednisolone at the dose of 1mg/kg per day.

Another 15-years-old-female presenting cysticercosis of the optic nerve is reported by Gurha et al [188] This patient presented with rapidly diminishing vision in the left eye, headache and papillitis. A magnetic resonance imaging revealed a cystic lesion at the entrance of the optic canal. Surgery performed was a transcranial orbitotomy which included deroofing of the optic canal and removal of the cyst from under the sheath of the optic nerve and the outcome was a remarkable visual recovery. At the same time a 15-year-old boy presented with diminution of vision which rapidly progressed to no perception of light. In the ocular fundus, a neuroretinitis-like picture was seen. On CT-scan and ultrasonography, an optic nerve swelling was detected with a shadow of scolex. Abnormal P-100 values of visual evoked potential can be useful for supporting a differential diagnosis.

This condition is often mistaken for optic nerve tumors and on neuroimaging the diagnosis is often delayed or missed. [197] However, imagenology studies based on contrast-enhanced MR imaging study and contrast-enhanced CT usually reveals a ring-enhancing cyst with a mural nodule located in the optic nerve although sometimes it only shows a thickened of the optic nerve with or without ring-enhancing lesion containing an eccentric nodule. [190,193, 197, 198] Ultrasonography can also help to determine the cause of optic neuritis due to the disorganization of the cyst with inflammation of the adjacent optic nerve. [187, 191, 193, 195, 197-201] and these investigations are useful to confirm: response to the treatment and patient's compliance. Other investigation to support the diagnostic process is an enzyme-linked immunosorbent assay test for cysticercosis. [190, 193, 195, 196]

Medical therapy in the form of steroids along with albendazol was ineffective. Surgical removal by lateral orbitotomy was done and a complete cyst with scolex was removed, which was confirmed histopathologically as a case of retrobulbar optic nerve cysticercosis. [189] Next patient, a 50-year-old woman with atypical optic neuritis was also treated with oral prednisolone and albendazole, with no improvement in vision [190] While other patients presenting optic nerve cysticercosis including bilateral optic nerve involvement improved dramatically with prednisone and albendazole. [191, 193,195]

4. Conjunctival cysticercosis

Ocular and extraocular cysticercosis are a commonly encountered manifestation of the disease caused by the cysticercus cellulosae. Any region of the eye may be afflicted including the subconjunctival space. The conjunctiva is a connection between the eyelids, sclera and cornea. It is the mucous membrane that lines the posterior surface of the eyelids (palpebral conjunctiva) and the anterior aspect of the globe (bulbar conjunctiva).

The host inflammatory response to cysticerci located into the conjunctival depends on the parasite's ability to evade host immunity; therefore, inflammation is restricted to degenerating cysts whose ability to evade host defenses is faltering. Lack of inflammation occurs with both healthy cysticerci (vesicular stage) and those that have involuted (inactive disease). Upon involution, cysts undergo granulomatous change and exhibit calcification. [70] It almost never happens in the conjunctiva region. Subconjunctival cysticercosis usually presents as a painful, yellowish, nodular subconjunctival mass with surrounding conjunctival congestion or may even present as an eyelid nodule or even as subconjuctival abscess from orbital myocysticercosis. [202] Patients presenting lacrimal canalicular obstruction have been reported as well. [85, 97]

The most common outcome is the spontaneous extrusion of the T solium cysticercus. [90-92, 94-96,98, 203] sometimes they got extruded from the orbit or from subconjunctival space but almost always associated with clinical improvement. [90]

Anterior subconjunctival cysts may be treated with excision biopsy .As the cyst is usually adherent to the adjacent muscle, excision may be difficult. Care must be taken to keep the extraocular muscle intact during dissection because an excessive intraoperative dissection of the sub conjunctival cyst may damage the extraocular muscle fibers, leading to postoperative diplopia and strabismus. [89, 99]

5. Extraocular muscle cysticercosis

Extraocular muscles differ histologically from most other skeletal muscles in that they are made up of two different types of muscle cells. Each muscle cell is composed of groups of myofibrils called sarcomeres. Fast-twitch muscle fibrils generate fast eye movements and are composed of well-defined myofibrils with well-developed sarcomeres while slow-twitch muscle fibrils generate slow or tonic eye movements and are composed of poorly defined myofibrils with poorly developed sarcomeres. Cholinergic motor neurons supply both types of muscle fibers. The innervation to fast-twitch fibrils is thick and heavily myelinated, with a single (en plaque) neuromuscular junction, whereas the innervation to slow-twitch fibrils is thin, with multiple grapelike clusters of neuromuscular junctions. [204] The eye's major blood supply comes from the ophthalmic artery. The lateral muscular branch of the ophthalmic artery supplies the lateral rectus, superior rectus, and superior oblique muscles. The medial muscular branch supplies the inferior rectus, medial rectus, and inferior oblique muscles. Medial and lateral muscular branches of the artery give rise to seven anterior ciliary vessels, which travel with the four rectus muscles to provide circulation for the anterior segment of the eye. Each rectus muscle has two anterior ciliary vessels, except for the lateral rectus muscle, which has 1 vessel. These vessels pass anteriorly to the episclera and supply the anterior segment of the eye, including the sclera, limbus, and conjunctiva. [204]

The extraocular muscles rotate the eyeball around vertical, horizontal and antero-posterior axes. Extraocular muscles other than the medial rectus and lateral rectus have more than one action due to the angle they make with the optical axis of the eye while inserting into the eyeball. The superior and inferior oblique muscles make an angle of 51 degrees with the optical axis.

As we before-cited, orbital cysticercosis is an uncommon presentation of cysticercosis even in endemic countries. In some South African provinces where it was seen before, it does exist at the present moment, and infestation of extraocular muscle remains exceedingly rare; but because of the versatility of the presentation, cysticercosis still should be considered in the differential diagnosis of many orbital disorders, especially in an endemic region and extraocular muscle cysticercosis should be considered in the differential diagnosis of recent acquired motility disorder or proptosis. According to several publications in the international medical literature and based on our experience we fully support that cysticercosis is a pleomorphic disorder whose presentation depends on a combination of inflammatory response, topography of the lesions, degree of parasitic load and sequelae of previous infestation as was established by others as well. [78, 205-208]

The rectus muscles are all approximately 40 mm long and each receives innervation from the undersurface (intraconal space) at the junction of the middle and posterior thirds of the muscle or 26 mm from the insertion

To achieve a better understanding of this variant of solium tapeworm infestation of the extraocular muscles, we have decided to merge the contents of sub chapter in accordance to the affected muscles after committing a first attention to the more important type of presentation: the proptosis.

Before continue, our readership should remember that other causes of thickening of the extraocular muscle such as: fatty infiltration of the muscle can also cause a bulging of the eye anteriorly out of the orbit (Graves-Basedow disease) but in those cases we prefer the medical term: exophthalmos. In other words, we reserve the medical terminology of exophthalmos for those cases of protrusion of the eyes related to endocrine dysfunction.

One of the primary symptoms of extraocular cysticercosis is double vision (diplopia) from misalignment of the visual axes, and the pattern of image separation is the key to diagnosing which particular cranial nerve (and extraocular muscle) is involved. Therefore, at this stage is important to know how to approach these patients. Our first recommendation is to break down between monocular (i.e. present with one eye closed) and binocular diplopia (far more common). For causes of monocular diplopia is important to check the ophthalmological function mainly. If binocular diplopia is present then is important to look for: variations on the quality of diplopia through the day (myasthenia gravis), associated endocrinopathy (Graves-Basedow disease), orbital fracture (most likely to cause inferior oblique palsy), orbital tumours, gaze palsy (progressive supranuclear palsy, brainstem disorders, Wernicke's, Miller-Fisher, cavernous sinus syndrome, etc.). If your patient complains of diplopia on looking in one diagonal direction, it is either the same-sided and oriented rectus muscle or the other-sided oppositely-oriented oblique muscle; e.g. diplopia on looking up and right, it is either right superior rectus or left inferior oblique. If your patient complaints of diplopia on looking down and left is either left inferior rectus or right superior oblique. Finally, if you cover up an eye when the patient is complaining of diplopia, the eye that, when covered, takes away the most peripheral image is the problem.

5.1. Proptosis of the eyes secondary to cysticercosis

We use the medical terminology of proptosis when there is a protrusion of one or both eyeballs by at least two millimeters but less than 18 mm, which can be congenital, familial, or due to a pathological condition not secondary to endocrinopathies.

Apart from extraocular cysticercosis as a cause of proptosis other etiologies include: leukemias, orbital cellulitis, meningioma of the sphenoid wing, dacryoadenitis, mucormycosis, dermoid, orbital fracture of the apex, floor, medial wall or zygomatic bone, Duane syndrome, cavernous sinus syndrome, congenital glaucoma, nasopharyngeal angiofibroma, Hand-Schuller-Christian disease, hemangioma, high altitude cerebral edema (proptosis), Beckwith–Wiedemann syndrome, aortic incompetence: manifests as a pulsatile pseudo proptosis, Wegener's granulomatosis and Pfeiffer syndrome.

Proptosis due to cysticercosis has been reported also in children, usually presenting progressive painful protrusion of the eye with redness, lacrimination and diminution of vision [206] but it is an uncommon cause of proptosis in all age groups with reported incidence varying from 0 to 20%, [208-213] some authors say that the commonest cause of proptosis is medial rectus cysticercosis [208] and the frequency of proptosis among other signs of orbital cysticercosis is around 20-30% preceded by ocular motility restriction (60-64%) and followed by diplopia (35-38%) and palpebral ptosis (12-16%). [77]

5.2. Levator palpebrae superioris muscle cysticercosis and palpebral ptosis

The Levator palpebrae superioris originates on the lesser wing of the sphenoid bone, just above the optic foramen. It broadens and becomes the Levator aponeurosis. This portion inserts on the skin of the upper eyelid, as well as the superior tarsal plate. It is a skeletal muscle. The superior tarsal muscle, a smooth muscle, is attached to the levator palpebrae superioris, and inserts on the superior tarsal plate as well. (See figure 7)

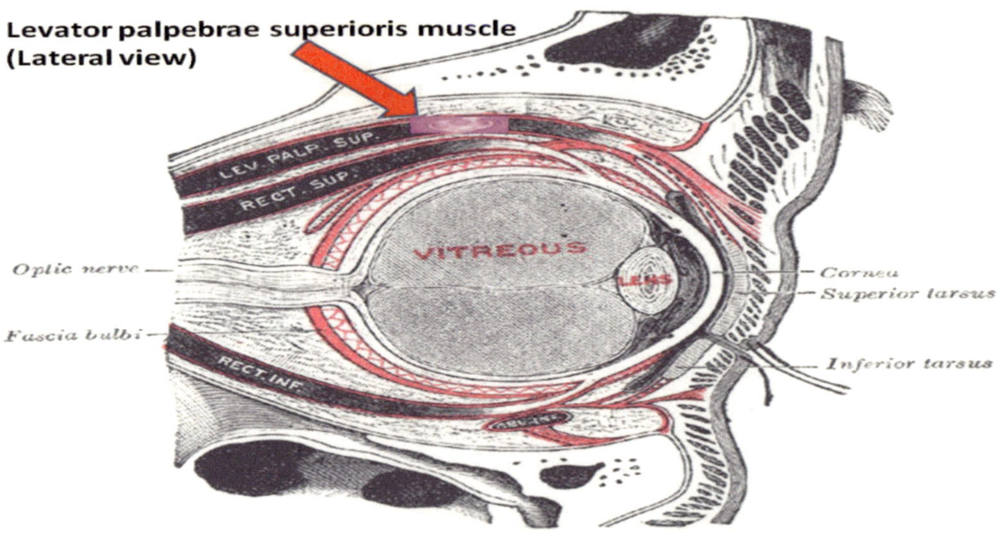

Figure 7. Representation of cysticercosis in the Levator palpebrae superioris.

It is well known that cysticercosis of the extraocular musculature is rare and within this group the affectation of the eyelid is about 0.6% [77] despite the number of patients reported in the medical literature. [214-217] The Levator palpebrae superioris muscle cysticercosis presenting clinically as ptosis is much more uncommon than other affected extraocular muscles. [218, 219]

Cysticercosis of the Levator palpebrae superioris, superior rectus, eyelid or anterior orbit are important differential diagnoses for acquiring ptosis. [219] Features suggestive of Levator palpebrae superioris myocysticercosis include a young patient from an endemic region with a suggestive exposure history, proptosis, mild lid edema or erythema and a palpable cystic eyelid mass. [136] Sekhar et al [78] reported that subconjunctival cyst might be related to ptosis and suggested that the surgical removal of the parasite is a good management.

Only six patients (all from India) have been reported in the medical literature, they had between 9 and 23 years of age and most of some of them complained of unilateral ptosis, inflammation of the upper eyelid and restricted ocular motility while another complained of mild upper eyelid discomfort without display or decreased vision and no lid erythema or edema plus full extraocular movements in all directions of gaze. [14, 29, 218, 219]

There are also other parasitic infestations that can induce ptosis. Echinococcosis [220] and trichuriasis [221] are the two widely mentioned parasitic infestations that can induce ptosis. Therefore neuroimaging studies are useful to distinguish myocysticercosis from other cystic lesions of the extraocular muscles, such as echinocococus granulosus (hydatid cyst), cystic tumors or extraocular myositis with cystic changes. A hydatid cyst lacks a scolex and does not usually demonstrate intense rim enhancement. However, CT may be preferable as intracranial CT can identify cerebral cysticercosis, which was as high as 16.7% in a case series of myocysticercosis. [155] The diagnosis by neuroimagen is important as myocysticercosis responds well to anti-helminthic therapy, while surgical excision is the primary treatment modality for hydatid cysts or tumors. Ultrasound and CT scan appear comparable in ability to detect the scolex. [29, 136]

In patients presenting fluctuating palpebral ptosis with negative neostigmine and electrophysiological tests (pseudo myasthenia) cysticercosis of midbrain should be investigated because focal encephalitis and edema at the midbrain may cause this symptomatology. [222]

Indeed, ocular cysticercosis is not a rare disease in the developing countries, and ptosis due to cysticercosis is sporadically reported [223] but it should keep it mind during the differential diagnosis of unilateral eyelid ptosis.

5.3. Superior rectus muscle cysticercosis

The superior rectus muscle is a muscle in the orbit. It is one of the extraocular muscles. It is innervated by the superior division of the oculomotor nerve (Cranial Nerve III). In the primary position (looking straight ahead), the superior rectus muscle's primary function is elevation, although it also contributes to intorsion and adduction.

Extraocular muscle cysticercosis is the most common site of this parasitic disease when involving the orbit. [224]

In some series of patients with extraocular cysticercosis, the superior rectus muscle is the most commonly affected (33.3%) compared other involved muscles. [77] and clinical features usually are painful unilateral ptosis, inflammation of the upper eyelid and some restriction on down gaze. Diagnosis is made by neuroimagen studies that show a well-defined ring-enhancing lesion in the superior rectus muscle. [14]

Angotti-Neto et al [224] reported a 38-year-old Brazilian female patient with extraocular muscle enlargement and a small cystic lesion near the insertion of the superior rectus muscle treated with oral prednisone for almost one year due to a non-specific inflammation of right orbit diagnosis later confirmed as superior rectus muscle cysticercosis. That report illustrates the consequences of delayed antiparasitic treatment leading to leading to marked hypertrophy and limitation of infraduction and later an incomplete recovery. It also serves to emphasize that cysticercosis should be included in the differential diagnosis of extraocular muscle enlargement, especially in cases of orbital inflammation non-responsive to corticosteroid treatment. Although the differential diagnosis of extraocular muscle enlargement is extensive, including Graves' orbitopathy, myositis, carotid cavernous fistula, lymphoma, metastatic and primary tumors, when associated with other clinical signs such as lid retraction or pain with eye movement, a correct diagnosis can usually be established. [225] Less frequent conditions include arteriovenous fistulas and malformations and orbital tumors. [226]

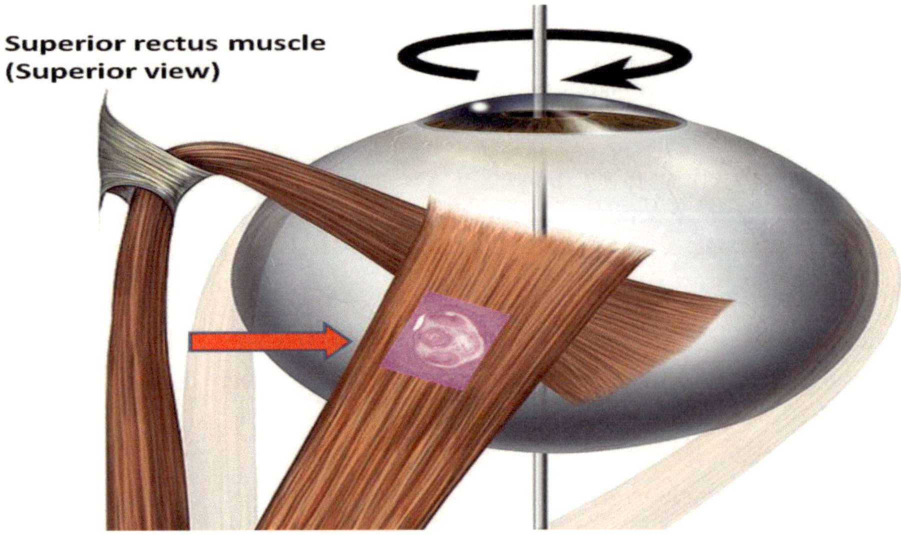

Figure 8. Cysticercus near to insertion of superior rectus muscle in the eyeball.

5.4. Inferior rectus muscle cysticercosis

The inferior rectus muscle is another muscle in the orbit. (See figure x) It depresses, adducts, and helps extort (rotate laterally) the eye. The inferior rectus muscle is the only muscle that is capable of depressing the pupil when it is in a fully abducted position.

An isolated paralysis of the inferior rectus muscle is often congenital in our experience. However, it may also occur following orbital trauma, especially after fracture of the orbital floor; from vascular disease; or in conjunction with myasthenia. [197] The diagnosis is made on the basis of the prism and cover test in the diagnostic positions and an examination of ductions and versions. The deviation is greatest on attempts to look downward with the affected eye in abduction (Fig. 9). The unopposed action of the antagonistic superior rectus muscle causes the paretic eye to be incyclotropic and hypertrophic in primary position. When the patient fixates with the paretic eye in primary position, pseudoptosis may occur in the sound eye, creating diagnostic problems. Ocular torticollis is a frequent occurrence but is not of diagnostic value since the head may be tilted to either side. [197]

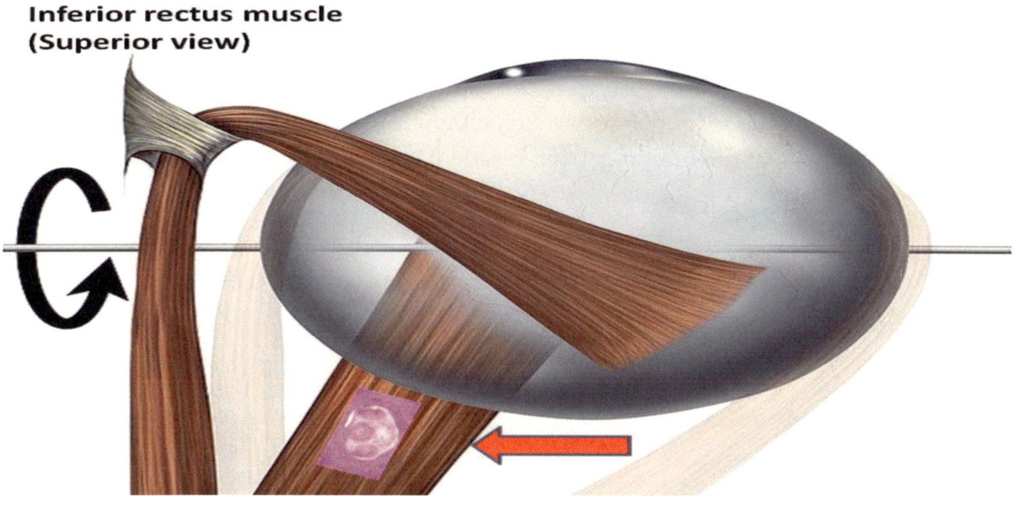

Figure 9. Representation of T solium cysticercosis in the inferior rectus muscle

The inferior rectus muscle was commonly involved in one study. [29] Inferior rectus cysticercosis like other the affected extraocular muscle typically shows fusiform enlargement of its belly and contain a well-defined, spherical cyst with a nodule attached to its wall. This nodule and the enlarged muscle show intense enhancement on the contrast-enhanced studies. [227, 228]

In Meher' series [227] about six patients presenting extraocular muscle cysticercosis two of them had inferior rectus muscle involvement and proptosis for the eyes but imaging studies of the brain showed no evidence of cerebral cysticerci in any of the patients and not palpable subcutaneous nodules were found.

Based on the clinical features of patients reported in the medical literature [229] and our observations, the commonest symptom and signs of the inferior rectus cysticercosis are eccentric proptosis and restriction of upward gaze no associated with loss of vision or painful eyes. MRI orbit is the investigation of choice which can reveal a cystic lesion in the belly of inferior rectus muscle, hypointense on T1 and hyperintense on T2 weighted images and a tiny eccentric hypointense speck suggestive of scolex can be seen.

Shadangi et al [229] have noticed that the cysticerci of the extraocular muscles travel forward, come to lie in a subconjunctival location and then extrude out spontaneously and they have adopted a policy to wait and watch in these cases. They avoid giving steroids and anthelmintic as these suppress inflammation and delay the movement of the cyst outward, and hence, its extrusion. Because delayed treatment can favored chronic inflammatory process, associated fibrosis and permanent damage on the physiology of the muscles, in our opinion, each patient should be assessed individually and a decision should be taken accordingly.

Isolated inferior rectus muscle palsy resulting from a nuclear third nerve lesion as the initial manifestation of multiple sclerosis has been reported in the medical literature. [230]

5.5. Superior oblique muscle cysticercosis

The superior oblique muscle, or obliquus oculi superior, is a fusiform muscle originating in the upper, medial side of the orbit (i.e. from beside the nose) which abducts, depresses and internally rotates the eye. It is the only extraocular muscle innervated by the trochlear nerve (the fourth cranial nerve).

The primary (main) action of the superior oblique muscle is intorsion (internal rotation), the secondary action is depression (primarily in the adducted position) and the tertiary action is abduction (lateral rotation).

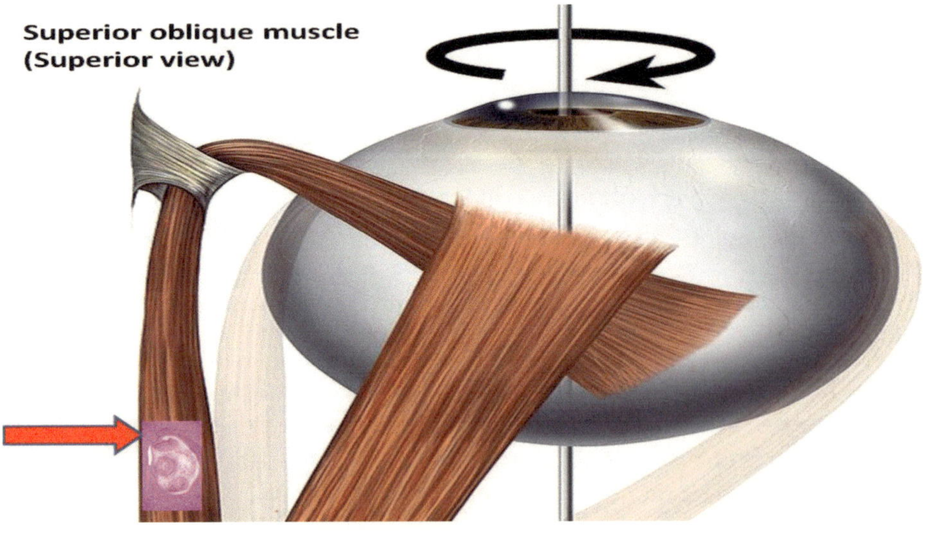

Figure 10. Superior oblique myocysticercosis

The depressing action of the superior oblique (making the eye look down towards the mouth) is most effective when the eye is in an adducted position. This is because as the eye is abducted (looks laterally), the contribution made by superior oblique to depression of the eye decreases, as the inferior rectus muscle causes this movement more directly and powerfully. The main muscle for abduction is the lateral rectus, so although superior oblique contributes to a downwards and lateral eye movement, testing this motion would not be specific enough as inferior and lateral recti muscles would also be tested. Therefore, during neurological examinations, the superior oblique is tested by having the patient look inwards and downwards, testing only the depressing action of the muscle. This is a source of confusion on the subject as although clinical testing asks the patient to adduct and depress the eye, anatomically the muscle depresses and abducts it.

The great importance of intorsion and extorsion produced by the two oblique muscles can only be understood when it is considered with regards to the other muscle actions present. The two obliques prevent the eye from rotating about its long axis (retina to pupil) when the superior and inferior rectus muscles contract. This is because the orbit does not face directly forwards- the centre-line of the orbit is a little over 20 degrees out from the mid-line. But because the eyes do face forwards, when acting alone, as well as making the eye look up, superior rectus causes it to rotate slightly about the long axis, so the top of the eye moves medially (intorsion). Similarly, in addition to making the eye look down, inferior rectus would cause the eye to rotate about the long axis so the top of the eye moves slightly laterally (extortion), if acting alone. Clearly this is undesirable as our vision would rotate when we looked up and down. For this reason, these two rectus muscles work in conjunction with the two obliques. When acting alone, superior oblique causes intorsion, inferior oblique, and extorsion. Hence, when inferior rectus contracts so we look down, superior oblique has also contracted to prevent extorsion of the eye, and when superior rectus contracts so we look up, inferior oblique contracts to prevent intorsion, thus the undesired rotatory actions of the inferior and superior rectus about the long axis of the eye are cancelled out. This keeps our vision horizontally level, irrespective of eye position in the orbit.

In one of the large series of patients presenting extraocular muscle cysticercosis (n=35) the average age was 19.6 years, no differences between female and males were found and the most common clinical feature was restricted ocular motility with diplopia and recurrent pain and redness. [194] In the superior oblique muscle cysticercosis are kept the same demographic and clinical feature described for other extraocular muscles. However, the lateral rectus, medial rectus and the superior oblique were affected to a greater extent and in all cases the extraocular muscle cysticercosis can be suspected in cases of acquired ocular motility disorder with recurrent ocular congestion. Perhaps the most interesting aspect of superior oblique cysticercosis is its clinical presentation as: Brown syndrome and Canine tooth syndrome.

Brown syndrome is defined as an ocular motility disorder, characterized by an inability to elevate the adducted eye actively or passively. In 1950, Harold W. Brown first published on an unusual motility disorder, characterized by the following: limited elevation in adduction; divergence in straight upgaze (V-pattern); same degree of limitation on versions, ductions, and forced ductions; widening of the palpebral fissure on adduction; normal or near normal elevation in abduction; restricted forced ductions to elevation in adduction; and compensatory chin elevation for binocular fusion.

Diplopia may occur when the patient looks up and to the contralateral side of the affected eye. Patients with congenital Brown syndrome rarely complain of diplopia, because most patients have developed suppression. The most common signs of Brown syndrome include:

supranasal orbital pain, tenderness. Limited elevation in adduction, an invariable sign, is the hallmark of Brown syndrome and pain that is associated with this ocular movement. The canine tooth syndrome is an ocular motility disorder comprising ipsilateral Brown's syndrome and superior oblique muscle dysfunction. Ocular motility shows ipsilateral deficit of elevation and depression, maximum in an adducted position. Typically this follows a dog bite (hence the name) that damages the trochlea and superior oblique muscle concurrently but it can be caused by trauma to the trochlear area, producing a "double Brown syndrome"; secondary to strengthening the superior oblique along with a residual superior oblique palsy, or a combination of local trauma to the trochlea causing restriction to upgaze along with closed head trauma producing a trochlear nerve disorder. Trochlear nerve palsy is the most common cause of vertical diplopia then apart from periocular pain, and lid swelling, an upgaze vertical diplopia can be present. [231-242]. Superior rectus muscle cysticercosis should be considered in the differential diagnosis of acquired motility disorder.

Lee and O'Halloran [239] described the case of a 5-year-old girl traumatized from a dog bite to the superior aspect of the orbit in the right eye. The dog's canine tooth penetrated deep into the posterior orbit and severed the attachment of the superior oblique muscle of the globe posterior to the trochlea leading to the clinical presentation before-cited.

The acquired Brown syndrome is known to occur after trauma, iatrogenic events, cysts of superior oblique muscle, tenosynovitis, and systemic lupus erythematosus. [238, 243,244] Although surgical excision and reconstruction of the superior oblique tendon has been reported [230] this aspect will be discussed under the subchapter of treatment.

Rao et al [238] reported seven patients presenting Brown syndrome secondary to superior oblique muscle cysticercosis. All patients had the ocular motility limitation, ie, limitation of elevation in adduction (characteristic of Brown syndrome) and associated pain and swelling in the superior nasal orbit.

5.6. Inferior oblique muscle cysticercosis

The inferior oblique muscle is a thin, 36 mm long narrow muscle placed near the anterior margin of the floor of the orbit. It originates a few millimeters behind the medial end of the inferior orbital rim just lateral to the lacrimal fossa and proceeds posteriorly and temporally at an angle of 51 degrees with the frontal plane passing beneath the inferior rectus (between the inferior rectus and the floor of the orbit) and inserting posterior to the equator on the inferior and lateral aspect of the globe. [204] Its actions are extorsion, elevation and abduction of the eye. The primary action is extorsion; secondary action is elevation; tertiary action is abduction (i.e. It extorts the eye and moves it upward and outwards). The field of maximal inferior oblique elevation is in the adducted position.

This muscle receives its innervation on its upper surface at the point where it passes beneath the lateral border of the inferior rectus, approximately 12 mm posterior to the lateral corner of the insertion of the inferior rectus. The inferior oblique muscle is unique in its anatomic relationships. This muscle behaves as though it has two potential insertions and two potential points of origin. Because the inferior oblique is innervated near its middle, it may be weakened either proximal or distal to its point of innervation.

The inferior oblique muscle is the only muscle that is capable of elevating the eye when it is in a fully adducted position. While commonly affected by palsies of the inferior division of the oculomotor nerve, isolated palsies of the inferior oblique (without affecting other functions of the oculomotor nerve) are quite rare and can be confused with Brown syndrome.

In a series of 25 patients with inferior oblique palsy studied by Pollard [245], all presented with a head tilt to the side of the paretic muscle. None of these patients complained of tilting images, but incyclotorsion was measurable in all cases. The most important conclusion from this study is that inferior oblique palsy is a benign entity, with none of these patients having a brain tumor, myasthenia gravis or cysticercosis.

While many vertical deviations that appear to be due to an inferior oblique palsy based on the results of the three-step test may be caused by inferior oblique weakness, skew deviation should also be considered in any patient with a history of head trauma, or other neurological findings. The cyclotorsion observed in inferior oblique palsy is opposite that seen by the ocular tilt reaction, and differentiates the two entities clinically. We postulate that these deviations are caused by damage to the otolithic projections that correspond to those from the ipsilateral posterior semicircular canal (on the side of the hypotropic eye). [246]

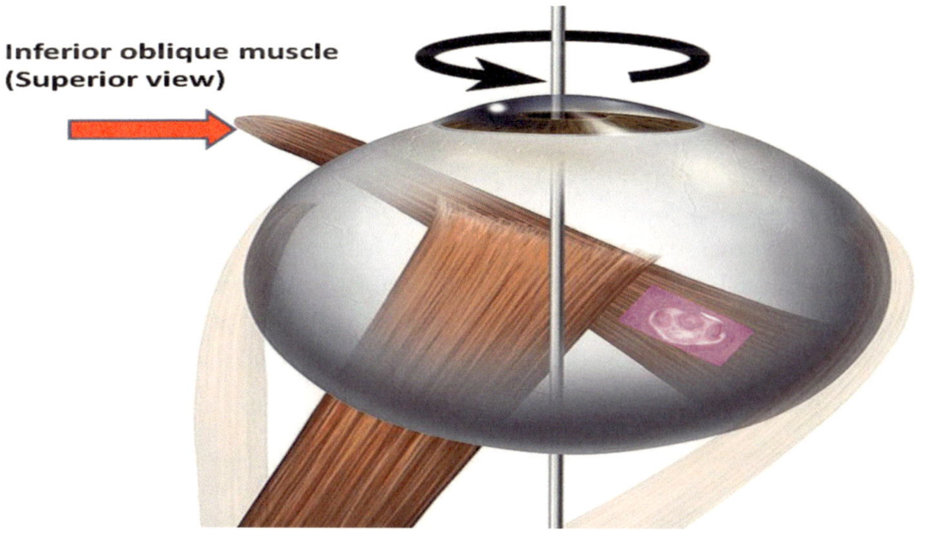

Figure 11. Illustration of inferior oblique muscle cysticercosis close to its insertion in the eyeball.

The common causes of inferior oblique muscle dysfunctions are facial trauma, endoscopic ethmoidectomy, superior oblique muscle palsy (overaction of the inferior oblique muscle), unilateral inferior oblique anterior transposition. [24, 247, 248] Overaction of the inferior oblique muscle is manifest by over the elevation of the adducted eye. It is a common enigma in the field of ocular motility and it may occur secondary to a weak contralateral superior rectus muscle or a weak ipsilateral superior oblique muscle. [248-250]

Based on our experience and an extensive review of the medical literature we conclude that cysticercosis of the inferior oblique muscle practically does not exist in human beings compare with other presentations. Despite the inferior oblique muscle has the same change to be infected by T solium like other extraocular muscles, we think it is rarer than the other because the inferior oblique is unique among the extraocular muscles in that, in many cases, weakening of this muscle, even with extensive surgery, seems to have relatively little effect on the movement of the globe or alignment of the eyes. Therefore isolated cysticercotic lesion on the inferior oblique muscle can be asymptomatic. Even in patients presenting a relatively uncommon inferior oblique paresis due to other causes, strabismus is much less than would occur after paresis of any of the other muscles. Effective weakening of this muscle could be made more difficult because of the unique anatomy. Likewise neurologically, the muscle innervation by the inferior branch of cranial nerve III makes isolated paralysis extremely uncommon. [250]

Of all the extraocular muscles supplied by the oculomotor nerve, the inferior oblique muscle is less likely to become paralyzed. The onset is usually congenital but the trauma has been mentioned as a cause. In primary position the affected eye may be hypotropic or the unaffected eye hypertrophic, depending on whether the patient fixates with the nonparalyzed or paralyzed eye. The greatest deviation occurs when the patient attempts to elevate the adducted paretic eye. Overreaction of the unopposed ipsilateral superior oblique muscle causes incyclotropia. In all patients whom we have evaluated, onset was congenital. As in the case of superior oblique paralysis, the anomalous head posture is more characteristic than in paralyses of the vertical rectus muscles. As a rule the head is inclined toward the paralyzed side, and the face is turned to the uninvolved side, but there are exceptions. The Bielschowsky head tilt test is positive on tilting the head to the normal side. The forced duction test is necessary in making this diagnosis, since the prevalence of Brown syndrome is far greater than paralysis of the inferior oblique muscle and since the defect of ocular motility is clinically similar. However, with Brown syndrome the involved eye is frequently depressed more severely in adduction than it is with inferior oblique paralysis.

5.7. Lateral rectus muscle cysticercosis

Each rectus muscle inserts at a different distance from the limbus. The lateral rectus muscle is one of six extraocular muscles that control the movements of the eye (abduction in this case) and the only muscle innervated by the abducens nerve, cranial nerve VI. Its function is to bring the pupil away from the midline of the body. It is tested clinically by asking the patient to look laterally.

As we before-mentioned the extraocular muscles have differences undoubtedly related to their very specialized function. Both skeletal and extraocular muscles have several types of twitch fibers, but the extraocular muscles are unique, having tonically contracting fibers not found in skeletal muscle. There are two muscle fiber layers in the medial and lateral recti. The shorter orbital layer inserts in the muscle pulley, and the longer global fibers insert into sclera at the muscle's *insertion*. The muscle fibers are long, traversing the entire length of the muscle, or in some cases, nearly so. The medial and lateral extraocular muscles have the lowest innervation ratio of any of the muscles of the body; that is, they have the *most* nerve fibers per muscle fiber which support the stringent requirements of accuracy of fixation and smoothness of following required to support a visual apparatus capable of both rapid, accurate movement and sustained fixation. There is evidence, not always corroborated but accumulating nonetheless, showing that the extraocular muscles participate in proprioception. Muscle spindles and other muscle sensors communicate by means of an *inflow* mechanism which is functional but apparently less powerful than the *outflow* mechanism generated from stimuli arising in the retina. [251]

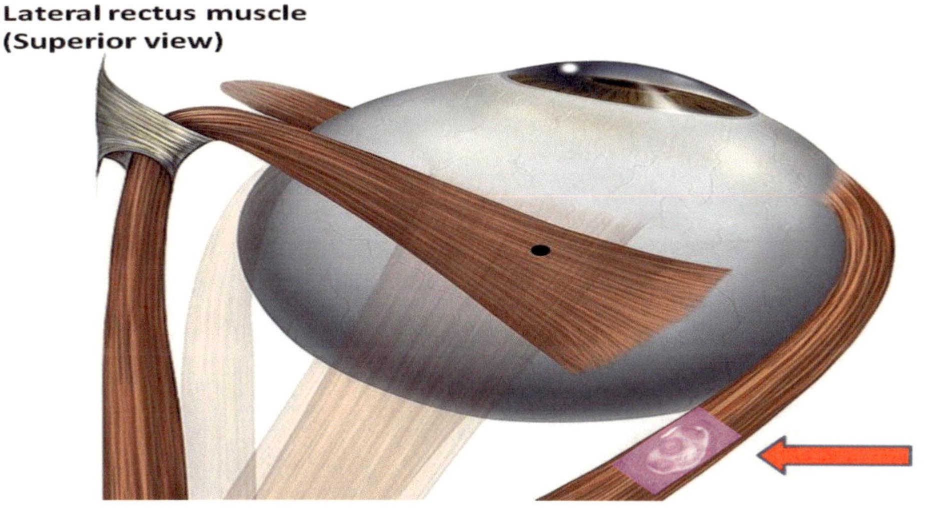

Figure 12. Illustration of the lateral rectus muscle myocysticercosis

Lateral rectus palsy is commonly seen in patients presenting intracranial hypertension due to NCC, because abducen nerves has the longest pathway along to the subarachnoid space and it can be damaged by raise intracranial pressure without focalizing the intracranial lesion. Like other extraocular muscles first clinical symptom is diplopia (horizontal) To differentiate horizontal diplopia secondary to abducen palsy from horizontal diplopia secondary to lateral rectus muscle cysticercosis is an easy task if other symptoms and signs of intracranial hypertension of orbital cysticercosis are present. In our series intracranial hypertension is most commonly seen in patients with intraventricular and subarachnoid NCC whom a complaint of epilepsy, headache, nausea, vomiting, and cognitive dysfunction and they can present meningeal sings and focal neurological signs. Patients with lateral rectus cysticercosis also complaint of proptosis of the affected eyes, painful eye movements and decrease visual acuity due to optic nerve damage. Imagenology studies are extremely useful to confirm the final diagnosis. [251]

With acquired sixth nerve paralysis it is essential to determine whether the restriction of abduction is caused by paralysis of the lateral rectus muscle, contracture of the medial rectus muscle or a combination of both conditions. The estimation of generating muscle force determines whether residual lateral rectus muscle function is present. [251]

To identify the cause of horizontal diplopia due to a lateral rectus muscle lesion or due to abducens palsy, imagenology studies are mandatory. Below, our readership can see the main differences in two well documented patients.

Abducens palsy is commonly seen as part of the clinical feature of intracranial hypertension because its long pathway across to the subarachnoid space but it is non useful as a focal neurological sing. Another multifactorial cause of abducens palsy is MÖBIUS syndrome which is characterized by congenital bilateral abducens paralysis associated with facial diplegia and microglossia.

In May 2012, the previous patient came to the department of ophthalmology in Nelson Mandela Academic Hospital complaining of pain on the left eye, horizontal diplopia, poor vision, and proptosis of the left eye. She was assessed by two of us (MCSC and HFS). Apart from CT scan findings, the ELISA test for Ig G antigen (*Tenia solium)* in the cerebro-spinal fluid was positive. She is still under medical treatment with prednisone and albendazol and responding well to the medications.

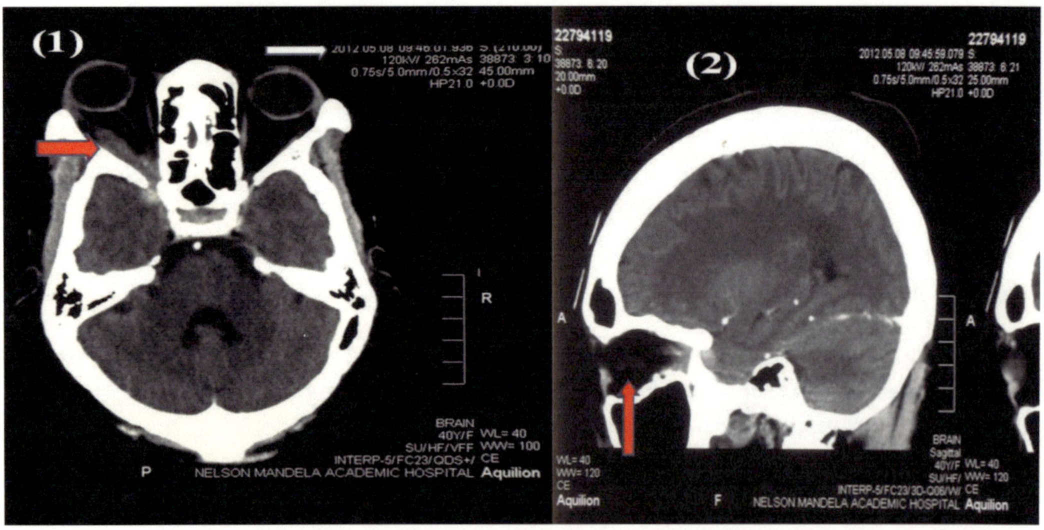

Figure 13. CT scan axial view (1) shows proptosis of the left eyes and lateral rectus myocysticercosis. Intramuscular cyst with "scolex" within is seen. Lateral view (2) shows enlargement of the lateral rectus muscle and an associated intraparenchymal neurocysticercosis (calcified lesions).

Another two patients from our series presented horizontal diplopia secondary to abducens palsy, headache and chronic seizure disorder came to Neurology clinic and CT scans of the brain confirmed intraventricular NCC (2) and subarachnoid NCC (1), in both patients ELISA tests for serum antigen and Western blot were positive for T solium.

Extraocular cysticercosis associated to disseminate cysticercosis including NCC can be seen. It was communicated by Patwardhan and Bhatti. [111] in India. They reported a young male patient presented with a complaint of blurring of vision in the left eye for a few days. Funduscopy examination showed vitreous haze, localized in the lower half, of the vitreous. A clearly defined, spherical, white mass somewhat resembling a dislocated lens, was seen in the vitreous body and anterior to the retina, freely mobile, lying in the lower temporal quadrant. This mass showed occasional contractile waves passing through it. Systemic examination showed the presence of subcutaneous nodules on the scalp , and neck. CT Scan confirmed multiple neurocysticercosis cysts involving superior and medial rectus bilaterally and right lateral rectus.

One or more extraocular muscles may be simultaneously involved, although a propensity for involvement of the superior muscle complex and the lateral rectus muscles has been most commonly reported. [90, 194] As we explained before, according to muscle involved, patients will present different clinical manifestations such as; Brown syndrome, Canine tooth syndrome, Duane retraction, Skew deviation, overreaction, different types of diplopia, painful proptosis. Also acquired strabismus, recurrent redness and some of the clinical signs in patients with orbital cysticercosis can be observed. [70]

5.8. Medial rectus muscle cysticercosis

The medial rectus muscle is a muscle in the orbit. The medial rectus is said to insert in the normal eye 5.5 mm from the limbus.

As with most of the muscles of the orbit, it is innervated by the inferior division of the oculomotor nerve (Cranial Nerve III).

This muscle shares an origin with several other extrinsic eye muscles, the annulus tendineus, or common tendon.

It is the largest of the extraocular muscles and its only action is adduction of the eyeball. Its function is to bring the pupil closer to the midline of the body. It is tested clinically by asking the patient to look medially.

In our experience, an isolated paralysis of the medial rectus muscle due to cysticercosis without involvement of other muscles is very uncommon. In this type of weakness or paralysis the greatest defect of ocular motility occurs when the affected eye goes to adduction position. In the differential diagnosis of an isolated medial rectus paralysis, internuclear ophthalmoplegia is listed.

Cysticercosis as a cause of medial rectus myositis have been reported by others [197, 208, 218, 221, 252- 256] most of patients presented headache, orthotropia in primary gaze, painful drooping of the eyelid, decrease visual acuity, and on examination of the ocular motility, abduction deficit with the resulting horizontal diplopia is found. Sometimes the head of patients turns to the non-paretic side to allow them to attain single binocular vision. The most common extra ocular muscle to get involved in cysticercosis is the medial rectus. [197]

Isolated medial rectus cysticercosis may be associated with ptosis and upper lid retraction on attempted adduction (aberrant regeneration) in patients with partial third nerve paralysis. Medial rectus cysticercosis must be distinguished from internuclear ophthalmoplegia (INO), caused by lesions in the medial longitudinal fasciculus. In this condition unilateral or bilateral limitation of adduction is associated with nystagmus of the abducting eye. Convergence may or may not be normal and we will discuss briefly about this matter below. A clinical picture similar isolated media rectus cysticercosis or INO can be caused by myasthenia gravis but a Tensilon test is diagnostic. Restriction of adduction may be caused by an excessively resected lateral rectus muscle.

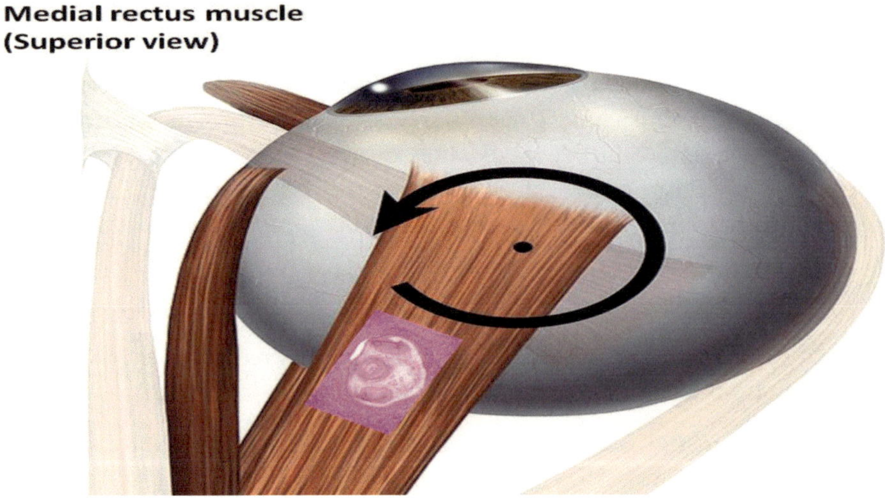

Figure 14. Medial rectus myocysticercosis

One of the most important differential diagnoses of medial rectus palsy cysticercosis is with isolated medial rectus palsy as a sign then clinically is easier to perform. There are an important number of publications related to isolated medial rectus palsy in of midbrain infarction but if impaired adduction of the ipsilateral eye is associated with a bilateral ptosis and normal pupil function midbrain infarction. [259-263]

6. Treatment of extraocular muscle cysticercosis

Contact B-scan ultrasonography was a diagnostic test of cysticercosis in 84.4% of patients [77] but the accuracy of a CT scan and MRI is more than 98% in our series.

Surgical excision of an extraocular muscle cyst had been described [77, 177, 194, 202]. In contrast to medical treatment, surgical excision is technically difficult due to the attachment of the cysts to underlying orbital structures, the amorphous consistency of degenerating cysticerci and the risk to neurovascular structures in the posterior orbit. [29] There is also a likelihood of postoperative restrictive myopathy arising from the fibrotic response in surgical excisions of large cysts or in cysts requiring extensive dissection from the underlying muscle. [215] The potential risk of damage to adjacent tissue and adhesion from surgical exploration should not be taken lightly, particularly when effective medical therapy is available. As a general consent medical treatment with albendazol and prednisone is the best choice taken by most of the authors and recommended duration of treatment varies from a few days to up to 6 weeks. [29, 95,155, 194,197, 204- 208, 218,219, 220, 223, 224, 227-232,237-240, 242, 252, 253,255, 264-266]

In some, cyst elimination rates were more than 90%, and time to recovery of ocular motility ranged between 0.5 and 35 month. [136, 155, 265]

Although oral albendazole and prednisone are efficient, a long history of disease can lead to important residual ocular motility restriction [220] and some author found that oral albendazole and prednisone are not effective thus their role in ocular cysticercosis need to be studied. [256]

In the next figure we summarize the frequency of affected extraocular muscle by cysticercosis.

In some, cyst elimination rates were more than 90%, and time to recovery of ocular motility ranged between 0.5 and 35 month. [136, 155, 265]

Although oral albendazole and prednisone are efficient, a long history of disease can lead to important residual ocular motility restriction [220] and some author found that oral albendazole and prednisone are not effective thus their role in ocular cysticercosis need to be studied. [256]

In the next figure we summarize the frequency of affected extraocular muscle by cysticercosis before medical treatment.

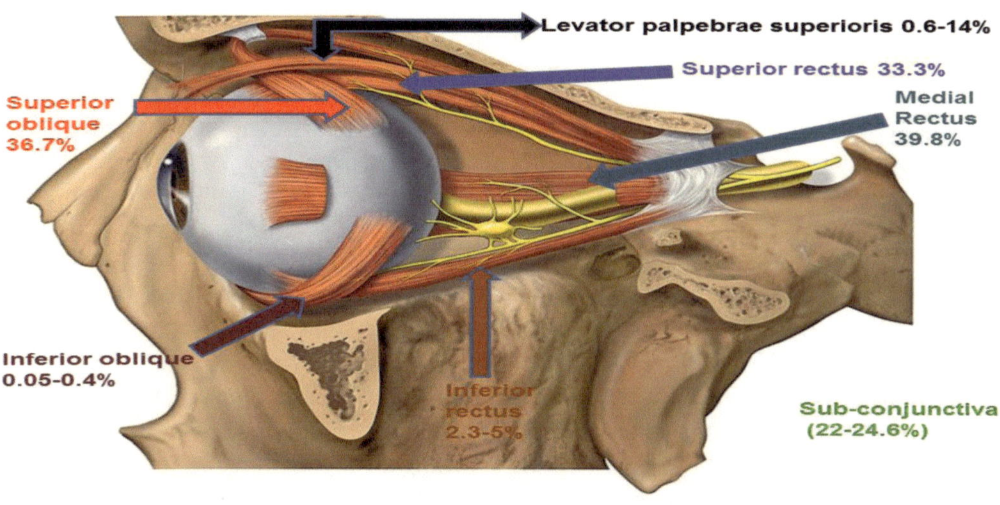

Figure 15. Distribution of extraocular myocysticercosis in the orbital cavity.

7. Conclusion

The cysticercosis of the orbit is an uncommon zoonotic parasitic disease. Its early diagnosis and appropriate treatment avoid the permanent loss of vision. The surgical treatment is the best choice in intraocular cysticercosis while medical treatment is the best choice for extraocular presentations including the extraocular muscles cysticercosis. The adequate knowledge of the anatomy and physiology of the intra orbital content contributes to a better diagnosis. Sometimes the patience helps resolve the conflicts that create the conjunctiva cysticercosis. It must take into account other processes that mimic the orbital cysticercosis in their differential diagnosis. Although it is a rare disease it is a challenge for those health professionals committed to the management of these patients.

Author details

Humberto Foyaca Sibat, María Carolina Salazar Campos
and Lourdes de Fátima Ibañez Valdés
Department of Neurology and Department of Ophthalmology, Nelson Mandela Academic Hospital, Faculty of Health Sciences, Walter Sisulu University, South Africa

Acknowledgement

For understanding my long nights at the computer, I'd like to thank my wife Lourdes de Fátima, who was worked with me on this project; to my first daughter Zayra Susana who died in 1979 but continues inspiring me from wherever she is; to my second daughter Lorna Maria who is a good lawyer and encourages me all the time to continue moving forward, and to my children Fatima Susana Adolfina (3 years old) and Thabo Humberto Jorge (4 years old) for helping me to find peace of mind, persistence and hope every time I needed. My father, my sisters, nephews, nieces, aunts, uncles, cousins and almost all members of my family contributed to this project in one way or another - to all of them: a great Thank You indeed.

8. References

[1] Sotelo J. Neurocysticercosis. Eradication of cysticercosis is an attainable goal. BMJ. 2003;326(7388):511–512.
[2] Hotez PJ; Bottazi ME, Franco-Paredes C, Ault SK, Periago MR. The Neglected Tropical Diseases of Latin America and the Caribbean: A Review of Disease Burden and Distribution and a Roadmap for Control and Elimination. PLoS Neglected Tropical Diseases 2008; 2: e300 doi:10.1371/journal.pntd.0000300.
[3] García HH, Gonzalez AE, Evans CA, Gilman RH; Cysticercosis Working Group in Peru. Taenia solium cysticercosis. Lancet. 2003; 362: 547-556.
[4] García HH, Del Brutto OH; Cysticercosis Working Group in Peru. Neurocysticercosis: updated concepts about an old disease. Lancet Neurol. 2005; 4:653-661.

[5] Román G, Sotelo J, Del Brutto O, Flisser A, Dumas M, Wadia N et al. A proposal to declare neurocysticercosis an international reportable disease. Bull World Health Organ 2000; 78: 399-406.

[6] Sawhney IM, Singh G, Lekhra OP, Mathuriya SN, Parihar PS, Prabhakar S. Uncommon presentations of neurocysticercosis. J Neurol Sci. 1998;154(1):94-100.

[7] Loo L, Braude A: Cerebral cysticercosis in San Diego: a report of 23 cases and review of the literature. Medicine (Baltimore) 1982;61:341-350.

[8] McComick G, Zec Chi-S, Heiden J. Cysticercosis Cerebri. Review of 127 cases. Arch Neurol 1982; 39:534-539.

[9] Carpio A. Neurocysticercosis: an update. Lancet Infect Dis 2002;2:751-762.

[10] Wadia N, Desai S, Bhatt M: Disseminated cysticercosis. New observations, including CT scan findings and experience with treatment by praziquantel. Brain 1988, 111:597-614.

[11] Bhalla A, Sood A, Sachdev A, Varma V. Disseminated cysticercosis: a case report and review of the literature Medical Case Reports 2008; 2:137-140. http://www.jmedicalcasereports.com/content/2/1/137 (accessed May 04, 2012).

[12] Foyaca-Sibat H, Ibanez-Valdes LdeF, Mashiyi MK. Disseminate Cysticercosis. One-day treatment in a case.Rev Electron Biomed / Electron J Biomed 2004;3:39-43. http://biomed.uninet.edu/2004/n3/foyaca-n.html (accessed 05 May,2012).

[13] Park SY, Min HK, Jung HK, Kwan YS. Disseminated cysticercosis. Journal of Korean Neurosurgical Society. 2011;49(3):190-193.

[14] Basu G, Surekha V, Ganesh A. Disseminated cysticercosis. Trop Doct. 2009;39(1):48-99.

[15] Pushker N, Bajaj MS, Balasubramanya R. Disseminated cysticercosis involving orbit, brain and subcutaneous tissue. J Infect. 2005;51(5):245-248.

[16] Narang P, Chhibbers S, Puri SK. Middle-aged man with altered behaviour and seizures. The British Journal of Radiology, 81 (2008), 984–986.

[17] Jakhere SG, Chemburkar VC, Yeragi BS, Bharambay HV. Imaging findings of disseminated cysticercosis with unusual involvement of spleen and pancreas. J Glob Infect Dis. 2011 Jul;3(3):306-308.

[18] Sandeep GJ, Vipul CC, Bhakti SY, Himanshu VB. Imaging Findings of Disseminated Cysticercosis with Unusual Involvement of Spleen and Pancreas. J Glob Infect Dis. 2011;3(3):306–308.

[19] Niakara A, Cisse R, Traore A, Niamba PA, et al. Myocardial localization of a disseminated cysticercosis. Echocardiographic diagnosis of a case. Arch Mal Coer Vaiss 2002;95(6):606-608.

[20] Blandon R, Leandro IM: Human Cardiac cysticercosis. Rev Med Panama. 2002;7- 40.

[21] Foyaca-Sibat H, L. Ibanez-Valdes L: Generalized Cysticercosis With Cardiac Involvement. The Internet Journal of Neurology. 2007 Volume 7 Number 2. http://www.ispub.com/journal/the-internet-journal-of-neurology/volume-7-number-2/generalized-cysticercosis-with-cardiac-involvement.html. (accessed 05 May 2012)

[22] Thomas MB, Thomas KM, Awotedu AA, Blanco-Blanco E, Anwary M. Cardiocysticercosis. S Afr Med J 2007;97(7):504-505.

[23] Eberly MD, Soh EK, Bannister SP, Taraf-Motamen H, Scott JS: Isolated Cardiac Cysticercosis in an adolescent; Pediatr Infect Dis J. 2008; 27(4); 369-71.

[24] Jain BK, Sankhe SS, Agrawal MD, Naphade PS. Disseminated cysticercosis with pulmonary and cardiac involvement. Indian J Radiol Imaging 2010;20:310-313.

[25] Scholtz L & Mentis H, Pulmonary cysticercosis. SAMT 1987 ;72(17) :573

[26] Mamere AE, Muglia VF, Simao GN, Belucci AD, Carlos dos Santos A, Trad CS, et al. Disseminated cysticercosis with pulmonary involvement. J Thorac Imaging 2004;19:109–111.

[27] Banu A, Veena N. A rare case of disseminated cysticercosis: Case report and literature review. Case Report. 2011;29(2):180-183.

[28] Sekhar GC, Honavar SG. Myocysticercosis: experience with imaging and therapy. Ophthalmology. 1999;106(12):2336-2340.

[29] Bhigjee AI. Disseminated cysticercosis. J Neurol Neurosurg Psychiatry 1999;66(4):545

[30] Thomas MB, Thomas KM, Awotedu AA, Blanco-Blanco E, Anwary M. Cardiocysticercosis. South Africa Medical Journal. 2007; 97(7): 504-505

[31] Sobnach S, Khosa SA, Pather S, Longhurst S, Kahn D, Raubenheimer PJ. First case report of pharyngeal cysticercosis. Trans R Soc Trop Med Hyg. 2009;103(2):206-208.

[32] White AC Jr. Neurocysticercosis: updates on epidemiology, pathogenesis, diagnosis and management. Ann Rev Med 2000;51:187-206.

[33] Foyaca-Sibat H. Epilepsy Secondary to Parasitic Zoonoses of the Brain, Novel Aspects on Epilepsy, Humberto Foyaca-Sibat (Ed.), ISBN: 978-953-307-678-2, InTech, Rijeka, 2011.

[34] Sarti E, Schantz PM, Plancharte A, Wilson M, Gutierrez R, Lopez AS, Roberts J, Flisser. Prevalence and risk factor for Taenia solium taeniasis and cysticercosis in humans and pigs in a village in Morelos, Mexico. Am J Trop Med Hyg 1992; 46:677-684.

[35] Garg RK. Neurocysticercosis. Postgrad Med J 1998; 74(872):321-326.

[36] Schantz PM, Moore AC, Muñoz JL, et al.: Neurocysticercosis in an Orthodox Jewish community in New York City. N England J Med 1992;327:692-696.

[37] Rousseau MC, Guillotel B, Delmont J. Neurocysticercosis in the South-East of France 1988-1998. Presse Med 1999;28(39):2141-2144.

[38] O'Neal S, Noh J, Wilkins P, Keene W, Lambert W, Anderson J, Compton Luman J, Townes J. Taenia solium Tapeworm Infection, Oregon, 2006-2009. Emerg Infect Dis. 2011 Jun;17(6):1030-1036.

[39] Kelesidis T, Tsiodras S. Extraparenchymal neurocysticercosis in the United States: a case report. Journal of Medical Case Reports 2011;5:359 .

[40] Serpa JA, Graviss EA, Kass JS, White AC Jr. Neurocysticercosis in Houston, Texas: an update. Medicine (Baltimore). 2011;90(1):81-86.

[41] Wallin M, Kurtzke J. Neurocysticercosis in the United States: review of an important emerging infection. Neurology 2004; 63: 1559-1564.

[42] Pawlowski ZS. Control of neurocysticercosis by routine medical and veterinary services. Trans R Soc Trop Med Hyg 2008;102:228-232.

[43] Takayanagui OM, Odashima NS. Clinical aspects of neurocysticercosis. Parasitol Int. 2006;55:S111–S115.

[44] Sánchez L, Abad L, Lozano E, Maldonado G. Neurocisticercosis intraventricular. Presentación de un caso localizado en el tercer ventriculo. Radiologia. 2002;44:309-313.

[45] Amaral L, Maschietto M, Maschietto R, Cury R, Ferreira NF, Mendonça R, et al. Unusual manifestations of neurocysticercosis in MR imaging : analysis of 172 cases. Arq Neuropsiquiatr. 2003;61:533–541.

[46] Sarti E. La taeniasis y cisticercosis en México (revisión bibliográfica). Salud Pública Mex 1986; 28:556-563.

[47] Rabiela MT, Lombardo L, Flores F. Cisticercosis cerebral. Estudio de 68 casos de autopsia. Patología (Mex) 1972; 10:27-40.

[48] Lopez-Hernández A, Garaizar C. Childhood Cerebral Cysticercosis: clinical features and computed tomographic findings in 98 Mexican children. Can J Neurol SC 1982;9:401-407.

[49] Flisser A. Neurocysticercosis in Mexico. Parasitol Today.1988; 4:131-137.

[50] Sotelo J, Penagos P, Escobedo F, Del Brutto OH: Short course of albendazole therapy for neurocysticercosis. Arch Neurol. 1988;45:1130-1133.

[51] Agapejev S. Epidemiology of Neurocysticercosis. in Brazil. Rev Inst Med Trop Sao Paulo 1996;38(3):207-216.

[52] Ramírez G, Pradilla G, Rodríguez M, González C. Cisticercosis. Estudio de 80 casos. Acta Med Colombiana 1986;11:62-73.

[53] Botero D. Cisticercosis en Colombia. Investigaciones realizadas hasta 1988. An Acad Med Medellin 1989;2(II):75-82.

[54] Takayanagui OM, Jardim E. Clinical aspects of nerocysticercosis: analysis of 500 cases. Arq Neuropsiquiatr 1983; 41(1):50-63.

[55] White AC Jr. Neurocysticercosis: updates on epidemiology, pathogenesis, diagnosis and management. Ann Rev Med 2000;51:187-206.

[56] Foyaca-Sibat H, Del Rio AR, Ibañez-Valdés LdeF, Vega-Novoa EC, Awotedu A. "Neuroepidemiological survey for Epilepsy and knowledge about neurocysticercosis at Sidwadweni location, South Africa" Electron J Biomed 2004;2(1):40-48. http://www.biomed.edu/2004/n1/foyaca.html

[57] Foyaca-Sibat H, Del Rio-Romero AH, Ibañez-Valdés LdeF, Vega-Novoa E. Neuroepidemiological Survey For Epilepsy And Knowledge About Neurocysticiercosis At Ngqwala Location, South Africa. The Internet Journal of Neurology 2005 3(2). http://www.ispub.com/journal/the_internet_journal_of_neurology/volume_3_number_2_31/article/neuroepidemiological_survey_for_epilepsy_and_knowledge_about_neurocysticiercosis_at_ngqwala_location_south_africa.html

[58] Foyaca-Sibat H, A. Del Rio-Romero, Ibañez-Valdés LdeF : Prevalence Of Epilepsy And General Knowledge About Neurocysticercosis At Ngangelizwe Location, South Africa . The Internet Journal of Neurology. 2005 Volume 4 Number 1. http://www.ispub.com/journal/the_internet_journal_of_neurology/volume_4_number_1_30/article/prevalence_of_epilepsy_and_general_knowledge_about_neurocysticercosis_at_ngangelizwe_location_south_africa.html

[59] Foyaca-Sibat H, Del Rio A: "Epilepsy, Neurocysticercosis and, Poverty at Mphumaze and Marhambeni Locations, in South Africa". The Internet Journal of Neurology (ISSN: 1531-295X). 2007;7(1):8-14.

http://www.ispub.com/journal/the_internet_journal_of_neurology/volume_7_number_1_7/article/epilepsy_neurocysticercosis_and_poverty_at_mphumaze_and_marhambeni_locations_in_south_africa.html

[60] Foyaca-Sibat H, Ibañez-Valdés LdeF, Del Rio IA: "Prevalence of Epilepsy and General Knowledge about Neurocysticercosis at Ngangelizwe Location, South Africa". The Internet Journal of Neurology.(ISSN: 1531-295X). 2005; 4(1):23-37. http://www.ispub.com/journal/the_internet_journal_of_neurology/volume_4_number_1_30/article/prevalence_of_epilepsy_and_general_knowledge_about_neurocysticercosis_at_ngangelizwe_location_south_africa.html

[61] Foyaca-Sibat H, Del Rio- Romero AI: "Prevalence Of Epilepsy In An Endemic Area For Neurocysticercosis In South Africa". The Internet Journal of Neurology.(ISSN: 1531-295X). 2008;9(1):8-18. http://www.ispub.com/journal/the_internet_journal_of_neurology/volume_9_number_1_6/article/prevalence_of_epilepsy_in_an_endemic_area_for_neurocysticercosis_in_south_africa.html

[62] Turkulov V, madle-Samardzija N, Canak G, Vukadinov J, Aleksic-Dordevic M. Clinical and diagnostic approaches to neurocysticercosis. Med Pregl 2001; 54(7-8):353-356.

[63] Chimelli L, Lovalho AF, Takayanagui OM. Neurocysticercosis: contribution of autopsies in the consolidated of mandatory notification in Ribeirao Preto-SP, Brazil. Arq Neuropsiquiatr 1998; 56(3B):577-584.

[64] Sanchez AL, Ljungstrom I, Medina MT. Diagnosis of human neurocysticercosis in endemic countries: clinical study in Honduras. Parasitol Int 1999;48(1):81-89.

[65] Foyaca-Sibat H, Ibañez-Valdés LdeF & J. Moré-Rodríguez : Parasitic Zoonoses Of The Brain: Another Challenger?. The Internet Journal of Neurology. 2010 Volume 12 Number 2. http://www.ispub.com/journal/the_internet_journal_of_neurology/volume_12_number_2_4/article/parasitic-zoonoses-of-the-brain-another-challenger.html

[66] Foyaca-Sibat H and Ibañez-Valdés L de F. (2011). Treatment of Epilepsy Secondary to Neurocysticercosis, Novel Treatment of Epilepsy, Humberto Foyaca-Sibat (Ed.), ISBN: 978-953-307-667-6, InTech, Available from: http://www.intechopen.com/articles/show/title/treatment-of-epilepsy-secondary-to-neurocysticercosis

[67] Foyaca-Sibat H.(2011). Epilepsy Secondary to Parasitic Zoonoses of the Brain. Novel Aspects on Epilepsy, Humberto Foyaca-Sibat (Ed.), ISBN: 978-953-307-678-2, InTech, Available from: http://www.intechopen.com/articles/show/title/epilepsy-secondary-to-parasitic-zoonoses-of-the-brain

[68] Murthy GR, Rao AV. Sub-conjunctival cysticercosis. Indian J Ophthalmol. Jul 1980;28(2):77-78.

[69] Menon-Mehta S. Ocular Cysticercosis Treatment & Management. eMedicine.2011http://emedicine.medscape.com/article/1204683-treatment

[70] Ziaei M, Elgohary M, Bremner FD. Orbital cysticercosis, case report and review. Orbit. Oct 2011;30(5):230-235.

[71] Ratra D, Phogat Ch, Singh M, Choudhari NS : Intravitreal cysticercosis presenting as neovascular glaucoma. Indian J Ophthalmol. 2010;58(1):70–73.

[72] Kruger-Leite E, Jalkh AE, Quiroz H, Schepens CL. Intraocular cysticercosis. Am J Ophthalmol 1985; 99(3):252-257.
[73] Topilow HW, Yimoyines DJ, Freeman HM, et al. Bilateral multifocal intraocular cysticercosis. Ophthalmology. 1981;88(11):1166-1172..
[74] Kapoor S, Kapoor MS. Ocular cysticercosis. J Pediatr Ophthalmol Strabismus. May-Jun 1978;15(3):170-173..
[75] Sharma T, Sinha S, Shah N, et al. Intraocular cysticercosis: clinical characteristics and visual outcome after vitreoretinal surgery. Ophthalmology. May 2003;110(5):996-1004.
[76] Rath S, Honavar SG, Naik M, Anand R, Agarwal B, Krishnaiah S et al. Orbital cysticercosis: clinical manifestations, diagnosis, management, and outcome. Ophthalmology 2010; 117(3):600-5, 605.
[77] Sekhar GC, Lemke BN. Orbital cysticercosis. Ophthalmology 1997; 104(10):1599-1604.
[78] Natarajan S, Malpani A, Kumar NP, Dutta B. Management of intraocular cysticercosis. Graefes Arch Clin Exp Ophthalmol 1999; 237(10):812-814.
[79] Reddy PS, Satyendran OM. Ocular cysticercosis. Am J Ophthalmol 1964;57:664-667
[80] Malik SR, Gupta AK, Choudhry S. Ocular cysticercosis. Am J Ophthalmol 1968;66:1168-1171
[81] Sen DK, Mathur RN, Thomas A. Ocular cysticercosis in India. Br J Ophthalmol 1967;51:630-632
[82] Rao N, Balakrishnan E. Cysticercosis of the eye. Orient Arch Ophthalmol 1967;5:249-252.
[83] Reddy CC, Gupta VP, Sarada P, Prabhakar V, Reddy DL, Anjaneyulu C. Ocular cysticercosis: A study of 15 cases. Indian J Ophthalmol 1980;28:69-72
[84] Sen DK Cysticercosis cellulosae in the lacrimal gland. orbit end eye lid Acta Ophthalmalogica 1980;58:144-147.
[85] Murthy GR, Rao AV. Sub-conjunctival cysticercosis. Indian J Ophthalmol. 1980;28(2):77-78.
[86] Sud RN, Grewal SS Spontaneous expulsion of subconjunctival cysticercosis cellulose, Afro Asian J Ophthalmology 1982;13:82-83.
[87] Nath K, Gogi R, Zaidi N, Johri A. Cystic lesions of conjunctiva (A clinico-pathological study). Indian J Ophthalmology 1983; 31 (1): 1-4.
[88] Honavar SG, Sekhar CG. Ultrasonological characteristics of extraocular cysticercosis. Orbit. Dec 1998;17(4):271-284.
[89] Bansal RK, Gupta A, Grewal S, Mohan K. Spontaneous extrusion of cysticercosis : Report of three cases. Indian J Ophthalmol 1992;40:59-60 Available from: http://www.ijo.in/text.asp?1992/40/2/59/24401
[90] Raina UK, Taneja S, Lamba PA, Bansal RL. Spontaneous extrusion of extraocular cysticercus cysts. Am J Ophthalmol 1996;121:438-41.
[91] Magu, S., Nada, M., Khurana, A.K., Chugh, J.P. Spontaneous extrusion of subconjunctival cysticercus cellulosae. British Journal of Ophthalmology. 2000;85(1): 116-117 .
[92] David S, Mathai E. Ocular cysticercosis-a review of 25 cases. J Assoc Physicians India 2000;48:704-707.

[93] Raina, U.K., Jain, S., Arora, R., Mehta, D.K., Sharma, V.Photographic documentation of spontaneous extrusion of a subconjunctival cysticercus cyst. Clinical and Experimental Ophthalmology. 2002; 30(5): 361-362.

[94] Mohan K, Saroha V, Sharma A, et al. Extraocular muscle cysticercosis: clinical presentations and outcome of treatment. J Pediatr Ophthalmol Strabismus. Jan-Feb 2005;42(1):28-33..

[95] Chand K, Srivastava SK. Spontaneous expulsion of subconjunctival Cysticercus cellulosae. MJAFI. 2006;62:188-9.

[96] Kaur A, Agrawal A, Agrawal PK, et al. Lacrimal canalicular obstruction by cysticercus cellulosae. Orbit. Jun 2006;25(2):163-165.

[97] Reddy B, Raj, Maurya, A.Spontaneous extrusion of subconjuntival cysticercosis. Annals of Ophthalmology. 2007;39(3): 241-242

[98] Mehdi G, Ansari HA, Akhtar K, Shukla M.Ocular manifestations of cysticercosis: a case report. Indian J Pathol Microbiol. 2007;50(2):345-346

[99] Lesh Jr. Ocular cysticercosis. Am J Ophthalmol 1949;32:523-526

[100] Duke-Elder S, Perkins ES. System of Ophthalmol. Diseases of uveal tract. CV Mosby: St. Louis; 1966;11:478-488.

[101] Hutton WL Vaiser A. Svnder WB. Pars plana vitrectomy for removal of intravitreous cysticercosis Am J Ophthalmol 1976;81:571-573

[102] Messner KH, Kammerer WS. Intraocular cysticercosis. Arch Ophthalmol. Jun 1979;97(6):1103-5.

[103] Wood TR, Binder PS. Intravitreal and intracameral cysticercosis. Ann Ophthalmol. Jul 1979;11(7):1033-1036

[104] Topilow HW, Yimoyines DJ, Freeman HM, et al. Bilateral multifocal intraocular cysticercosis. Ophthalmology. Nov 1981;88(11):1166-72. (repetido en 77)

[105] Welsh NH, Peters AL, Crewe-Brown W, Blignaut P, Donnoli P, da Souza BS, et al Ocular cysticercosis. A report of 13 cases. S Afr Med J 1987;71:719-722

[106] Susanna S, King W, Alan H, Friedman, Fredrick AJ. Infectious causes of posterior uveitis. In : principles and practice of Ophthalmology-clinical practice. Albert DM, [108]

[107] Seo MS, Woo JM, Park YG. Intravitreal cysticercosis. Korean J Ophthalmol. Jun 1996;10(1):55-59

[108] Adegbehingbe BO, Soetan EO, Adeoye AO. Case report: intraocular cysticercosis. West Afr J Med. Dec 2003;22(4):354-355.

[109] Natarajan S, Malpani A, Kumar Nirmalan P, Dutta B. Management of intraocular cysticercosis. Graefes Arch Clin Exp Ophthalmol. Oct 1999;237(10):812-4.

[110] Patwardhan N, Bhatti SS. Intra-ocular cysticercosis. A case report. Journal of the Bombay Ophthalmologists' Association. 2000;10(3):161-164.

[111] Sharma T, Sinha S, Shah N, et al. Intraocular cysticercosis: clinical characteristics and visual outcome after vitreoretinal surgery. Ophthalmology. May 2003;110(5):996-1004

[112] Ziaei M, Elgohary M, Bremner FD. Orbital cysticercosis, case report and review. Orbit. 2011 Oct;30(5):230-235.

[113] Honavar SG, Sekhar CG. Ultrasonological characteristics of extraocular cysticercosis. Orbit. 1998;17(4):271-284.

[114] Kaur A, Agrawal A, Agrawal PK, et al. Lacrimal canalicular obstruction by cysticercus cellulosae. Orbit. 2006;25(2):163-165.

[115] Pushker, N., Bajaj, M.S., Betharia, S.M. Orbital and adnexal cysticercosis. Clinical and Experimental Ophthalmology. 2002; 30(5): 322-333.

[116] Madigubba S, Vishwanath K, Reddy G, Vemuganti GK. Changing trends in ocular cysticercosis over two decades: An analysis of 118 surgically excised cysts. Indian J Med Microbiol 2007;25:214-219. Available from: http://www.ijmm.org/text.asp?2007/25/3/214/34761 (Accessed on June 09, 2012)

[117] Schmidt M, Schmidt T, Ugi I.Orbital metastasis of kidney carcinoma. Klin Monbl Augenheilkd. 1994 Jul;205(1):40-43.

[118] Konya E, Hara Y, Umekawa T, Uejima S, Sugiyama T, Kurita T. Two cases of renal cell carcinoma detected by metastasis to another organ. Hinyokika Kiyo. 1997;43(9):647-650.

[119] Zdinak LA, Nik NA, Hidayat AA, Hargett NA. Renal medullary carcinoma metastatic to the orbit: a clinicopathologic report. Ophthal Plast Reconstr Surg. 2004 Jul;20(4):322-5.

[120] Sharma K, Verma A, Rathi B, Kumar R, Kanaujia V. Metastatic tumor of orbit presenting as pulsatile proptosis. Ann Ophthalmol (Skokie). 2006 Spring;38(1):69-72.

[121] Shome D, Honavar SG, Gupta P, Vemuganti GK, Reddy PV. Metastasis to the eye and orbit from renal cell carcinoma--a report of three cases and review of literature. Surv Ophthalmol. 2007 Mar-Apr;52(2):213-23.

[122] Mudiyanselage SY, Prabhakaran VC, Davis GJ, Selva D. Metastatic renal cell carcinoma presenting as a circumscribed orbital mass. Eur J Ophthalmol. 2008;18(3):483-485.

[123] Mancini V, Battaglia M, Lucarelli G, Di Lorenzo V, Ditonno P, Bettocchi C, Selvaggi FP. Unusual solitary metastasis of the ciliary body in renal cell carcinoma. Int J Urol. 2008 ;15(4):363-365.

[124] Preechawai P, Amrith S, Yip CC, Goh KY.Orbital metastasis of renal cell carcinoma masquerading as cysticercosis. Orbit. 2008;27(5):370-373.

[125] Alasil T, Khazai B, Loredo L, Rauser ME. Renal cell carcinoma metastasis to the ciliary body responds to proton beam radiotherapy: a case report. J Med Case Rep. 2011;3;5:345

[126] Zubler MA, Rivera R, Lane M. Hepatoma presenting as a retro-orbital metastasis. Cancer. 1981;48(8):1883-1885.

[127] Wakisaka S, Tashiro M, Nakano S, Kita T, Kisanuki H, Kinoshita K. Intracranial and orbital metastasis of hepatocellular carcinoma: report of two cases. Neurosurgery. 1990 ;26(5):863-866.

[128] Font RL, Maturi RK, Small RG, Garcia-Rojas M. Hepatocellular carcinoma metastatic to the orbit. Arch Ophthalmol. 1998 Jul;116(7):942-945.

[129] Barbat V, Morin Y, Metge F, Hamard H. Hepatocellular carcinoma: a case revealed by metastatic orbital tumor. Rev Med Interne. 2000;21(1):86-90.

[130] Gupta R, Honavar SG, Vemuganti GK. Orbital metastasis from hepatocellular carcinoma. Surv Ophthalmol. 2005;50(5):485-489.

[131] Fonseca Júnior NL, Frizon L, Paves L, Wolosker AM, Manso PG. An unusual orbital metastatic lesion: the only finding in a case of hepatocellular carcinoma: case report. Arq Bras Oftalmol. 2008 Nov-Dec;71(6):865-867.

[132] Danis P.: Intraocular cysticercus. Arch Ophthalmol 91: 238-9 1974.

[133] George T, Mathai A, Challa JK, Braganza A, Thomas R.Intravitreal cysticercosis: w did it get there?. Aust N Z J Ophthalmol. May:26(2): 159-60, 1998.

[134] Bajaj MS, Pushker N.: Optic nerve cysticercosis. Clin Experiment Ophthalmol. Apr; 30 (2): 140-3, 2002.

[135] Pushker N, Bajaj MS, Chandra M, Neena. Ocular and orbital cysticercosis. Actathalmol Scand. 2001;79 (4):408-413.

[136] Sharma T, Sinha S, Shah N et al.: Intraocular cysticercosis: clinical characteristics visual outcome after vitreoretinal surgery. Ophthalmology. May; 110(5); 996-1004,2003.

[137] Sachdeva RS, Manchada SK,et al: Freely mobile cysticercus in the anterior chamber. Indian J Ophthalmol 43: 135-6, 1995.

[138] Barraquer J: Lens extraction and extraction of the cysticercus. Annual meeting of AAO and Otolaringology. New York Oct 23, 1963.

[139] Gross J, Gross FJ, Friedman A. Sistemic Infectious and Inflammatory Diseases. In Tasman w and Jaeger EA, eds. Duane`s Clinical Ophthalmology .Philadelphia. JB Lippincott 1995.

[140] Wender JD, Rathinam SR, Shaw RE, Cunningham ET Jr. Intraocular cysticercosis: case series and comprehensive review of the literature. Ocul Immunol Inflamm. 2011;19(4):240-245.

[141] Chung GW, Lai WW, et al.: Magnetic resonance imaging in the diagnosis of subretinal cysticercosis. Am J Ophthalmol 2002;134 (6): 931-932.

[142] Chowdhary A, Bansal R, Singh K, Singh V.: Ocular cysticercosis- -a profile. Trop Doct. 2003;33(3): 185-188.

[143] David S, Mathai E.: Ocular cysticercosis: a review of 25 cases. J Assoc Physicians India. 2000;;48(7):704-707.

[144] Cano MR.: Ocular Cysticercosis. In Ryan SJ: Retina third edition volume II, Medical Retina. St Louis Mosby chapter 92 (1553-1556) 2001.

[145] George T, Mathai A, Challa JK, Braganza A, Thomas R.: Intravitreal cysticercosis: How did it get there?. Aust N Z J Ophthalmol. 1998;26(2):159-160.

[146] Sloan L et al: Evaluation of enzyme-linked immunoassay for serological diagnosis of cysticercosis. J Clin Microbiol 1995;33:3124.

[147] Sabrosa NA, Zajdenweber M.: Nematode infections of the eye: toxocariasis, onchocerciasis, diffuse unilateral subacute neuroretinitis and cysticercosis. Ophthalmol Clin North Am. 2002;15(3): 351-356.

[148] Sachdeva RSD, Manchanda SK, Abrol S, Wadhwa SC, Ramachandran KA. Freely mobile cysticercus in the anterior chamber. Indian J Ophthalmol 1995;43:135-136.

[149] Wender JD, Rathinam SR, Shaw RE, Cunningham ET Jr. Intraocular cysticercosis: case series and comprehensive review of the literature. Ocul Immunol Inflamm. 2011;19(4):240-245.

[150] Malik SRK, Gupta AK, Chowdhary S. Ocular cysticercoisis. Am J Ophthalmol 1968;66:1168-1171

[151] Mathur RN, Abraham L. Cysticercosis of the eye. Arch Ophthalmol 67:562-563, 1962

[152] Gemmel MA. Immunology and regulation of cestode zoonosis. In: Immunology of Parasitic Infections, 2nd ed., Cohen S, Sadun EH, eds. London, Blackwell Scientific Publication, 1982

[153] Chandra A, Singh MK, Singh VP, et al. A live cysticercosis in anterior chamber leading to glaucoma secondary to pupilary block. J Glaucoma. Mar 2007;16(2):271-273.

[154] Adegbehingbe BO, Soetan EO, Adeoye AO. Case report: intraocular cysticercosis. West Afr J Med. 2003;22(4):354-355.

[155] SihotaR, Honavar SG. Oral albendazole inthe managementofextraocular cysticercosis. Br J Ophthalmol 1994;78:621-3.

[156] Kruger Leite E, Jalkh AE, Quiroz H Scheppens; CL Intraocular cysticercosis Am J Ophthalmol 1985;99: 252-257

[157] Mais FA. Cryosurgery in ocular cysticercosis. Rev Bras Ophthalmol. 1969;28:99–106

[158] Wittig EO. Ocular cysticercosis—an epidemiological study. Arq Neuropsiquiatr. 2001;59:696–701

[159] Graefe's Archive for Clinical and Experimental Ophthalmology. August 1996, Volume 234, Issue 8, pp 515-520

[160] Proctor N. Tapeworm cyst infestation. Med Proc 1964; 10: 168-171.

[161] Pammenter MD, Rossouw EV. Serological tests for the diagnosis of cysticercosis. S Afr Med j 1984;65:875-878.

[162] Keane JR. Neuro-ophthalmologic signs and symptoms of cysticercosis. Arch Ophthalmol 1982; 100: 1445-1448.

[163] Foyaca-Sibat H Cowan LD, Carabin H, Serrano-Ocaña G, , Krecek RC, Willingham A. "Accuracy of serological exam for the diagnosis of neurocysticercosis in outpatients with epilepsy, Eastern Cape Province, South Africa" PLOS Negleted Trop.Dis.Dec.2009;3(3):1-7

[164] Welsh N, Proctor E. Taenia solium in the anterior chamber. Aust j Ophthalmol . 1977; 1: 73-76.

[165] Aracena T, Roca FP. Macula and peripheral subretinal cysticercosis. Ann Ophthalmol 1981; 13: 1265-1267.

[166] Santos R, Chavarria M, Aguirre A. Failure of medical treatment in two cases on intraocular cysticercosis. Amy Opthalmol 1984;97:249-250

[167] Hutton WL Vaiser A. Svnder WB Pars plana vitrectomy for removal of intravitreous cysticercosis Am J Ophthalmol 1976;81:571-573

[168] Das JC, Chaudhuri Z, Bansal RL, et al. Viscoexpression of anterior chamber cysticercus cellulosae. Indian J Ophthalmol. Jun 2002;50(2):133-135.

[169] Beri S, Vajpayee RB, Dhingra N, et al. Managing anterior chamber cysticercosis by viscoexpression: a new surgical technique. Arch Ophthalmol. 1994;112(10):1279-1280.

[170] Atul K, Kumar TH, Mallika G, et al. Socio-demographic trends in ocular cysticercosis. Acta Ophthalmol Scand. 1995;73(5):438-441.

[171] Agarwal B, Vemuganti GK, Honavar SG. Intraocular cysticercosis simulating retinoblastoma in a 5 year old child. Eye. 2003;17:447–449.

[172] Luger MH, Stilma JS, Ringens PJ, van-Baarlen J.: In-toto removal of a subretinal Cisticercosis celulae by pars plana vitrectomy. Br J Ophthalmol. 1991;75(9): 561-563.

[173] Bartholomew RS.: Subretinal cysticercosis. Am J Ophthalmol. 1975;79:670 –673.

[174] Zinn KM, Guillory SL and Friedman AH.: Removal of intravitreous cysticerci from the surface of the optic nerve head: a pars plana approach. Arch Ophthalmol 1980;98:714-716.

[175] Santos R, Dalma A, Ortiz E, et al. Management of subretinal and vitreous cysticercosis: role of photocoagulation and surgery. Ophthalmology. Aug 1979;86(8):1501-1507.

[176] Jain IS, Dhir SP, Chattopadhaya PR, Kumar P. Ocular cysticercosis in North India. Indian J Ophthalmol. 1979;27(2):54-58.

[177] Messner KH, Kammerer WS. Intraocular cysticercosis. Arch Ophthalmol. 1979;97(6):1103-1105.

[178] Patnaik B, Kalsi R. Intraocular cysticercosis in the non-pork eaters. Indian J Ophthalmol 1979;27:203-205 Available from: http://www.ijo.in/text.asp?1979/27/4/203/32629

[179] Segal P, Mrzyglod S, Smolarz-Dudarewicz J. Subretinal cysticercosis in the macular region. Am J Ophthalmol 1964; 57:655.

[180] Gupta A, Gupta R, Pandav SS, Dogra MR, Joshi K.Successful surgical removal of encapsulated subretinal cysticercus. Retina 1998;18:563-566.

[181] Lombardo J. Subretinal cysticercosis. Optometry and vision science 2001; 78: 188-94.

[182] Barkeh H, Wong S, Muhaya M. A Rare Case of Subretinal Cysticercosis. Med J Malaysia. 2005;60(5):650-652.

[183] Shea M, Maberley AL, Walters J, Freeman RS, Fallis AM. Intraretinal larval trematode. Trans Am Acad Ophthalmol Otolaryngol. 1973;77(6):784-791.

[184] BawaYS, Wahi PL. Cysticercosis cellulosae of the optic disc with generalized cysticercosis· Br J Ophthalmol. 1962; 46(12):753–755.

[185] Madan VS, Dhamija RM, Gill HS, Boparai MS, Souza PD, Sanchete PC, Bhardwaj JR. Optic nerve cysticercosis: a case report. J Neurol Neurosurg Psychiatry. 1991 May; 54(5): 470–471.

[186] Bousquet CF, Dufour TF, Derome PC. Retrobulbar optic nerve cysticercosis. Case report. J Neurosurg. 1996;84(2):293-296.

[187] Tandon R, Sihota R, Dada T, Verma L. Optic neuritis following albendazole therapy for orbital cysticercosis. Aust N Z J Ophthalmol. 1998 Nov;26(4):339-341.

[188] Gurha N, Sood A, Dhar J, Gupta S Optic nerve cysticercosis in the optic canal. Acta Ophthalmol Scan1999;77(1):107-109

[189] Betharia SM, Tandon R, Thanikachalam S, Ramkrishna K, Sen S, Kashyap S, Vashishta S. Retrobulbar optic nerve cysticercosis with surgical removal: a case report. Orbit 1999;18(4):311-316

[190] Menon V, Tandon R, Khanna S, Sharma P, Khokhar S, Vashisht S, Garg I.ticercosis of the optic nerve. J Neuroophthalmol. 2000 Mar;20(1):59-60.

[191] Gulliani, B. P; Subhash D; Malik MS; Jain DC.Bilateral Cysticercosis of the Optic Nerve. Journal of Neuro-Ophthalmology: 2001;21(3):217-218

[192] Verma L, Agarwal T, Kulkarni A, Mahajan H, Tandon R. Optic Nerve Cysticercosis. Arch Ophthalmol. 2002;120(10):1408-1409.

[193] Bajaj MS, Pushker N. Optic nerve cysticercosis. Clin Experiment Ophthalmol. 2002 Apr;30(2):140-144

[194] Sundaram PM, Jayakumar N, Noronha V. Extraocular muscle cysticercosis - a clinical challenge to the ophthalmologists. Orbit. Dec 2004;23(4):255-262.

[195] Sudan R, Muralidhar R, Sharma P. Optic nerve cysticercosis: case report and review of current management. Orbit. 2005;24(2):159-162.

[196] Venkatesh R, Ravindran RD, Bharathi B, Sengupta S. Optic nerve cysticercosis. Ophthalmology. 2008;115(11):2094.
[197] Taksande B,Jajoo U, Yelwatkar S, Ashish J. Unusual presentation of orbital cysticercosis-ptosis, diminution of vision and medial rectus weakness: a case report. Cases J. 2009; 2: 7025. This article is available from: http://casesjournal.com/casesjournal/article/view/7025
[198] Chandra S, Vashisht S, Menon V, Berry M, Mukherji SK.Optic nerve cysticercosis: imaging findings. AJNR Am J Neuroradiol. 2000;21(1):198-200.
[199] Goyal, J. L.; Das, S.; Kumar, S.; Chauhan, D.; Baheti, U.; Sangit, V. et al. Retrobulbar Cysticercosis Masquerading as Optic Nerve Glioma. Orbit;2007;26(1):
[200] Chung GW, Lai WW, et al.: Magnetic resonance imaging in the diagnosis of subretinal cysticercosis. Am J Ophthalmol 2002;134(6):931-932.
[201] Wender JD, Rathinam SR, Shaw RE, Cunningham ET Jr. Intraocular cysticercosis: case series and comprehensive review of the literature. Ocul Immunol Inflamm. 2011;19(4):240-245.
[202] Grover AK, Puri P. Orbital myocysticercosis presenting as subconjunctival abscess. Ind J Ophthalmol. 1996;44:229–231
[203] Baskararajan G. Srinivasan A. Sivarama Zuleramanian P. Thivagarajan S Case of cysticercosis; presenting with persisiten diplopia and spontaneous extrusion. Indian J Ophthalmal 1981;28:219-220.
[204] Graham RH. Extraocular Muscle Anatomy. Medscape. Jun 2011 Available at the URL: http://emedicine.medscape.com/article/1189799-overview (last review Jul 05,2012)
[205] DiLoreto DA, Kennedy RA, Neigel JM, Rootman J. Infestation of extraocular muscle by Cysticercus cellulosae. Br J Ophthalmol. 1990;71:751–752
[206] Menon V, Kumar G, Prakash P. Cysticercosis of extraocular muscles. J Pediatr Opthalmol Strabismus. 1994;31:126–129
[207] Madan N, Chopra K, Popli V. Proptosis as a Manifestation of Cysticercosis. Indian Pediatric. 1995;32:914-917.
[208] Ursekar MA, Dastur DK, Manghiani DK, Ursekar AT. Isolated cysticercal infestation of extraocular muscles: CT and MR findings. AJNR Am J Neuroradiol. 1998;19:109–113
[209] Trivedi N, Malthus RN. CT evaluation of proptosis. Proceedings of the 44th Annual Conference of AH India Oph- thalmological Society 1968, pp 45.
[210] Vashisht S, Hemlata RK, Dayal Y, Bhargav. Orbital lesion. A CT Study. ISRI1.986;4: 40.
[211] Pupo PP. Cystecercosis of the nervous system—Clinical manifestations. Revropsychiatr 1964;27:70-82.
[212] Canelas HM. Neurocysticercosis. Its incidence, diagnosis and clinical forms. In: Tropical Neurology. Eds Ven Bogasert L, Pereyrakafer J, Poch CW. Buenos Aires, Lopezco, 1963, pp 149-162.
[213] Powell ST, Proctor SM. Wilmost AJ, et al. Cysticercosis and epilepsy in Africans. A clinical and serological study. Ann Trop Med Parasitol 1966, 60:150- 153.
[214] Jampol LM, Caldwell JBH, Albert DM. Cysticercus cellulosae in the id. Arch Ophthalmol 1973;89:319–320
[215] Perry HD, Font RL. Cysticercosis of the eyelid. Arch Ophthalmol;96:1255–1257

[216] Sen DK. Cysticercus cellulosae in the eyelid, orbit and lacrimald. Acta Ophthalmol (Kbh) 1980;58:144–147

[217] Sing G, Kaur J. Cysticercosis of the eyelid. Ann Ophthalmol 1982;47–950

[218] Kundra R, Kundra SN. Uniocular ptosis due to cysticercosis of extraocular muscle. Indian J Pediatr. 2004;71(2):181-182.

[219] Chan EW, Looi A. Cysticercosis of the Levator Palpebrae Superioris. Annals Academy of Medicine. 2010;39(12):938-940.

[220] Basset D, Girou C, Nozais IP, et al. Neotropical echinococcosis in Suriname: Echinococcus oligarthrus in the orbit and Echinococcus vogeli in the abdomen. Am J Trop Med Hyg 1998; 59:787-90.

[221] Kamath KR. Severe infection with Trichuris trichiura in Malaysian children. A clinical study of 30 cases treated with stilbazium iodine.Am J Trop Med Hyg 1973; 22:600-605.

[222] Netravathi N, Banuprakash AS, Khamesra R, Singh NH. Cysticercosis of midbrain presenting with fluctuating ptosis. Ann Indian Acad Neurol. 2011;14(3):208–210.

[223] Wiwanitkit S, Wiwanitkit V. Cysticercosis and ptosis. Ann Indian Acad Neurol 2012;15:68

[224] Angotti-Neto H, Gonçalves AC, Moura FC, Monteiro ML. Extraocular muscle cysticercosis mimicking idiopathic orbital inflammation: case report. Arq Bras Oftalmol. 2007;70(3):537-539.

[225] Monteiro ML. Liposarcoma of the orbit presenting as an enlarged medial rectus muscle on CT scan. Br J Ophthalmol. 2002;86(12):1450.

[226] Trokel SL, Hilal SK. Recognition and differential diagnosis of enlarged extraocular muscles in computed tomography. Am J Ophthalmol, 1979; 87(4): 503-512.

[227] Meher A. Ursekar, Darab K. Dastur, Daya K. Manghani, and Atul T. Ursekar. Isolated Cysticercal Infestation of Extraocular Muscles: CT and MR Findings. Am J Neuroradiol 1998;19:109–113.

[228] DiLoreto DA, Kennedy RA, Neigel JM, Rootman J. Infestation of aocular muscle by Cysticercus cellulosae. Br J Ophthalmol 1990;74:751–752

[229] Shadangi P, Saggar V,et al; Isolated Cysticercosis Of Inferior Rectus Muscle Presenting With Eccentric Proptosis.- A rare case report and treatment review. Journal of Clinical and Diagnostic Research. 2010;4(3):2536-2539.

[230] Lee AG; Tang RA, Wong GOD, Schiffman JS, Singh S. Isolated Inferior Rectus Muscle Palsy Resulting From a Nuclear Third Nerve Lesion as the Initial Manifestation of Multiple Sclerosis. Journal of Neuro-Ophthalmology 2001;20(4):246-247

[231] Ellis FH, Helveston EM. Superior oblique palsy: diagnosis and classification. Int Ophthalmol Clin 1976; 16: 127-135.

[232] Brooks AM, Essex WB, West RH: Cysticercosis of superior oblique muscle. Aust J Ophthalmol 1983;11:119-122.

[233] Mafee MF, Folk ER, Langer BG, Miller MT, Lagouros P, Mittleman D. Computed tomography in the evaluation of Brown syndrome of the superior oblique tendon sheath. Radiology, 1985;154(3): 691-695.

[234] Ozkan SB, Aribal ME, Sener EC, Sanac AS, Gurcan F. Magnetic resonance imaging in evaluation of congenital and acquired superior oblique palsy. J. Pediatr. Ophthalmol. Strabismus. 1997; 34(1): 29-34.

[235] Wright KW. Brown's syndrome: Diagnosis and management. Trans. Am. Ophthalmol. Soc., 1999; 97:1023-1029.

[236] Thorne JE, Volpe NJ, Liu GT. Magnetic resonance imaging of acquired Brown syndrome in a patient with psoriasis. Am. J. Ophthalmol. 1999;127(2): 233-235

[237] Pramod K. Pandey P, Chaudhuri Z, Bhatia A.Extraocular muscle cysticercosis presenting as brown syndrome. Am J Ophthal 2001;131(4):526-527.

[238] Bajaj MS, Pushker N, Sen S, et al. Cysticercosis of superior oblique muscle: surgical excision and reconstruction of superior oblique tendon. Can J Ophthalmol 2002; 37(7):423-426.

[239] Rao VB, Sahare P, Varada V. Acquired brown syndrome secondary to superior oblique muscle cysticercosis. J. Am. Assoc. Pediatr. Ophthalmol. Strab. 2003;7(1):23 – 27.

[240] Venkateshwar B, Rao VB, Prashant P, Sahare P, Varada VV. Acquired brown syndrome secondary to superior oblique muscle cysticercosis. J AAPOS 2003;7(1):23-27. Available at the URL://pubget.com/paper/12690365/Acquired_brown_syndrome_secondary_to_superior_oblique_muscle_cysticercosis (Last revision on July, 03, 2012)

[241] Lee WB, O'Halloran HS.A report of canine tooth syndrome. Orbit 2004;23(1):53-57.

[242] Pandey PK, Bhatia A, Garg D, Singh R.Canine tooth syndrome due to superior oblique myocysticercosis. J Pediatr Ophthalmol Strabismus. 2006;43(3):185-187.

[243] Case report: tenosynovitis of the left superior oblique muscle. Ophthalmology Times Europe. 2006. Available at the URL: http://www.oteurope.com/ophthalmologytimeseurope/mail/emailContent.jsp?id=314314

[244] Alonso-Valdivielso JL, Alvarez Lario B, Alegre López J, Sedano Tous MJ, Buitrago Gómez A. Acquired Brown's syndrome in a patient with systemic lupus erythematosus. Ann Rheum Dis. 1993; 52(1):63–64.

[245] Pollard ZF. Diagnosis and treatment of inferior oblique palsy. J Pediatr Ophthalmol Strabismus. 1993;30(1):15-18.

[246] Donahue S, Lavin PJM, Mohney B, Hamed L. Skew deviation and inferior oblique palsy. Amer J Ophthal 2001;132(5):751-756

[247] Hüseyin B, Cem M, Soner D. Inferior Oblique Paresis, Mydriasis, and Accommodative Palsy as Temporary Complications of Sinus Surgery. Journal of Neuro-Ophthalmology 2004;24(3):225-227.

[248] Parks M, Mitchell P .Oblique Muscle Dysfunctions. Chapter 17. Full text available the URL: http://www.oculist.net/downaton502/prof/ebook/duanes/pages/v1/v1c017.html#ove

[249] Kim M, Lee YC. A Case of Contralateral Pseudo Inferior Oblique Overaction after Unilateral Inferior Oblique Anterior Transposition. J Korean Ophthalmol Soc. 2000;41(9):2018-2023.

[250] Surgical anatomy of the inferior oblique. Paralysis. Cyber-Sight. Orbis/Telemedicine. Available at the URL:://telemedicine.orbis.org/bins/volume_page.asp?cid=1-2161-2163-2177

[251] Sixth Nerve Paralysis: Diagnosis. Paralysis. Cyber-Sight. Orbis/Telemedicine. Available at the URL:://www.cybersight.org/bins/volume_page.asp?cid=1-12628-351-355-521

[252] Stewart CR, Salmon JF, Murray AD, Sperryn C. Cysticercosis as a cause of severe medial rectus muscle myositis. Am J Ophthalmol.1993;116(4):510-511.

[253] Wong YC, Goh KY, Choo CT, Seah LL, Rootman J. An unusual cause of acquired horizontal diplopia in a young adult. Br J Ophthalmol. 2005;89(3):390–391.

[254] Khwaja GA, Singh AC, Chaudhry Neera, Gupta Meena, Chowdhury D. Recurrent Headache and Unilateral Ptosis. JIACM. 2008;9(3):218–220.

[255] Taksande B,Jajoo U, Yelwatkar S, Ashish J. Unusual presentation of orbital cysticercosis-ptosis, diminution of vision and medial rectus weakness: a case report. Cases J. 2009; 2: 7025. This article is available from: http://casesjournal.com/casesjournal/article/view/7025

[256] Tuli N. A Non Responding Case Of Extraocular Muscle Cysticercosis Mimicking As Pseudo-Tumor Orbit In A Child. The Internet Journal of Ophthalmology and Visual Science. 2010;7(2)

[257] Medial Rectus Muscle Paralysis. Cyber-Sight. Orbis/Telemedicine. Available at the URL://www.cybersight.org/bins/volume_page.asp?cid=1-12628-351-355-515&lang=1 (accesed on July 08, 2012)

[258] Castro O, Johnson LN, Mamourian AC. Isolated inferior oblique paresis from brain-stem infarction. Perspective on oculomotor fascicular organization in the ventral midbrain tegmentum. Arch Neurol 1990;47:235-237

[259] Kwon JH, Kwon SU, Ahn HS, Sung KB, Kim JS. Isolated superior rectus palsy due to contralateral midbrain infarction. Arch Neurol 2003;60:1633-1635.

[260] Rabadi MH, Beltmann MA. Midbrain infarction presenting isolated medial rectus nuclear palsy. Am J Med 2005;118:836-837.

[261] Lee DK, Kim JS. Isolated inferior rectus palsy due to midbrain infarction detected by diffusion- weighted MRI. Neurology 2006;66:1956-1957

[262] Bal S, Lal V, Khurana D, Prabhakar S. Midbrain infarct presenting as isolated medial rectus palsy. Neurol India 2009;57:499-501

[263] Sarwal A. Isolated medial rectus palsy in midbrain infarction. Amer Acad Neurol. 2009; 10: 200. Available at the URL: http://www.aan.com/globals/axon/assets/6555.pdf (accessed on July 08, 2012)

[264] Puri P, Grover AK. Medical management of orbital myocysticercosis: a pilot study. Eye 1998;12:795–799

[265] Pandey PK, Chaudhuri Z, Sharma P, Bhomaj S. Extraocular muscle cysticercosis:a clinical masquerade.J Pediatr Ophthalmol Strabismus 2000;37:273-278.

[266] Jethani J.Outcome of treatment of extraocular muscle cysticercosis. J Pediatr Ophthalmol Strabismus. 2005;42(5):263-264

Chapter 7

What is a Low Frequency of the Disseminated Cysticercosis Suggests that Neurocysticercosis is Going to Disappear?

Humberto Foyaca Sibat and Lourdes de Fátima Ibañez Valdés

Additional information is available at the end of the chapter

http://dx.doi.org/10.5772/51395

1. Introduction

The zoonotic infections that affect the man can be caused by viruses (rabies, avian influenza, immunodeficiency virus from apes [VIS]), bacteria (brucellosis, salmonellosis), parasites (leishmaniasis and schistosomiasis, neurocysticercosis, toxocariasis) and other non-conventional agents such as prions (bovine spongiform encephalopathy and a variant of Jakob-Creutzfeldt disease) on which enough has been written[1].

There are 1407 pathogens that affect humans (excluding the ectoparasites), more than half (816) are zoonotic and 73% (130) cause zoonotic diseases that affect community health [2]. Parasitic diseases have occurred through the times more deaths and economic damage to humanity that all the genocidal wars together. Parasitic infections previously seen only in developing tropical settings can be currently diagnosed worldwide due to travel and population migration. Generally in countries with little socio-economic development is where parasitic diseases are presented with greater frequency, still this is offered by climatic conditions warm or temperate zone and by the lack of education for health in the population; because in the developed countries social, medical and economically, parasitic diseases have been eradicated or have very little significance [3].

Neurocysticercosis (NCC) is the parasitic disease more frequent of the CNS and the causal agent of the same is the larval stage of the T solium cysticerci when invades brain of a human being that has swallowed the viable eggs from food or contaminated liquids, from a carrier, by infection secondary to a reverse peristalsis or by the well-known fecal-oral route [4-6]. The man is in turn the only known host for the adult form of the parasite. This disease is a serious health problem for many third-world countries of Asia, Africa, and Latin America; moreover, a growing number of cases are being reported in many highly developed countries in Europe and North America, notwithstanding the foregoing, the

INTECH
open science | open minds

© 2013 Foyaca Sibat and de Fátima Ibañez Valdés, licensee InTech. This is a paper distributed under the terms of the Creative Commons Attribution License (http://creativecommons.org/licenses/by/3.0), which permits unrestricted use, distribution, and reproduction in any medium, provided the original work is properly cited.

incidence and prevalence accurate of this disease have not been confirmed from well-designed studies. Disseminated cysticercosis (DCC) was reported in 1912 by doctors of the English Navy stationed in India. Priest in 1926, describes a British soldier patient presenting an inflammation of the skeletal muscles, seizures, mental dulling and a large amount of subcutaneous nodules distributed throughout the body [7]. An intensive search performed in 1988 revealed 22 cases [7] and only 16 additional cases were reported until 2006 reported in the international medical literature most of them from India. [8]. It is considered that cysticercosis (CC) is a major problem for public health in several developing countries where the social, economic and cultural conditions favor the maintenance of this zoonotic disease and it is seen as a growing community problem in those developed countries with a high rate of immigrants from endemic areas. WHO includes the NCC between neglected diseases that cause a significant impact on the economy in several regions of the world. It affects 4% of the population in endemic areas [4, 9] and is the main cause of symptomatic epilepsy worldwide [1, 10-15] but where the hygiene habits-food and sometimes religious trends can determine the incidence and prevalence of the disease [1].

Based in our experience and according to this review of the literature we can say that in regions where the CC is endemic, the presence of late onset seizures in subjects older than 25 years of age is highly suggestive of NCC what had already been established since 1982 [16]. In the published series, the age group most commonly affected by the NCC, is the group of 35 to 63 years [18-20]. The males are most affected than females in the majority of the studios [17-19]. In 2003, Mafojane [20] reported a high prevalence in children and young South Africans in a region where the CC virtually does not exist.

Probably, there is a progressive decrease incidence of DCC based in our local perception and disseminated cysticercosis is always associated with NCC but it does not mean that the NCC is on the way to disappear completely in the next decade. In this chapter we will present a bibliographic investigation on the DCC, its prevalence in our region, and our arguments on the because we are going to spend many years before that the DCC eradicated from the face of the earth.

The pathogenesis and clinical manifestations of CC depend on the number, size, location, evolutionary state of the parasite and the host's immune response [1,5,10-15, 21-23]. In the above-mentioned studies, appear only the seizures and the headache as initial clinical manifestations while in others it is reported: meningitis, dementia, intracranial Hypertension, psychiatric symptoms, ischemic stroke, and radicular compression [10-15,17, 24-30]. It is important to note that the headache is not the most frequent clinical manifestation of the NCC in the majority of published studies but that occupies the second place; only in one of the studies consulted is presented as the main reason for consultation [19]. In the majority of the series, the frequency of headache varies from 4.6 % to 61.5 % [19,23-24]. While the frequency of seizures as a form of presentation of the NCC ranges from 54.3 % to 62.5 % in general series [12, 23, 27, 31-34]. In children the frequency of seizures to be the initial manifestation is higher, ranging from 72% to 94.8 % according to other authors [29, 35]. In summary, the majority of published studies confirm that the epilepsy and headache were the most frequent clinical manifestations of the NCC [1,10-15, 17, 24, 27-30,

36]. These manifestations begin between one and 35 years after the exposure to the parasite, as demonstrated in patients from the British army stationed in India where it is defined exactly the time of exposure to the parasite and the onset of clinical manifestations. The average life Expectancy of the parasite is estimated to be between four and five years [37]. The epilepsy secondary to NCC (ESNCC) responds well to first line antiepileptic drugs (AED) [1,10-15, 19,24, 28,31, 33, 38]. Other AED as the levetiracitam has also shown good results, but its high cost and lack of availability in the public sector and the primary health care system make it considered without practical usefulness for the control of the ESNCC [1]. Patients with DCC can present: refractory epilepsy, neuropsychiatric disturbances, pseudo hypertrophy in the four limbs and affectation of any other organ or system [8]. However, a fairly typical manifestation of the DCC is the subcutaneous cyst that occurs as a asymptomatic nodule. These subcutaneous nodules can be slide easily in the muscle tissue and measure up to 1.5 cm in diameter. In the case of patients who have suffered from the disease for more than five years, usually these are calcified [39].

Recently, Bielsa-Fernández [40] reported a patient carrier of severe rheumatic polymyalgia of the trunk and limbs with serological surveys negative for the CC and two muscle biopsy confirmed encapsulated nodules with diffuse calcification, compatible with parasitic diseases, whose state of calcification prevented identify the characteristics of the parasite. Logically, the presence of active NCC leaves no doubt about the nature of the subcutaneous nodules and reinforces the importance of bearing in mind the diagnostic criteria of Del Brutto for the correct differential diagnosis [41].

The main characteristic the DCC is structural epilepsy due to neurocysticercosis and the pseudo-hypertrophy in the four members and the allocation of any other organ or system [8]. However, a manifestation fairly typical of the DCC may be subcutaneous cyst that occurs as a nodule asymptomatic. These subcutaneous nodules can be sliders in the muscle and measure up to 1.5 cm. In the case of patients who have had for more than 5 years cysticerci, these are calcified [39]. A few months ago, Bielsa-Fernández [40] reported a female patient with a severe rheumatic polymyalgia of the trunk and limbs with serological studies for the CC negative and two muscle biopsy confirmed two nodes encapsulated with diffuse calcification, compatible with parasitosis, whose calcification of the content made it difficult determine the type of parasite. Logically, the presence of NCC active leaves no doubt about the nature of the subcutaneous nodules.

The pharmacological treatment of DCC reported good results for some patients with subcutaneous and muscular involvement if the CNS is not severely affected [41, 42]. On the other hand, have been confirmed cases with DCC and chronic liver disease in which case even if the ELISA test was suggestive, the final diagnosis was obtained by CT scans of the brain [43], and have been reported cases with unilateral eye lesion [44], and even bilaterally [80], thyroid involvement [8, 45] , pancreatic enzyme alterations [46] or without clinical or biochemical alterations of pancreatic function [47], spleen damage [47,47], cardiac [8, 48-53], even without associated DCC [52], lung [45, 53-55], joints [56] and muscles of the face and neck [44, 48]. There is not reported cases of DCC without involvement of CNS and its frequency may be the expression of an increase or decrease in the overall prevalence of porcine cysticercosis in general [1]. The host inflammatory response depends on the parasite's ability to evade host immunity. Usually both 'healthy' (active) and 'involuted' (inactive) cysticerci lack inflammatory response, which is restricted to 'currently degenerating' cysts whose ability to evade host defenses is becoming faulty. Involution of cysts implies granulomatous inflammation [56].

Epilepsy is the most common neurological manifestation of DCC in our region and it has been well documented in previous publication. [41,50] However seizures disorder in HIV patients present special problem with regard to choice of antiepileptic drugs (AED) and the potential for drug-drug interactions with antiretroviral (ARV) treatments also in our region. Newer AEDs with simpler pharmacokinetic profiles may be the preferred agents, particularly when protease inhibitors form part of ARV regimens. Seizures in NCC are easily controlled with the first line AEDs. Although there has been some debate about the value of anti-parasitic drugs in NCC, accumulating data suggest that the use of these agents in active disease decreases the risk for development of chronic epilepsy [57].

2. Methodology

In this chapter we included only cases reported to the medical literature, therefore no major ethical problems are afforded. Nevertheless, in order to protect all subjects participating in our studies, as part of a general measure aimed at protecting patients selected it was agreed that the principal investigator (HFS) and collaborators (LdeFIV) should adopt a program of basic training on the protection of human beings and animals participating in research studies and obtain the corresponding certificate which was done. All protocols were approved by the Review Committee from the University of Transkei and the Walter Sisulu University plus their respective Committee on Medical Ethics and the numbers of references are the following: Mthatha Hospital (UGH: 0001/99, letter of approval by the Director of Medical Services), University of Transkei (UNITRA:0018/05), and Walter Sisulu University (IRB) and their respective Ethics Committee (WSU:0068/09). The model of informed consent was signed by all participants in the first contact as a prerequisite to participate. To illiterate patients were explained the objectives of the study, the procedures which were to be subjected and their risks and the model of consent was signed by a family member, relative or a witness. To all patients we explained their rights to participate or not, with the assurance that in any case, this would not cause change in management or the attention of the same or other rights of any patient, their rights on anonymity (personal data replaced by keys), and to keep any information in strict confidentiality. In this chapter we did not use any graphical or written confidential information from patients reported by other author.

3. Results

3.1. Disseminated cysticercosis in South Africa

The former Transkei is the poorest region in South Africa and it was a well known batustan during the apartheid régimen before 1994. To the population of Xhosa origin were assigned the regions of the Ciskei and Transkei and Transkei is termed as an independent state in

1974 but was only recognized by South Africa with whom confronted territorial disputes between 1974 and 1978. The natural history of the NCC must be viewed within the historical context of this region in order to understand why the NCC has been confined almost to the former Transkei (currently region C and D of Eastern Cape Province), still the only endemic area of the country from where they come from all the sick people who could be diagnosed in the rest of the country.

Human cysticercosis appears to be most prevalent in Eastern Cape Province particularly in the poor, former black homeland, rural areas of Transkei, where pigs are allowed to roam freely and sanitation facilities are inadequate or nonexistent. Pig keeping and pork consumption have increased significantly during the past decade especially in rural smallholder communities, primarily due to the lack of grazing land for ruminants and the recognition of farmers of a quicker and more impressive return on their investment from raising pigs.

The first inform about patients presenting DCC in South Africa was made by Schultz and Mentis [58] In 1987. They reported a 48-year-old black man with two month history of a painless mass on the left side of his neck. He also complained of mild attacks of paroxysmal dyspnoea at night and progressive deafness of his left ear. On direct questioning the patient referred few grand mal seizures during the 6 years before admission. No other complaints or previous illnesses of note were elicited. The patient was born in Transkei (near to Mthatha) and had travelled throughout many parts of the country seeking work. On examination he appeared healthy and was of normal build. The pulse rate was 72/min, blood pressure 110/60 mmHg and temperature 37,2°C. Numerous subcutaneous nodules, ranging from one to three centimeter in diameter, which were well circumscribed and freely movable, could be palpated all over the neck, chest and legs. A bigger mass was palpable inferior to the left ear, extending down the left side of the neck. There was conduction deafness of the left ear. On chest auscultation a few fine crepitations were audible at the bases of both lungs, chest radiography revealed multiple nodular opacities; computed tomography of the brain, neck, thorax and upper abdomen revealed extensive organ involvement, including brain, thyroid, lungs, pancreas, kidney, spleen and muscle; and biopsies of two of the subcutaneous nodules were histologically pathognomonic of cysticercosis. The patient received praziquantel (Biltricide; Bayer-Miles) 1, 75 g twice daily and prednisone 20 mg per day for 4 weeks. He was reassessed radiologically after 4 weeks. There was marked regression in the size and numbers of nodules in the lung fields. Clinically, most of the subcutaneous nodules had disappeared. This is the only report in the international medical literary on CCD with so large involvement of organs and systems including the kidneys.

Bhigjee in 1999 [59], reported the second patient presenting DCC in South Africa. His patient was an Indian male presenting generalized subcutaneous and muscular nodules and neurocysticercosis. Diagnosis was confirmed by plain X-rays of the soft tissues in upper and lower limbs and CT scan of the brain where multiple bilateral active and calcify cysticerci on both cerebral hemisphere were found. (Figure 1)

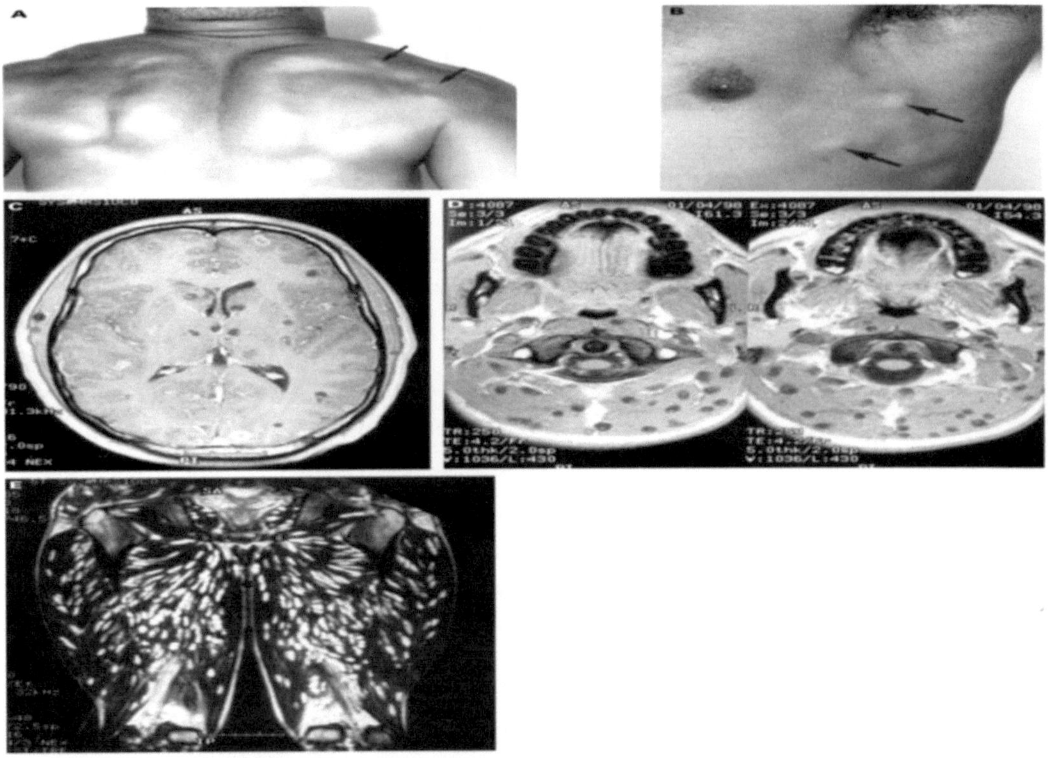

Figure 1. Shows generalized subcutaneous and intramuscular calcified nodules on lower limbs and intraparenchymal neurocysticercosis in vesicular, colloid and calcified stages. (Source: J Neurol Neurosurg Psychiatry 1999; 66(4): 545. Bhigjee A).

Five years later we reported a 42-year-old man (third report) admitted at Nelson Mandela Academic Hospital Mthatha in South Africa. He presented a history of recurrent generalized tonic-clonic epileptic seizures of six years duration, disseminated nodules all over the body of two-year duration and headache. On general examination multiple subcutaneous and intramuscularly, mobile, no tender nodules, measuring from 0.7 to 2.5 cm, were palpable on the chest, back, abdomen, and proximal regions of the four limbs. (Figure 2-3-4) Respiratory and cardiovascular system were normal except for a bradycardia of 42 bpm. A computed tomography (CT) scan of the brain showed multiple active and calcified lesions. Biopsy of the subcutaneous nodules confirmed the diagnosis of cysticercosis (Figure 3). A detailed neurological examination revealed unremarkable findings. Laboratory data were normal, ELISA test and IgG for cysticercosis were strongly positive. ECG and cardiac ultrasound confirmed: sinus bradicardia, II grade heart block, and calcifications in papillary muscles and upper septum respectively. CT Scan of the brain (Figure 4) shows bilateral cysts in different active stages and calcified NCC. [41]

We referred this patient to the cardiology clinic in our hospital for assessment of bradycardia and some findings were reported later by other authors [60]. Patient felt dizzy on getting up suddenly from a supine position. His pulse rate was 41/min, irregular and his blood pressure 76/124 mmHg. An electrocardiogram (ECG) showed sinus bradycardia with complete heart block (Figure 5). The patient was initially treated only with prednisolone, and anti-helminthic treatment was deferred fearing peri-cystic inflammation and aggravation of the conduction abnormalities. Five days later praziquantel 50 mg/kg/day for 14 days were added to the treatment regimen. Repeat ECG after a week of treatment showed sinus rhythm with a heart rate of 70/min. Diagnostic criteria for disseminated cysticercosis for this patient is based on the presence of NCC, subcutaneous, and muscular cysticercosis simultaneously.

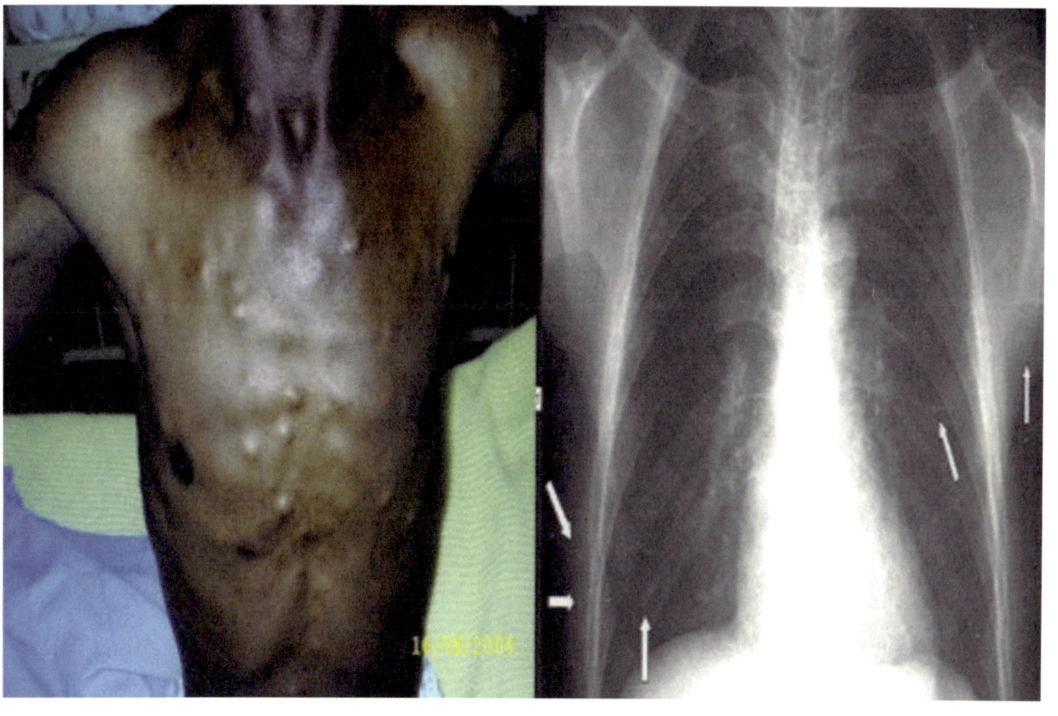

Figure 2. Multiple subcutaneous nodules on the chest wall and a few calcified lesions on chest X-ray. (Photo taken by H Foyaca-Sibat. Source: Foyaca et al., Rev Electron Biomed / Electron J Biomed 2004;3:39-43. Written patient consent is obtained).

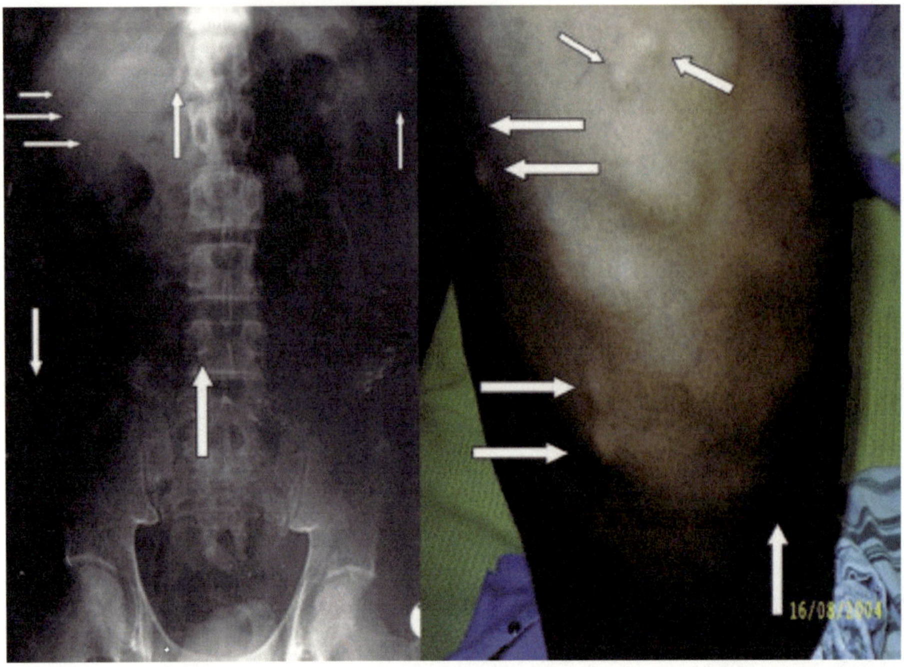

Figure 3. Multiple calcified subcutaneous and paravertebral nodules. (Photo taken by H Foyaca-Sibat. Source: Foyaca et al., Rev Electron Biomed / Electron J Biomed 2004;3:39-43. Patient written consent is obtained).

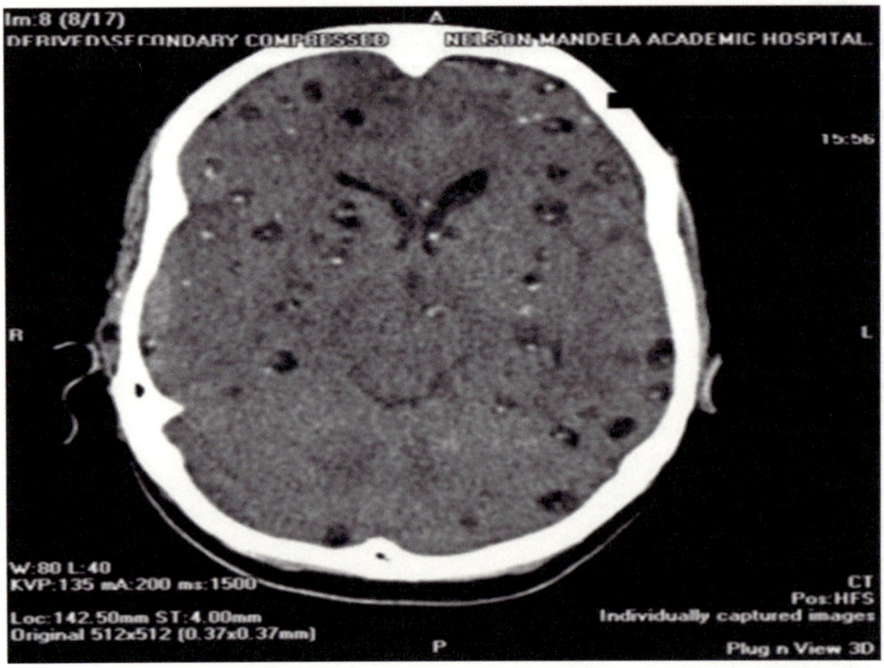

Figure 4. CT scan of the brain showing multiples intraparenchymal cysticerci in vesicular, colloid and calcified stages.

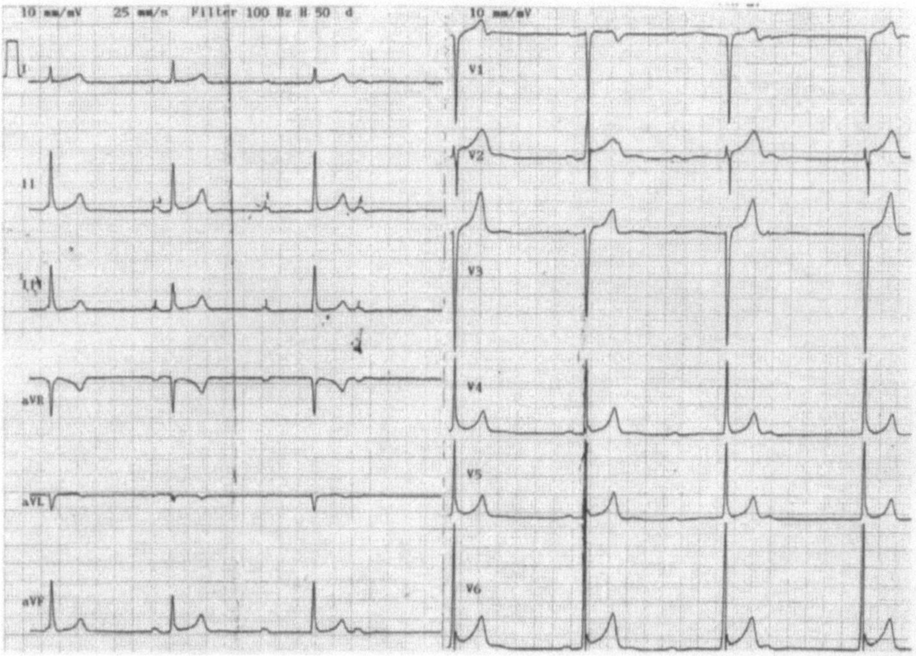

Figure 5. shows sinus bradycardia with complete heart block.[60]

The principal electrocardiographic (ECG) alterations are first-degree atrioventricular (AV) block, low QRS (QRS interval of the ECG) voltage, and primary T-wave changes (as can seen in Chagas' disease).

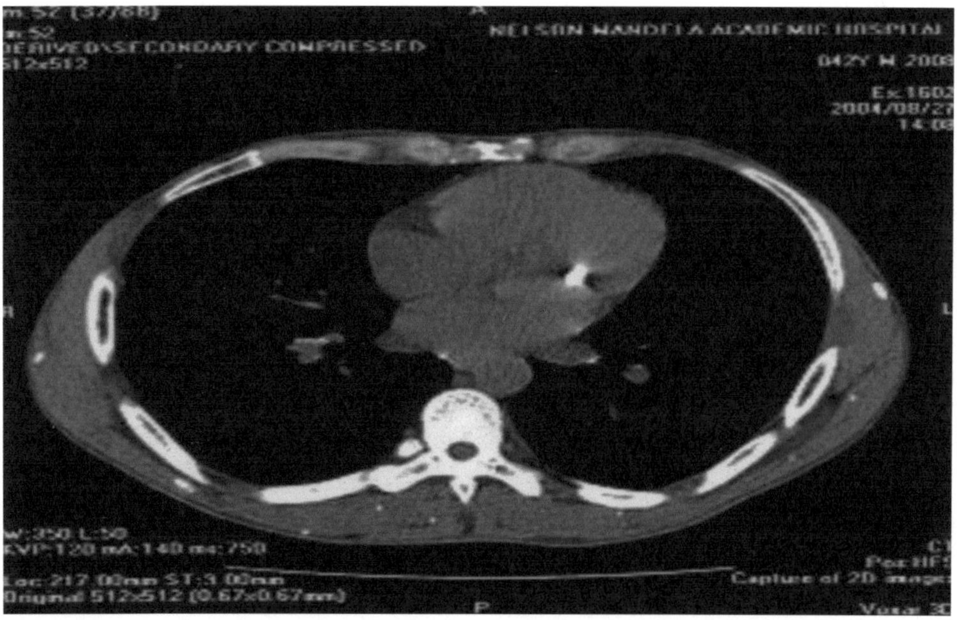

Figure 6. CT scan of chest confirmed the presence of cysts within the myocardium.[60]

In 2007, we reported a 48-year-old African male patient (Fouth patient) admitted at Nelson Mandela Academic Hospital in Mthatha, South Africa presenting a history of recurrent generalized tonic-clonic epileptic seizures with urinary incontinence of five years duration. Patient reported to have fitted at home with three episodes on the day of admission and sustained burns on the right leg while he was unconscious (Figure 7).

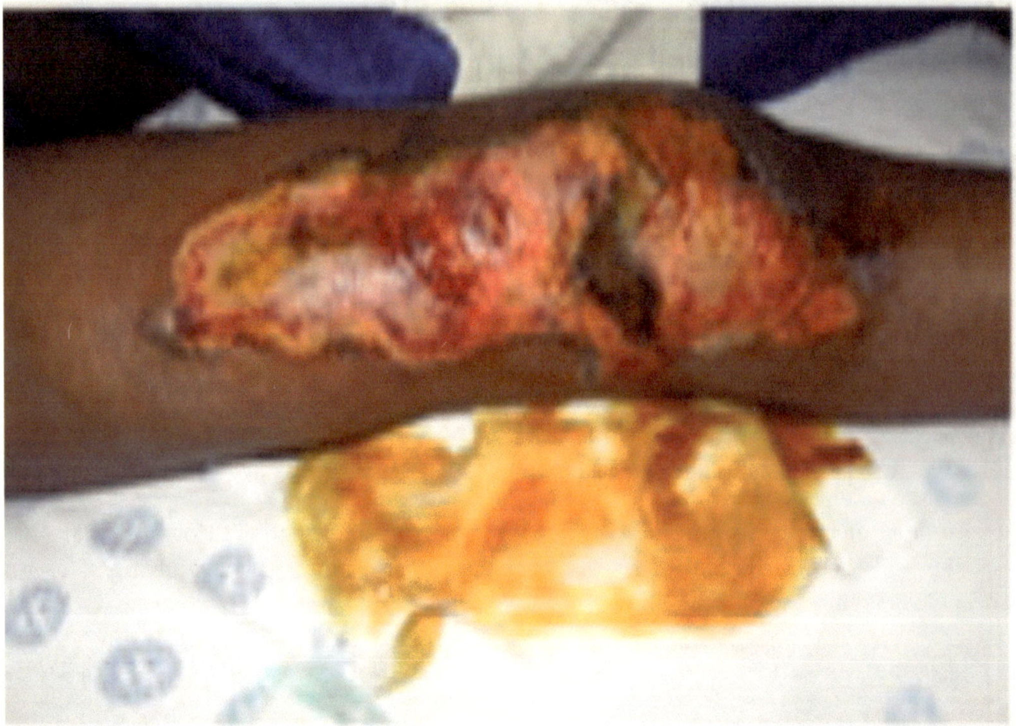

Figure 7. Show a burning lesion acquired during tonic-clonic generalized epileptic seizure. (Photo taken by H Foyaca-Sibat. Source: H. Foyaca-Sibat & L. Ibanez-Valdes: Generalized Cysticercosis With Cardiac Involvement. The Internet Journal of Neurology. (ISSN: 1531-295X) 2007; 7(2):6-11.

Burn is a frequent accident for epileptic peoples while they having epileptic seizures in rural areas when electricity is not available and they need to keep small fire inside the room as alternative way to survive during the winter. Unfortunately, there is not sustainable solution for this problem at the present moment.

This patient was on oral carbamazepine 200mg three times a day, but he discontinued treatment 2 weeks back because medication was not available at the nearest medical clinic. On general examination multiple subcutaneous and intramuscularly, mobile, no tender nodules, measuring from 0.7 to 2.5 cm, were palpable on the chest, back, abdomen, proximal regions of the four limbs and hemi-face (Figure 8-12). Respiratory and cardiovascular system were normal except for a bradicardia of 46 beat per minute. A detailed neurological examination revealed unremarkable findings. Laboratory data included routine blood test

(FBC, U&E, glucose, urinalysis) were normal, erythrocyte sedimentation rate and cardiac enzymes were also normal. ELISA test and IgG for cysticercosis were strongly positive.

Plain chest X-rays and X-rays of long bones showed multiple "cigar-shape calcifications" (Figure 11) and abdomen ultrasound confirmed multiple subcutaneous cystic lesions seen with centric enhancing form remembering the typical "dot-in-hole". ECG and cardiac ultrasound confirmed: sinus bradicardia, II grade heart block and calcifications in papillary muscles and upper septum respectively (Figure 7). CT scan of the brain showed bilateral cystic lesions in vesicular and colloid stages, and calcified NCC [50]. Plain X-ray studies of the muscles are also useful to identify the typical "cigar-shape" calcifications on the subcutaneous tissue, and if any query arise then a positive serological test for T solium (antigen/antibody) will help while the final diagnosis is confirmed by biopsy of the subcutaneous nodules or confirming NCC by imagenology.

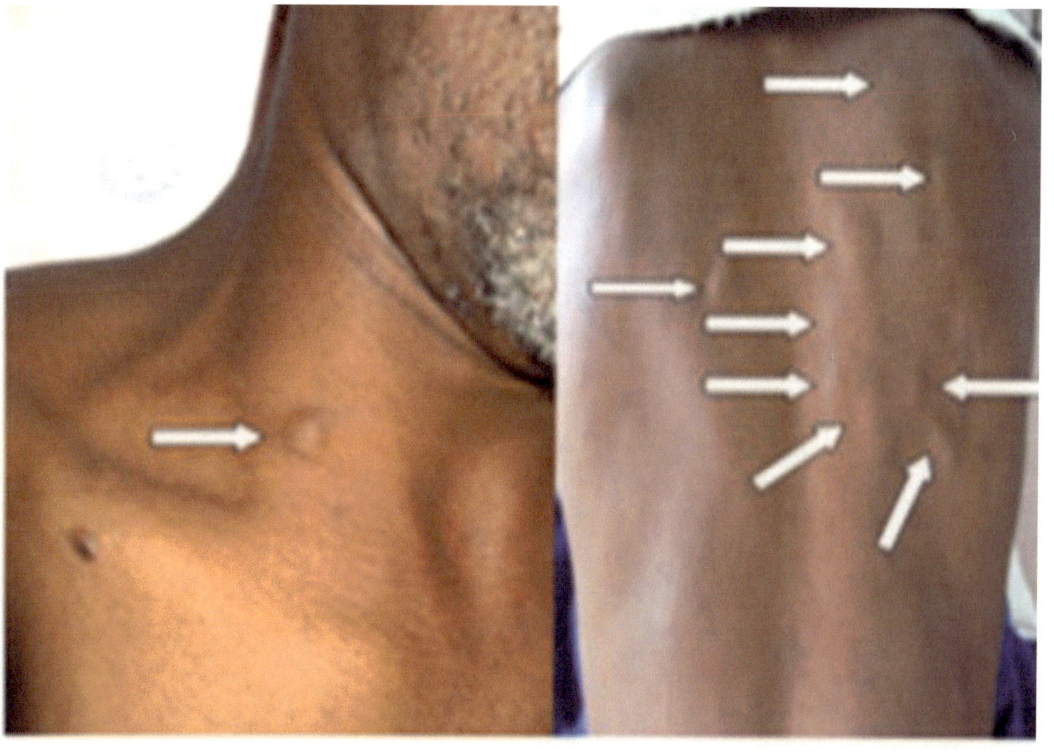

Figure 8. Show subcutaneous nodule on the right lateral aspect of the neck and multiple subcutaneous nodules in the upper back mainly on the right side. (Photo taken by H Foyaca-Sibat. Source: H. Foyaca-Sibat & L. Ibanez-Valdes: Generalized Cysticercosis With Cardiac Involvement. *The Internet Journal of Neurology*. 2007 Volume 7 Number 2.)

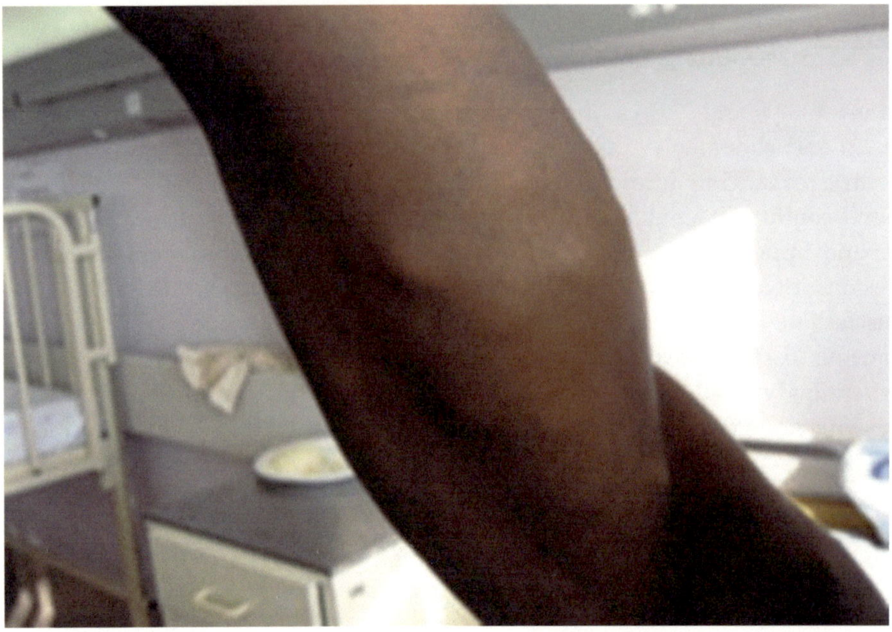

Figure 9. Shows multiple subcutaneous nodules in the left arm some of them were located in the biceps brachialis. (Photo taken by H Foyaca-Sibat. Source: H. Foyaca-Sibat & L. Ibanez-Valdes: Generalized Cysticercosis With Cardiac Involvement. *The Internet Journal of Neurology*. 2007 Volume 7 Number 2.)

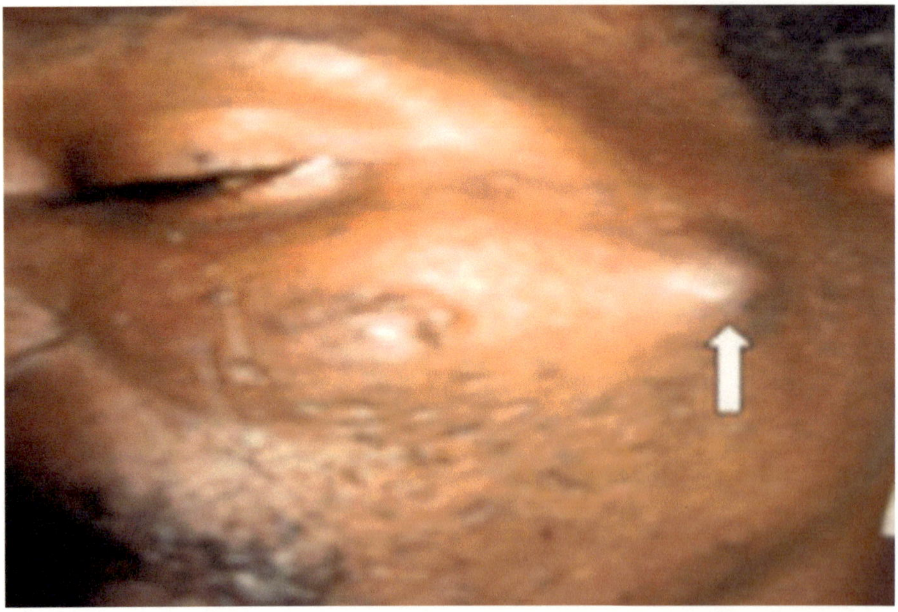

Figure 10. Shows a nodular lesion in the left hemiface at the zigomatic arch level removed by surgical procedure and histological examination confirmed subcutaneous cysticercosis (Photo taken by H Foyaca-Sibat. Source: H. Foyaca-Sibat & L. Ibanez-Valdes: Generalized Cysticercosis With Cardiac Involvement. *The Internet Journal of Neurology*. 2007 Volume 7 Number 2. Patient written consent is obtained)

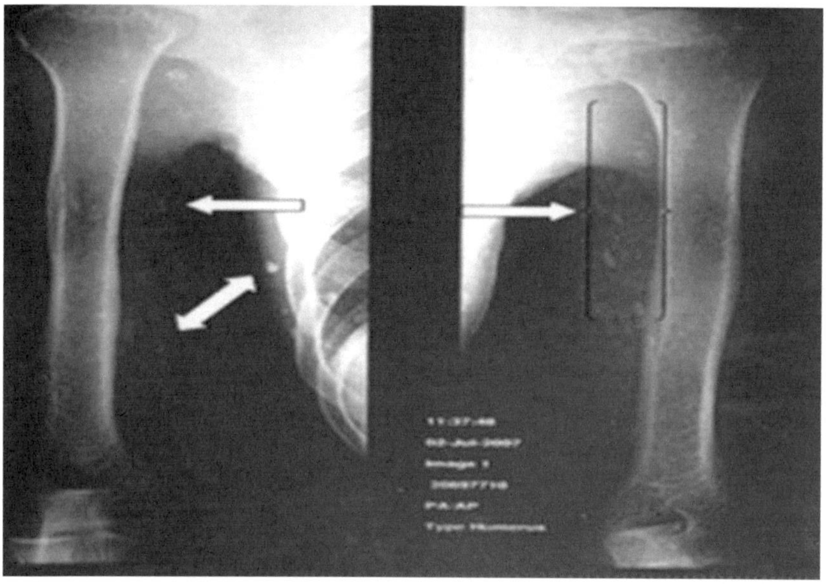

Figure 11. Plain X-ray of the chest and upper limbs show multiple subcutaneous and intramuscular "cigar-shape" calcifications.

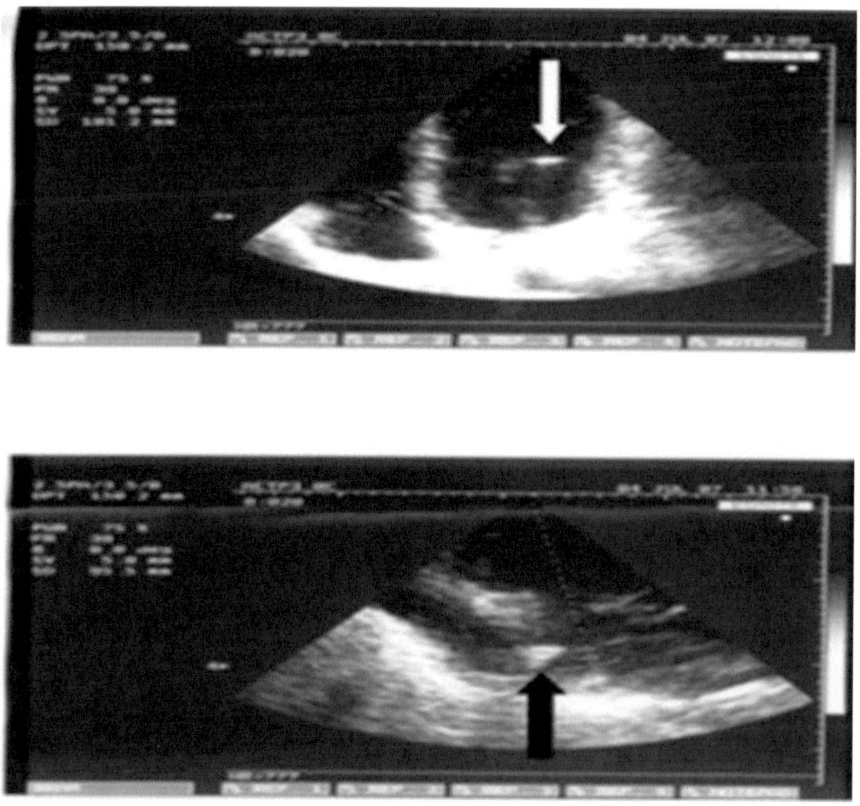

Figure 12. Cardiac ultrasound shows cysticercus in the cardiac muscle.

Ultrasography to diagnose subcutaneous cysticercosis was introduced a few years ago and from the beginning we also found some limitations to differentiated cysticercosis from lymphadenopathies, neurofibromas, and epidermoid cysts [41] however at the present moment is possible to confirm a diagnosis for subcutaneous nodules showing the scolex inside. Echocardiogram has a hight level of accuracy in cardiocysticercosis and we could confirm it in patients.

All South African patients presenting CCD also suffrering of symptomatic epilepsy because all had cerebro-cortical lesions caused by *T. solium.*

4. Disseminated cysticercosis and epilepsy

Epilepsy is also the most common clinical manifestation of NCC in our region [61-64] and it prevalence has been well documented in several communities of Eastern Cape Province in South Africa. [65-71]. While disseminated cysticercosis is an exceptional expression of CC characterized by high morbidity due to massive symptomatic parasite burden in the central nervous system, striated muscles, subcutaneous tissues and other organs. Less than 50 such cases have been reported worldwide and fewer than 10 children. In 2010, Kumar and collaborators [72] reported their findings on whole-body MRI as a diagnostic tool for extensively disseminated cysticercosis in a child and highlighted its role in diagnosis and management of this pleomorphic disease. Unfortunately, MRI is not available for most of patients with CCD worldwide and it can not replace the traditional way of diagnosis based on CT scan of the brain for NCC and plain X-ray for muscular and subcutaneous cysticercosis. Diagnosis of NCC can be made by Del Brutto's recommendation [73] but novel criterias suggested by Carpio in this boork, should be considerd

5. The disseminated cysticercosis going to disappear in the near future?

Before moving to another topic we would like to answer that research question.

We are convinced that CC will be eradicated from our planet, but today this is far from happen especially in some countries of Sub-Saharan Africa, Asia and Latin America, where there are communities who live, or have lived, either by choice (peoples living in voluntary isolation) or by circumstance, without significant contact with globalized civilization, therefore their current epidemiological situation is unknown and we even don't know how many peoples are infected by parasites.

We know that *T. solium* infested man long before there was any evidence of animal domestication (See chapter 1) [74, 75] by which we can assume that even in communities where very backward the taming of animals there is no zoonotic diseases may be acquired by other means.

For the other hand, there is an important number of hidden groups of peoples such as: racist groups and racist activists; drug traffickers in prisons; natives from the Central African Rain Forest; male and female prisoners and guards from a number of prison colonies; nationalists expressing anti-Semitic sentiment and young people participating in radical social and political mobilization among others [76]. How many of these hidden groups suffer of *T. solium* cysticercosis? We do not know.

In our opinion, even when the poverty disappear from underdeveloped countries and every person get a proper access to clean and safe water, living in very good hygienic conditions under an ideal health education and primary health care sustainable system program, we could not proclaim that the CC has been eradicated because of that important number of human beings sharing our planet whose epidemiological situation remain unknown. We are aware about an important number of individuals that still remains in that situation.

Congo region is included in our Cysticercosis Working Group for Eastern and Southern Africa (CGWESA). The Bambuti are pygmy hunter-gatherers, and are one of the oldest indigenous people of the Congo region of Africa. They are composed by bands which are relatively small in size, ranging from 15 to 60 people. The Bambuti population totals about 30,000 to 40,000 people. The forest where they live is a moist, humid region strewn with rivers and lakes. Disease is prevalent in the forests and can spread quickly, killing not only humans, but plants, and animals, the major source of food, as well. Their animal foodstuffs include crabs, shellfish, ants, larvae, snails, pigs, antelopes, monkeys, fishes, and honey. The vegetable component of their diet includes wild yams, berries, fruits, roots, leaves, and cola nuts [77]. Anyone is infected by *T. solium*?, Who knows? We do not know.

Many parts of the Americas are still populated by indigenous Americans; some countries have sizable populations, especially Bolivia, Peru, Mexico, Guatemala, Colombia, and Ecuador. Some indigenous peoples still live in relative isolation from Western society, and a few are still counted as uncontacted peoples [78]. Most uncontacted communities are located in densely forested areas in South America and New Guinea. Knowledge of the existence of these groups comes mostly from infrequent and sometimes violent encounters with neighboring tribes, and from aerial footage. Isolated tribes may lack immunity to common diseases, which can kill 50 to 80 per cent of their people after contact [79] but nobody knows how many parasites are affecting them.

The Sentinelese continues to actively and violently reject contact. They live on North Sentinel Island, a small and remote island which lies to the west of the southern part of South Andaman Island. They are thus considered the most isolated people in the world, and they are likely to remain so [73]. The current epidemiological situation on parasitic zoonoses of Sentinel is still unknown.

In Paraguay remains perhaps as many as 300 Totobiegosode who have not been contacted; they belong to the Ayoreo ethnicity, which numbers around 2,000. As of 2006, the presence of five uncontacted groups was confirmed in Bolivia; three more uncontacted groups are believed to exist. On January 18, 2007, the National Indian Foundation reported that it had confirmed the presence of 67 uncontacted tribes in Brazil, up from 40 in 2005. With this reported increase, Brazil has surpassed the island of New Guinea as the region having the highest number of uncontacted tribes. Ecuador continues to be the country with the largest number of uncontacted people killed since 2000. After Brazil and New Guinea (Papua New

Guinea and Iriyan Jaya), Peru has the largest number of uncontacted tribes in the world [79] and there is not available information about their current situation related to incidence or prevalence of infectious diseases.

Today there are more than 150 million tribal peoples worldwide, including at least 70 uncontacted tribes, living in 60 countries. Some organization such as: Survival International supports these endangered tribes on a global level, with campaigns established in America, Africa and Asia [80, 81]. In our opinion, many of them can be parasitized by *T. solium* as was the *H ergatus* more than a million of the year ago (See chapter 1).

Due to globalization, a growing number of uncontrolled immigrants from an endemic area in Latin America come to the USA every day, significantly increasing the number of cases of NCC in the country especially in Texas and California [82-91] where a total of 1494 patients with NCC were confirmed between 1980 and 2004 of which 66% suffered from epilepsy, 16% had a obstructive hydrocephalus and the 15% headache due to intraparechymal NCC (91 %), intraventricular (6 %) or subarachnoid (2 %) either because travelled to endemic areas, were of Hispanic origin or had any contact with carriers of the parasite [92-93]. In Latin America has been described the existence of NCC in 18 countries with an estimated 350,000 patients infected by the complex CC/TE. In 2008, Pawlowski stipulated that in the world would have approximately 2.5 million people infected T solium and at least 20 million with CC [70].

Disseminate presentations of cysticercosis is not common in our region, only six patients were previously confirmed and four of them reported to the medical literature [41, 50, 58, 59]. Typical manifestation is subcutaneous cyst present as nodules that tend to be asymptomatic [41, 50]. The natural history of the infection remains unknown up to date. However, is well known that most cysticercus complete their development within two to four months after larval entry living there months to years, and their locations in order of frequency are the central nervous system, subcutaneous tissues, striated muscle, heart, orbits, and other tissues. Human cysticercosis is acquired after eating food contaminated with fertilized eggs excreted in the feces of Taenia's carriers. In humans the most common routes of infection (cysticercosis) are ingestion of *T .solium* eggs from contamined food and fecal-oral auto-infestation in patients harbouring the adult parasite in their intestines. While the cysts can develop in most human tissue, they have a predilection for CNS. Cysticercosis is estimated to affect approximately 50 million people worldwide and is common in rural South Africa [1, 10-15, 61-71].

6. Disseminated cysticercosis with involvement of other organs

6.1. Cardiocysticercosis

The vast majority of patients with DCC reported to international medical literature are from India and although CC can affect almost any tissue the most frequently reported are the central nervous system and skeletal muscles [41,50,58]. Myocardial cysticercosis is rare [94,95] but its diagnosis is easier with modern radiological tools [95-97] . We will see in more detail the most important features of the cysticercosis of the cardiac muscle followed by cysticercosis in the lungs and the combination of both presentations.

As before-mentioned DCC means distribution of cysticerci along to the brain, skeletal muscles and subcutaneous tissues. In this part of the chapter we will discuss about other organs affected.

Long before the emergence of computerized tomography knew each other from the first cases with cardiocysticercosis with other associated diseases of the heart in living patients [98], even with silent presentation [99] or disorders of cardiac conduction [100]. The lack of brain imaging studies did not confirm the presence of associated NCC in those cases. Spent 10 years and then was possible achieve a better image of the heart and confirm best results with the use of praziquantel in this type of presentation associated with DCC [101]. Some parasites may directly or indirectly affect various anatomical structures of the heart, with infections manifested as myocarditis, pericarditis, pancarditis, or pulmonary hypertension. In other situations, parasitic infections may have more direct effects on various structures of the heart (myocardium, pericardium, endocardium, or the cardiac vasculature). The involvement of the myocardium may lead to myocarditis or different types of cardiomyopathies (i.e., dilated or restrictive). When the pericardium is affected, it may lead to pericarditis, pericardial effusion, cardiac tamponade, or constrictive pericarditis. Due to growing migration, population displacement, and travel, clinicians anywhere around the globe must be aware of the potential cardiac manifestations of parasitic diseases [57,102].

The myocardial inflammatory response is variable, resulting in granuloma formation and fibrosis, which subsequently leads to arrhythmias and conduction abnormalities either spontaneously or during treatment [57,103-105].

Cardiac involvement in cysticercosis was thought to be rare, but autopsy studies have shown a prevalence of 20 to 25% in patients with concomitant documented neurocysticercosis [104,105]. Cardiac cysticercosis is often asymptomatic and discovered during cardiac surgery or at autopsy. Cysticerci are usually multiple and randomly distributed in cardiac tissues, including the subpericardium, subendocardium, and myocardium [104]. Rarely, a single cardiac cyst may be present [102]. The computed tomography and ultrasonographic studies have demonstrated a fundamental importance in the diagnosis of cysticercosis of the heart according with results reported by other authors [57,106-108] and own personal experience [41, 50].

The DCC also affects children severely, an example of that is in the five years old patient reported by Asrani [108] in 2004, who presented subcutaneous swellings all over her body. The swellings were each between 0.5 and 2 cm in size. There were only 1 or 2 to start with on the back of the neck, and then they gradually increased to involve the chest, head, neck, arms, and legs in 2 to 3 months. These swellings were accompanied by onset of abnormal behavior in the form of irritability, talkativeness, disobeying commands, and bladder incontinence (secondary enuresis). Also, there was abnormal weight gain of 10 kg. The patient also had decreased vision for one month. Examination revealed multiple subcutaneous nodules between 0.5 and 2 cm in size over the forehead, abdomen, back, and legs. She weighed 29 kg (19 kg in a previous month). Her vision was 6/30 according to the Snellen chart. The patient was referred for sonography of the abdomen. The abdominal visceras on examination with a 3.5-MHz convex transducer were unremarkable, but the abdominal wall showed some tiny cystic lesions. Further examination using a high-frequency 7- to 12-MHz linear transducer (HDI 3000; Philips Medical Systems, Andover, MA) showed innumerable oval to circular, 0.5- to 1.5-cm, predominantly anechoic lesions in the subcutaneous tissues and abdominal wall muscles. Similar lesions were distributed over the back, neck, thighs, calves, legs, axillae, forearms, and arms. Sonography of the tongue also revealed similar multiple lesions. There was no increased vascularity surrounding these lesions on color Doppler examination. Only the palms and soles seemed to be uninvolved. A sonographic diagnosis of disseminated muscular cysticercosis was made. Whole-body contrast-enhanced computed tomography (CT) confirmed the sonographic findings and showed the classic "starry night" in the brain. The entire muscular system and the subcutaneous tissue had hypodense, nonenhancing, approximately 1-cm lesions without calcification, suggesting that all the cysts were live. Magnetic resonance imaging (MRI) of the brain,orbit, and musculoskeletal system showed multiple hyperintense lesions on transverse relaxation time (T2)-weighted images.

A biopsy of the subcutaneous nodules showed classic cysts with a central scolex. Multiple ocular cysts were also found on ocular examination. After this, the patient started receiving steroids and anthelminthic agents. Within 4 weeks of starting treatment, the patient's weight decreased by 10 kg (to 19 kg again). She became quiet and began obeying commands. Her vision became 6/12 (Snellen chart). Echocardiography revealed extensive myocardial involvement. The major differential diagnosis is hydatid cyst, which is usually larger and multilocular. Antihelminthic treatment may result in pericystic inflammatory reaction which might worsen the clinical state [109].

Other parasite can also affect the myocardium and the pericardium as we have previously pointed out, and that the most widely studied parasitic infection affecting the heart is Chagas' disease or American trypanosomiasis but African trypanosomiasis may also cause a myocarditis. The protozoan parasite, Entamoeba histolytica rarely causes a pericarditis while Toxoplasma gondii may cause myocarditis, usually in immunocompromised hosts. The larval forms of the tapeworms Echinococcus and *T. solium* may cause space occupying lesions of the heart. Severe infection with the nematode Trichinella spiralis may cause myocarditis [110].

Not always cardiocysticercosis is part of the disseminated cysticercosis as reported by Eberly and collaborators and it may occur as an isolated infection of the left ventricle [111].

In 2009, Shogan [112] reported a 17-year-old boy from Cameroon presenting a sessile cystic cardiac mass. A CT scan revealed a 1.0 × 1.5 cm nonenhancing, exophytic, ovoid mural-based fluid density in the left ventricle along the endocardial surface of the anterior wall near the anteroseptal basal region. On T1-weighted MR images, the mass was hypointense. On T2-weighted MR images, the mass was hyperintense, with a rounded hypointense signal visible at the posterior wall of the cyst. One internal septation of the mass was noted. After gadolinium administration, no enhancement was present. The patient underwent biopsy of the mass. Histologic evaluation showed a fluid-containing cystic structure, which exhibited a single protoscolex consistent with a cysticercus. These authors mentioned that involvement of the heart by *T. solium* is very rare and is usually diagnosed postmortem. After review the international medical literature we agree it is rare but diagnosis of cardiocysticercosis is made accurately in most of patient seeking for medical attention. Shogan's report is extremelly uncommon because his patient had not an associated DCC or NCC [112], but without doubt the cardiocysticercosis must always be borne in mind in patients with similar presentations and because it is commonly associated with intraparenchymal NCC therefore to look for epilepsy is strong recommended. (See figure 13)

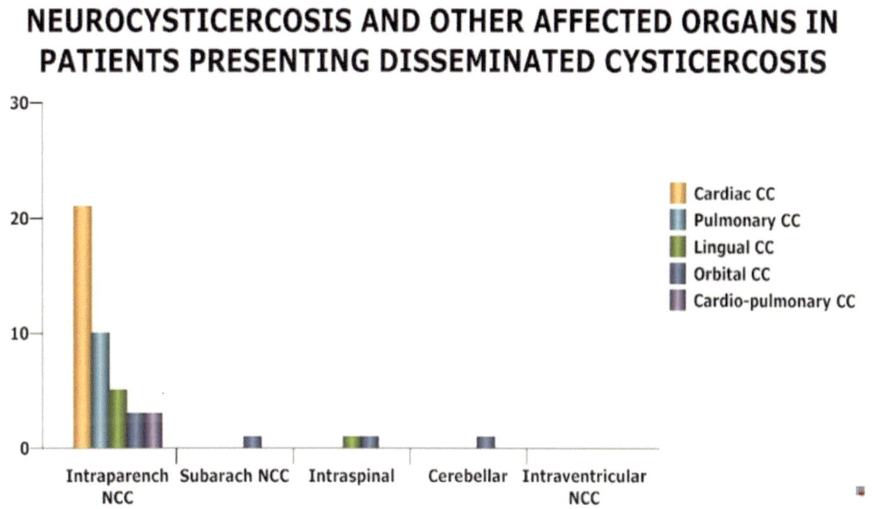

Figure 13. Graphical representation of other affected organs and location of cysticerci in the CNS.

6.2. Pulmonary cysticercosis

Most of patients presenting pulmonary cysticercosis have multiple rather than solitary pulmonary nodules (a "spot" on the lung that is less than 3 cm or 1½ inches in diameter by chest X-ray).

The differential diagnosis of multiple pulmonary nodules is large and includes congenital and inherited disorders, malignancy, infectious etiologies, noninfectious granulomatous and inflammatory conditions, among many others. Disseminated cysticercosis with pulmonary involvement should be suspected in any patient presenting with multiple pulmonary nodules who is an immigrant from an endemic region or an individual who has resided in one of the countries where cysticercosis is endemic [113].

Taking into consideration that the only infectious disease causing multiple pulmonary nodules and associated cutaneous manifestation are: blastomycosis, coccidiomycosis, tuberculosis and cysticercosis then the differential diagnosis of pulmonary cysticercosis is very easy if DCC/NCC complex is present.

In 1971, Bassermann [114] found some radiographic problems in pulmonary cysticercosis because at that time computed tomography system was not available. Siemens Medical Solutions (then known as Siemens Medical Engineering) presented the first machine commercially available in May 1974. Therefore confirmation of NCC by imagenology was not done. Other authors studied patients with pulmonary cysticercosis at different times and all of them agree that this is an uncommon condition [115-119].

Schotz and Mentis [116] in 1987 reported a 48-years-old black man admitted to hospital with a 2-month history of a painless mass on the left side of his neck. He also complained of mild attacks of paroxysmal dyspnoea at night and progressive deafness of his left ear. On direct questioning the patient referred a few grand mal seizures during the six years before admission. No other complaints or previous illnesses of note were elicited. The patient was born in Transkei (near to Mthatha in South Africa) and had travelled throughout many parts of the country seeking work, which he secured in the gold mines mainly. He ate a variety of meats including pork and smoked and drank excessively at times.On examination he appeared healthy and was of normal build. The pulse rate was 72/min, blood pressure 110/60 mmHg and temperature 37,2°C. Numerous subcutaneous nodules, ranging in size from 1 cm to 3 cm in diameter, which were well circumscribed and freely movable, could be palpated all over the neck, chest and legs. A bigger mass was palpable inferior to the left ear, extending down the left side of the neck. There was conduction deafness of the left ear. On chest auscultation a few fine crepitations were audible at the bases of both lungs. Computed tomography of the brain, neck, thorax and upper abdomen revealed extensive organ involvement, including brain, thyroid, lungs, pancreas, kidney, spleen and muscle; and biopsies of two of the subcutaneous nodules were histologically pathognomonic of *T. solium* cysticercosis. The patient received praziquantel (Biltricide; Bayer-Miles) 1,75 g twice daily and prednisone 20 mg per day for 4 weeks. He was reassessed radiologically after 4 weeks. There was marked regression in the size and numbers of nodules in the lung fields. Clinically, most of the subcutaneous nodules had disappeared. Authors highlighted that the radiological appearance of cysticercosis in the lung cannot be differentiated from other parasitic infections, e.g. echinococcosis, pentastomiasis, paragonimiasis and histoplasmosis, or conditions such as tuberculosis, alveolar carcinoma and metastases due to the varying reaction of the lung tissue and difference in size of the larvae [114]. Pulmonary sparganosis should be exluded from the list of differential diagnosis as well [120]. Although rare, pulmonary cysticercosis does occur and in developing countries should not be overlooked in the differential diagnosis of multiple lung opacities.

From our knowledge, this is the only patient with renal involvement reported to the medical literature ever.

From one case reported in Korea, authors concluded that the presence of cysticerci are difficult to discern from pulmonary infiltrates, because other parasitic infestations or tuberculosis, as well as metastatic lesions, produce similar chest X-ray findings and similar clinical symptoms (as before-mentioned) and they suggest open lung biopsy for confirmation, for treatment PZQ (50 mg/kg per day for 15 days) and to consider pulmonary cysticercosis as a diagnostic possibility in patients with nodular infiltrates in the lungs, especially in endemic areas, until such infiltrates are otherwise explained [118].

In 2011, a radiologist from Punjab, India [119] reported a well documented 28-year-old man presented with a history of fever, dry cough, headache and decreased responsiveness over 7 days. One year previously, he had suffered seizures and was hospitalised in another centre with an initial diagnosis of NCC and received treatment for it. MRI at that time depicted numerous ring enhancing lesions with eccentric scolex ('cyst with dot' appearance) in the cerebral hemispheres, subarachnoid space and orbits. The patient had a history of pork intake and intravenous drug misuse. Physical examination at the time of admission revealed small, movable, painless subcutaneous nodules that were palpable over the arms, axillae and trunk. No abnormalities were noted on auscultation of the lungs. Blood and urine cultures were negative. Sputum analysis was normal. A chest x-ray revealed small nodules in both lungs. This is the first report about pulmonary cysticercosis in a patient presenting DCC and subarachnoid NCC.

Next patient was reported by Strawter et.al., [113] a few weeks ago. They studied a 31-year-old incarcerated Hispanic male presented with a nonproductive cough for several months and one episode of blood tinged sputum. He admitted to weight loss and night sweats, headaches, and visual disturbances. He was an immigrant from Honduras and lived in Arizona for the past 15 years. He had chronic hepatitis C infection and was receiving treatment with pegylated interferon-alfa-2a (IFN-α) and ribavirin. His symptoms began one month after initiating antiviral therapy.They confirmed pulmonary nodules with cutaneous manifestations and concluded that: Disseminated cysticercosis with pulmonary involvement should be suspected in any patient presenting with multiple pulmonary nodules who is an immigrant from an endemic region or an individual who has resided in one of the countries where cysticercosis is present or when NCC is well documented. Lung are the second thoracic organ affected by *T solium* cysticercosis preceded by the heart (See Figure 14)

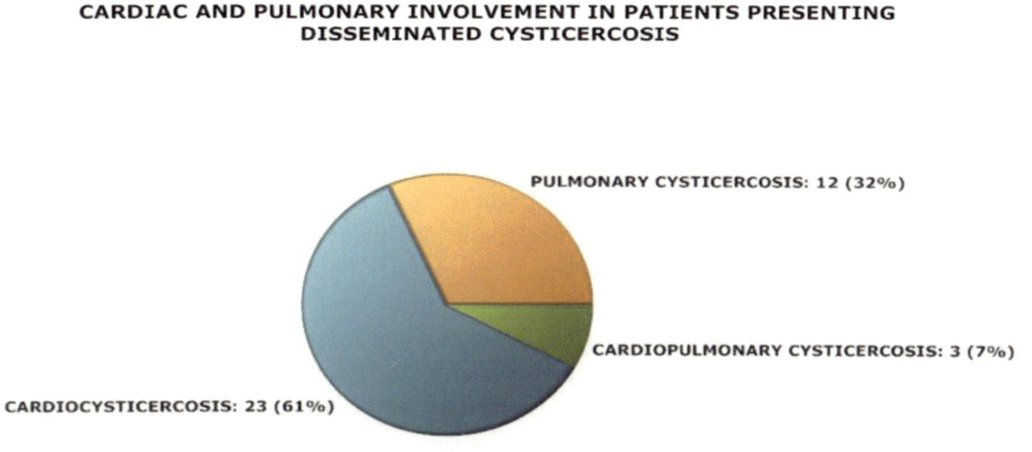

Figure 14. Thoracic organs involved in disseminated cysticercosis

6.3. Cardio-pulmonary cysticercosis

The heart and the lungs are the thoracic organs more frequently affected by parasitic infections. The involvement of the heart may be part of a more generalized illness, as is the case with human African trypanosomiasis [102] and other parasitic diseases as before-cited. The first case reported under this condition presented a massive cardiopulmonary cysticercosis and an associated leukemia. [121] being this one the only patient presenting this type of co-morbidity. Bastos et al., [122] from Brazil reported another patient and highlighted the importance of imagenology (CT scan) of the chest for confirmation of diagnosis based on their findings: multiple pulmonary, cardiac and chest wall nodules concluding that cysticercosis should be considered in the differential diagnosis of multiple pulmonary nodules, mainly in those patients with similar lesions in the cardiac muscle and/or in the chest wall which made the overall diagnosis easy to perform.

Other important contribution is made by Jain et al., [123]. They reported a 19-year-old boy from Mumbai (India) who presented with a history of headache and vomiting for six months, seizures for three months, and decreased vision and bilateral proptosis (right more than left) for one month. The patient was apparently asymptomatic six months back. The patient was a vegetarian. Examination revealed subcutaneous nodules over the right eyelid, with mild proptosis of both eyes. Using the Snellen chart, his vision was found to be 6/30 in the right eye and 7/30 in the left eye. Neurological examination did not reveal any abnormality. All the laboratory investigations were normal. The patient was referred for MRI of the brain, which revealed multiple 3–8 mm-sized cystic lesions with T2-hypointense foci within both cerebral hemispheres, cerebellum, extraocular muscles of both orbits and soft tissues of the neck. Similar lesions were distributed in the muscles and adjacent subcutaneous tissues of the back, abdominal wall, thighs, calves, legs, forearms and arms as well as the extradural spinal space. Multiple cystic lesions were seen in both lungs and in the cardiac muscles. Hyperintense nodules were also seen in the pancreas. For further evaluation, a high-resolution CT (HRCT) of the lungs was performed, which revealed bilateral multiple, randomly distributed, 3-8 mm nodules. A B-scan USG was performed, which revealed a large intravitreal cyst within the right eye, with a tiny hyperechoic scolex. The left eye was normal. On superficial probe evaluation of the heart and pericardium through a parasternal window, using a high-frequency 7 to 12 MHz linear transducer (HDI 3000; Philips Medical Systems, Andover, MA, USA), there were multiple oval to circular, 0.5–1.5-cm sized, predominantly anechoic lesions in the heart muscle. Later, a dedicated 2D echocardiography was performed, which revealed multiple disseminated cysticerci involving the muscle of the heart. On the basis of these imaging findings, a diagnosis of disseminated cysticercosis was made. The patient also had right bundle branch block on electrocardiogram; however, other functional parameters such as ejection fraction, valve function, systolic function and chamber size were normal on 2D echocardiography. A final diagnosis of cysticercosis was made and this was confirmed on muscle biopsy. Because drug-induced inflammation due to praziquantel may cause irreversible damage in cases with ocular lesions, this medication was not given, and the patient was treated symptomatically with antiepileptic drugs, steroids, and diuretics. To the best of our knowledge, this is the best documented patient presented with disseminated cysticercosis with cardiac, pulmonary, pancreatic, spinal, extradural, and ocular involvement reported in the international medical literature up today and clearly demonstrate the extent to which cysticercosis can be disseminated and almost all probable combination of involved organs.

Although this report does not describe the state of the evolutionary of cysticercus, it is logical to assume that a parasitic infection of this magnitud is due to uninterrupted ingestion of *T. solium* eggs which is only possible under deplorable sanitary conditions. Such a quantity of larvae of *T. solium* solium when driving through the bloodstream in a young patient allows its dissemination almost uniformly throughout the body including the CNS. This aspect will be discussed below.

6.4. Orbital cysticercosis

In the next chapter we will refer more details to the ocular cysticercosis according to their different locations within and outside of the eyeball but without exceeding the limits of the orbital cavity. In this chapter we will review only the clinical features of the ocular cysticercosis associated with damage to other organs as part of the disseminate cysticercosis, based on the results published in the international medical literature.

Almost all patients presenting cysticercotic orbital involvement and associated DCC were from India as we show below. Cheung et al., [124] in 1987 reported a patient with disseminated cysticercosis involving orbit, tongue, parotid glands, epicardial fat tissue, muscles, and subcutaneous tissues confirmed by MRI. This was the first communication on combination of cysticercosis of the orbit, parotid gland and epicardial fat. Cysticercosis of the eyelid was studied by Gupta et al., [125]. One of the youngest patient (5-years-old) ever studied was reported by Asrani and Morani [108] their patient apart from cardiocysticercosis (before-mentioned) also presented multiple orbital cysts with decreased visual acuity and neuropsychiatric manifestations. Despite this ocular involvement this patient received anthelmintic agents and not further complications were informed. Combination of epilepsy, DCC, proptosis of the eyes, fever and arthralgia can be seen [8]. Disseminated cysticercosis can cause intravitreal lesions with exudative retinal detachment and bilateral extra ocular muscular damage at the same time [126] or afect only the brain, orbits, subcutaneous tissue [127, 128] the eyes, tongue and spinal cord [127] or the tongue, eyes, face and scalp muscles [130], and an extensive involvement of both orbits [131]; face, scalp muscles, subconjuctival cysts in the eyes and cysticercotic encephalitis [132], cardiopulmonary cysticercosis plus proptosis of the eyes, extra ocular muscles of both orbits, extradural spinal, and cerebellar involvement [123] and other combinations such as: subarachnoid NCC, Brown syndrome, different extra ocular muscles involvement, mimicking idiopathic orbital inflammation, retina involvement , and canine tooth syndrome have been reported to the medical literature [119, 133-138].

6.5. Other organs affected

As we have seen, the disseminate cysticercosis (muscular and subcutaneous tissue) is always associated with the NCC and in addition, it can be associate to heart, lung, eyes, spleen, pancreas, parotid, liver, kidneys and pharynx involvement. Here we will discuss about some cases presenting this modalities of DCC.

Other presentations of the DCC include epilepsy with extensive muscular involvement, predominantly [139-144], associated liver damage [145], epilepsy with damage of the soft tissues of the scalp plus supra and infratentorial lesions; spinal cord [129] epilepsy and DCC with huge muscle involvement [146-148], vocal cord [149], thyroid gland [150], the tongue [129,151], spleen and pancreas [46]; or even without neurological symptoms [152] or immunocompromised patient [153].

Cysticercosis of the pharynx the kidneys have been reported in South Africa only [58, 61], as we have mentioned previously that serves to highlight that these two locations must also keep in mind when planning to perform clinical investigations for this type of patient. Most of isolated damaged organs by CC without dissemination of cysticerci throught the subcutaneous tissues are not associated with NCC and when it happen then extraparenchymal location can be seen. Because only anecdotic reports to the medical literature are available at the present moment (See figure 15) we can not arrive to solid conclusions and only advices are suggested.

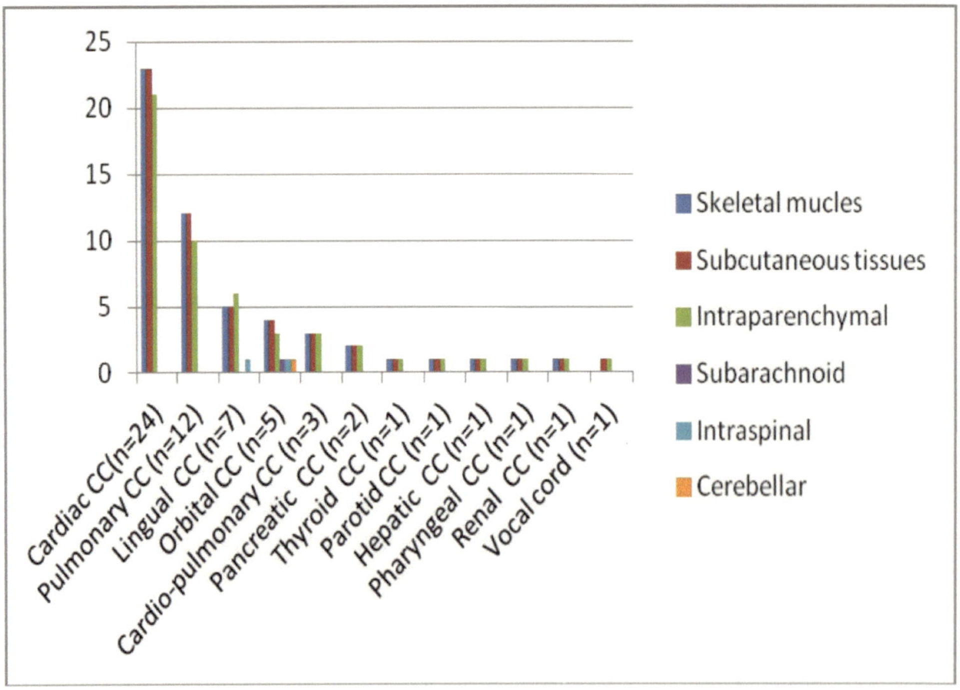

Figure 15. Graphic representation of number of patients with cysticercosis in different organs as part of disseminated cysticercosis with involvement of the central nervous system at different levels.

India has the highest prevalence of disseminate cysticercosis worldwide (Figure 17). Given the fact that cysticercosis is an endemic disease in India and that WB-MRI is now available on most modern MRI scanners, especially in academic institutions, Goenka and Kumar [154,

155] believe that awareness about this technique may enable to his fellow colleagues to explore its valuable potential in disseminated cysticercosis. Most of patients presenting DCC are from India (New Delhi) as can be seen in the figure 16 but even there, the number of well documented patient is still no enough to design an accurate clinical trial looking for a medication of choice for this condition. Based on our experiency, to combine Praziquantel and Albendazole with steroids provide good results if there is not involvement of the heart, the eyes or massive NCC.

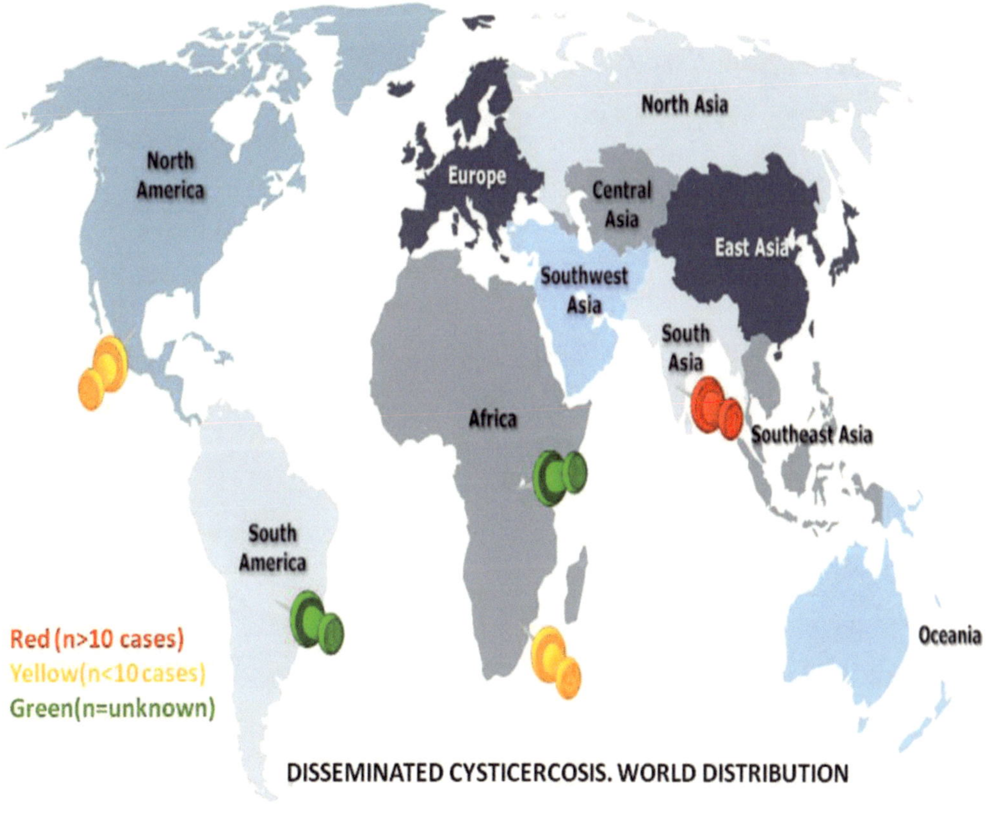

Figure 16. Distribution of disseminated cysticercosis worldwide.

As noted in the previous map there are two large areas in Latin America and Africa where the disease is may be present but the ignored epidemiological conditions of those not having established contact with the civilized world make impossible to predict the possible number of patients although by photos published in Internet we could not identified anyone.

7. Mortality rate in disseminated cysticercosis

The mortality rate for the cysticercosis is widespread and extremely low, in our series was always below 0.05 % in the past 15 years.

Based on our experience and in the cases reported in the international medical literature the causes of death are almost always related to the NCC and anecdotal cases secondary to pancreatic or cardiopulmonary complications.

The most frequent cause of death related to the NCC in patients with CCD is the intraventricular NCC with intracranial hypertension by obstructive hydrocephalus, the subarachnoid NCC with cerebrovascular complications, the NCC of the insula with associated neurogénic heart or sudden unexpected death and the massive NCC. When there are more than a thousand cysts in the brain the mortality rate is extremely high (see figure 17).

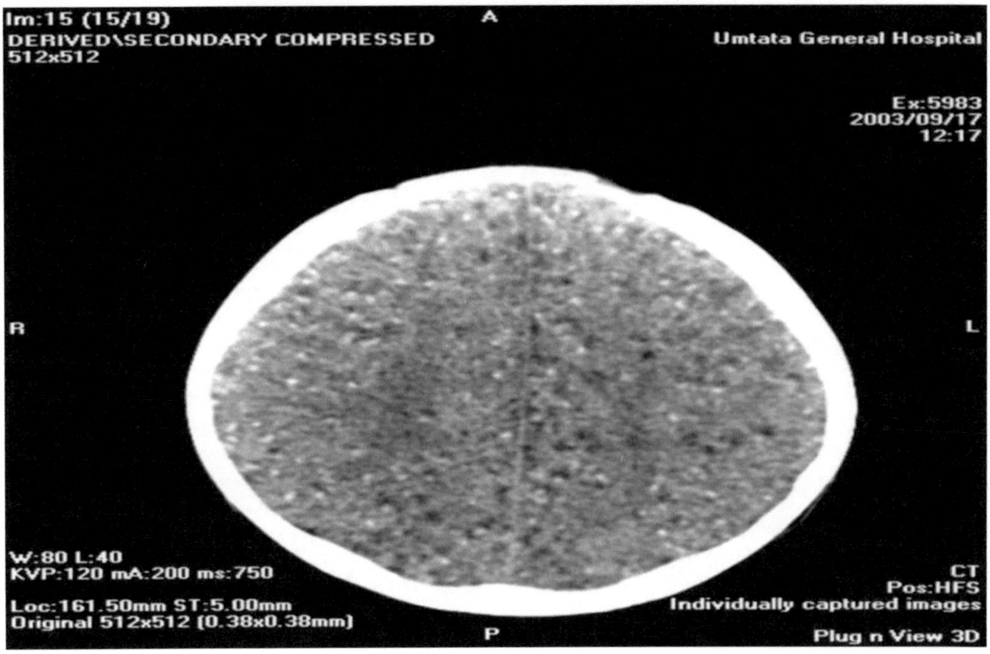

Figure 17. CT scan of the brain showing massive neurocystciercosis.

8. Why some cisticercus move to one path while other move to another one?

The cerebellar lesions are an expression of this type of distribution as they generally cisticercotic lesions in the posterior fossa are only seen when there are massive infestations or when the cysticerci traveling through a non-laminar flow secondary to vascular lesions not described in the medical literature (See figure 18).

We think this situation happen because of the haemodynamic characteristic of the blood flow can change in different blood vessel. Let us to explain what probably happen when cysticerci coincide in the same place at the same time. When between two cysticercus in movement speed gradient exists, or is that a moves faster than the other, they develop friccian forces acting tangentially to the same. The friction forces are trying to introduce rotation between the cysticerci in motion, but simultaneously the viscosity seeks to prevent rotation. Depending on the relative value of these forces can be produce different flow states. When the gradient of speed is low, the inertia force is greater than the friction, the cysticerci move but do not rotate, or they make it but with very little power, the final result is a movement in which the particles follow paths defined, and all of the particles that pass by a point in the field of flow follow the same trajectory. This type of flow was identified by O. Reynolds and is called "laminar", meaning that the particles are moving in the form of layers or sheets. The increase of velocity gradient increases the friction between neighboring cysticercus to the fluid, and these become a significant energy of rotation, the viscosity loses its effect, and due to the rotation of the cysticercus change trajectory. Going from one path to another, the cysticerci collide and change course in erratic. This type of flow is called "turbulent". Turbulent flow can also be due to abnormalities in the wall of blood vessels.The turbulent flow is characterized by:

- The cysticercus in the fluid does not move along with defined trajectories.
- The action of the viscosity is negligible.
- The cysticerci in the fluid possess appreciable energy of rotation, and they move erratically colliding with each other.

When entering the fluid articles to layers of different speed, its linear time increases or decreases, and the particles of the neighboring does so in a manner that is contrary. When the forces of inertia of the fluid in movement are very low, the viscosity is the dominant force and the flow is laminar. When dominated by the forces of inertia the flow is turbulent.

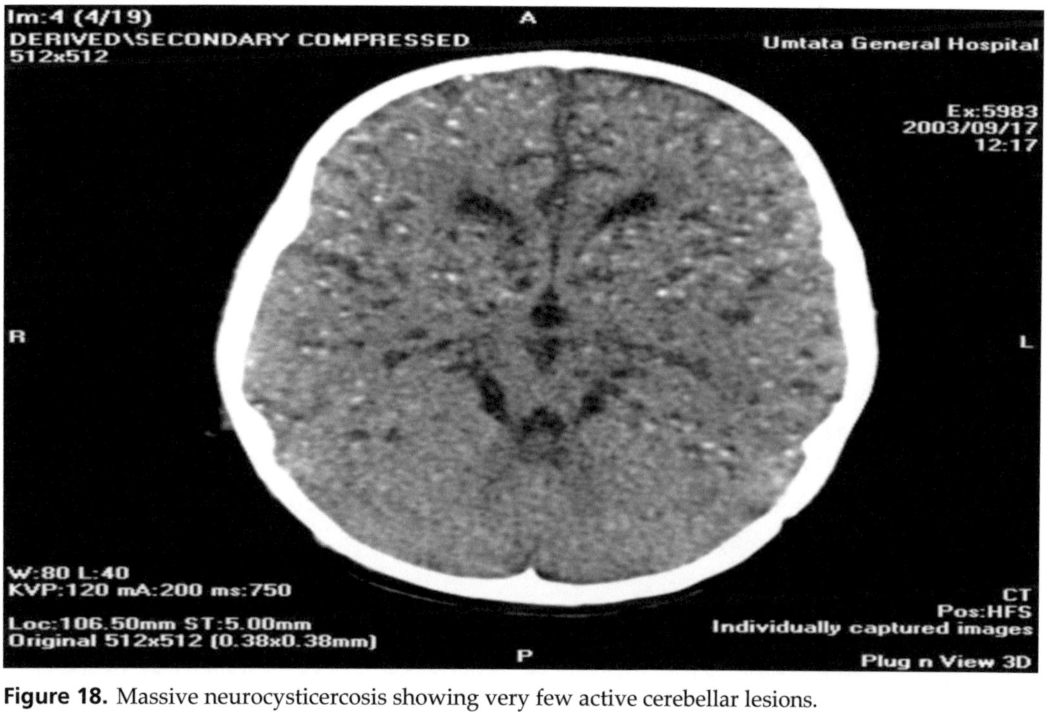

Figure 18. Massive neurocysticercosis showing very few active cerebellar lesions.

9. Conclusion

The disseminated cysticercosis is a rare disease and the largest number of cases have been confirmed and published in India. Disseminated cysticercosis is accompanied by neurocysticercosis especially in its intraparenchymal localization but other locations are possible. There have been no reported cases of neurocysticercosis intraventricular associated to disseminated cysticercosis.

Apart from the subcutaneous tissue, muscles and the brain, the organ most frequently affected is the heart and the disorder of cardiac conduction is the main problem. Orbital cysticercosis (intra or extra ocular) is not associated with the disseminated cysticercosis in South Africa while in India makes it with more frequency.

At the present time, DCC seems to be not associated to HIV infections.

The low prevalence of the disseminated cysticercosis does not mean that cysticercosis is about to disappear in the near future.

It is possible that the defining characteristics of blood flow may be determined by the erratic locations of cysticerci, but well designed hemodynamic studies are needed to demonstrate this hypothesis.

Author details

Humberto Foyaca Sibat and Lourdes de Fátima Ibañez Valdés
Walter Sisulu University, Faculty of Health Sciences, Nelson Mandela Academic Hospital, Department of Neurology, Mthatha, South Africa

Acknowledgement

We like to thanks to all veterinarian researches working on this field.

We also want to thank to all radiologists and radiographers from Nelson Mandela Academic Hospital and Inkhosi Albert Luthuli Central Hospital in South Africa for their contribution to this study.

Special thanks are due to the Cuban Ministry of Health and Institute of Tropical Medicine "Pedro Kouri", and authorities of Nelson Mandela Academic Hospital, School of Medicine, Faculty of Health Sciences and Directorate: Research Development from Walter Sisulu University for their kind support. Finally, we would like to declare our eternal and deepest gratitude to Lorna María Foyaca García, Fátima Susana Foyaca Ibañez and Thabo Humberto Foyaca Ibañez for their delight support.

Hereby, we acknowledge financial support from the South African Medical Research Council. The founder had no role in study design, data collection and analysis, decision to publish, or preparation of the manuscript

10. References

[1] Foyaca-Sibat H. Epilepsy Secondary to Parasitic Zoonoses of the Brain, Novel Aspects on Epilepsy, Humberto Foyaca-Sibat (Ed.), ISBN: 978-953-307-678-2, InTech, Rijeka, 2011.

[2] Woolhouse M.E.J, Gowtage-Sequeria S. Host range and emerging and reemerging pathogens. *Emerg Infect Dis.* 2005;11:1842-1847.

[3] Bautista IR. Neurocisticercosis una realidad y sus limitantes en el diagnóstico. SIRIVS. Curso: Investigación II. Maestría en Salud Animal. Universidad Nacional Mayor de San Marcos Facultad de Medicina Veterinaria.2008

[4] Garg RK. Neurocysticercosis. *Postgrad Med J* 1998; 74(872):321-326.

[5] White AC Jr. Neurocysticercosis: updates on epidemiology, pathogenesis, diagnosis and management. *Ann Rev Med* 2000;51:187-206.

[6] Uddin J, Gonzalez AE, Gilman RH, Thomas LH, Rodriguez S, Evans CA, Remick DG, Garcia HH, Friedland JS. Mechanisms regulating monocyte CXCL8 secretion in neurocysticercosis and the effect of antiparasitic therapy. J Immunol. 2010;185(7):4478-4484.

[7] Wadia N, Desai S, Bhatt M: Disseminated cysticercosis. New observations, including CT scan findings and experience with treatment by praziquantel. *Brain* 1988, 111:597-614.

[8] Bhalla A, Sood A, Sachdev A, Varma V. Disseminated cysticercosis: a case report and review of the literature *Medical Case Reports* 2008; 2:137-140. http://www.jmedicalcasereports.com/content/2/1/137 (accessed May 04, 2012).

[9] Sarti E, Schantz PM, Plancharte A, Wilson M, Gutierrez R, Lopez AS, Roberts J, Flisser. Prevalence and risk factor for *Taenia solium* taeniasis and cysticercosis in humans and pigs in a village in Morelos, Mexico. *Am J Trop Med Hyg* 1992; 46:677-684.

[10] Foyaca-Sibat H, Ibañez-Valdés L de F. Clinical trial of praziquantel and prednisone in rural patients with neurocysticercosis presenting recurrent epileptic attacks The Internet Journal of Neurology 2002;2):41-50. http://www.ispub.com/journal/the_internet_journal_of_neurology/volume_1_number_2_39/article/clinical_trial_of_praziquantel_and_prednisone_in_rural_patients_with_neurocysticercosis_presenting_with_recurrent_epileptic_attacks.html

[11] Foyaca-Sibat H, "Tapeworm and the brain" Journal of Sciences of Africa 2002;1:5-12. http://www.scienceofafrica.co.za/2002/june.worn.htm

[12] Foyaca-Sibat H, Ibañez-Valdés LdeF "Neurocysticercosis in HIV-positive patients" The Internet Journal of Infectious Diseases 2003:2(2):15-23.

[13] Foyaca-Sibat H, Ibañez-Valdés LdeF & J. Moré-Rodríguez : Parasitic Zoonoses Of The Brain: Another Challenger?. The Internet Journal of Neurology. 2010;12(2). http://www.ispub.com/journal/the_internet_journal_of_neurology/volume_12_number_2_4/article/parasitic-zoonoses-of-the-brain-another-challenger.html

[14] Foyaca-Sibat H and Ibañez-Valdés L de F. editor . Treatment of Epilepsy Secondary to Neurocysticercosis, Novel Treatment of Epilepsy. InTech, Rijeka, 2011

[15] Foyaca-Sibat H and Lourdes de Fátima Ibañez Valdés L de F (2011). Clinical Features of Epilepsy Secondary to Neurocysticercosis at the Insular Lobe, Novel Aspects on Epilepsy. InTech, Rijeka, 2011.

[16] McComick G, Zec Chi-S, Heiden J. Cysticercosis Cerebri. Review of 127 cases. *Arch Neurol* 1982; 39:534-539.

[17] Pfuetzenreiter MR, de Avila-Pires FD. Clinical manifestations in patients with computerized tomography diagnosis of Neurocysticercosis. Arq Neuropsiquiatr 1999;57(3A):653-658.

[18] Agapejev S. Epidemiology of Neurocysticercosis. in Brazil. *Rev Inst Med Trop Sao Paulo* 1996;38(3):207-216.

[19] Doder R, Madle-Samardzija N, Canak G, Vukadinov J, Tukulov V, Singhi sincerely. Neurocysticercosis-5 years′ experience at the Clinic for Infectious Diseases. *Med Pregl* 2002; 55(11-12):523-527.

[20] Mafojane NA, Appleton CC, Krecek RC, Michael LM & Willingham AL, III The current status of neurocysticercosis in Eastern and Southern Africa. *Acta Tropica* 2003;87: 25–33.

[21] Villa AM, Monteverde DA, Rodríguez W, Boero A, Sica RE. Neurocysticercosis in a hospital of the city of Buenos Aires: study of 11 cases. *Arq Neuropsiquiatr* 1993;51(3):336-336.

[22] García HH, Gonzalez AE, Evans CA, Gilman RH; Cysticercosis Working Group in Peru. Taenia solium cysticercosis. *Lancet.* 2003; 362: 547-556.

[23] García HH, Del Brutto OH; Cysticercosis Working Group in Peru. Neurocysticercosis: updated concepts about an old disease. *Lancet Neurol.* 2005; 4:653-661.

[24]] Takayanagui OM, Jardim E. Clinical aspects of nerocysticercosis: analysis of 500 cases. Arq Neuropsiquiatr 1983; 41(1):50-63.

[25] Takayanagui OM. Neurocysticercosis: I.Clinical and laboratory course of 151 cases. *Arq Neuropsiquiatr 1990; 48(1):1-10.*

[26] Takayanagui OM, Leite JP. Neurocysticercosis. *Rev Soc Bras Med Trop* 2001;34(3):283-290.

[27] Pitella JEH. Neuro schistosomiasis. *Brain Pathol 1997;*7:649-662.

[28] Sanchez, A.L.; Lindback, J.; Schantz, P.M.; Sone, M.; Sakai, H.; Medina, M.T. & Ljungstrom I. A population based case-control study of *Taenia solium* taeniosis and cysticercosis. *Ann Tropical Medical Parasitology* 1999;93: 247-258.

[29] Morales NM, Agapejev S, Morales RR, Padula NA, Lima MM. Clinical aspects of neurocysticercosis in children. *Pediatr Neurol* 2000; 22(4):287-291.

[30] Varma A, Gaur KJ. The clinical spectrum of Neurocysticercosis in the Uttraranchal region. *Assoc Physicians India* 2002;50:1398-1400.

[31] Scharf D. Neurocysticercosis. Two hundred thirty-eight cases from a California Hospital. *Arch Neurol* 1988; 45:777-780.

[32] Foyaca-Sibat H, Del Rio- Romero AI: Prevalence of Epilepsy in an Endemic Area For Neurocysticercosis In South Africa. *The Internet Journal of Neurology*.2008;9(1):8-18. http://www.ispub.com/journal/the_internet_journal_of_neurology/volume_9_number_1_6/article/prevalence_of_epilepsy_in_an_endemic_area_for_neurocysticercosis_in_south_africa.html

[33] Turkulov V, Madle-Samardzija N, Canak G, Vukadinov J, Aleksic-Dordevic M. Clinical and diagnostic approaches to neurocysticercosis. *Med Pregl* 2001; 54(7-8):353-356.

[34] Sotelo J, Guerrero V, Rubio F. Neurocysticercosis: a new classification based on active and inactive forms. *Arch Intern Med.* 1985;145:442–445.

[35] Singh G. Neurocystycercosis in South-Central America and the Indian subcontinent. A comparative evaluation. *Arq Neuropsiquatr* 1997; 55(3A):349-356.

[36] Del Brutto OH. Neurocysticercosis. *Rev Neurol* 1999; 29(5):4456-4466.

[37] Salata et al. Parasitic Infections of the Central Nervous System p 821. In Aminoff MJ et al., (eds) the Neurology and General Medicine. Churchill Livingstone, Philadelphia 2001

[38] Sotelo J, Penagos P, Escobedo F, Del Brutto OH: Short course of albendazole therapy for neurocysticercosis. *Arch Neurol* 45:1130-1133, 1988.

[39] Flisser A. Cisticercosis subcutáneo. *Ciencias,* UNAM 2011. http://hydra.fciencias.unam.mx:8080/xmlui/handle/123456789/62343?show=full (accessed May 04, 2011)

[40] Bielsa-Fernández MV. Hallazgo incidental de cisticercosis generalizada *Rev Gastroenterol* (Mex) 2011;76(2):169-170.

[41] Foyaca-Sibat H, Ibanez-Valdes LdeF, Mashiyi MK. Disseminate Cysticercosis. One-day treatment in a case.Rev Electron Biomed / Electron J Biomed 2004;3:39-43. http://biomed.uninet.edu/2004/n3/foyaca-n.html (accessed 05 May, 2012).

[42] Park SY, Min HK, Jung HK, Kwan YS. Disseminated cysticercosis. *Journal of Korean Neurosurgical Society.* 2011;49(3):190-193.

[43] Basu G, Surekha V, Ganesh A. Disseminated cysticercosis. Trop Doct. 2009;39(1):48-99.

[44] Pushker N, Bajaj MS, Balasubramanya R. Disseminated cysticercosis involving orbit, brain and subcutaneous tissue. *J Infect.* 2005;51(5):245-248.

[45]] Narang P, Chhibbers S, Puri SK. Middle-aged man with altered behaviour and seizures. The British Journal of Radiology, 81 (2008), 984–986.

[46] Jakhere SG, Chemburkar VC, Yeragi BS, Bharambay HV. Imaging findings of disseminated cysticercosis with unusual involvement of spleen and pancreas. *J Glob Infect Dis.* 2011 Jul;3(3):306-308.

[47] Sandeep GJ, Vipul CC, Bhakti SY, Himanshu VB. Imaging Findings of Disseminated Cysticercosis with Unusual Involvement of Spleen and Pancreas. *J Glob Infect Dis.* 2011;3(3):306–308.

[48] Niakara A, Cisse R, Traore A, Niamba PA, et al. Myocardial localization of a disseminated cysticercosis. Echocardiographic diagnosis of a case. Arch Mal Coer Vaiss 2002;95(6):606-608.

[49] Blandon R, Leandro IM: Human Cardiac cysticercosis. Rev Med Panama. 2002; 27:37-40.

[50] Foyaca-Sibat H, L. Ibanez-Valdes L: Generalized Cysticercosis With Cardiac Involvement. The Internet Journal of Neurology. 2007 Volume 7 Number 2. http://www.ispub.com/journal/the-internet-journal-of-neurology/volume-7-number-2/generalized-cysticercosis-with-cardiac-involvement.html. *(accessed 05 May 2012)*

[51] Thomas MB, Thomas KM, Awotedu AA, Blanco-Blanco E, Anwary M. Cardiocysticercosis.S Afr Med J 2007;97(7):504-505.

[52] Eberly MD, Soh EK, Bannister SP, Taraf-Motamen H, Scott JS: Isolated Cardiac Cysticercosis in an adolescent; Pediatr Infect Dis J. 2008; 27(4); 369-71.

[53] Jain BK, Sankhe SS, Agrawal MD, Naphade PS. Disseminated cysticercosis with pulmonary and cardiac involvement. Indian J Radiol Imaging 2010;20:310-313.

[54] Scholtz L & Mentis H, Pulmonary cysticercosis. SAMT 1987 ;72(17) :573

[55] Mamere AE, Muglia VF, Simao GN, Belucci AD, Carlos dos Santos A, Trad CS, et al. Disseminated cysticercosis with pulmonary involvement. J Thorac Imaging 2004;19:109–111.

[56] Banu A, Veena N. A rare case of disseminated cysticercosis: Case report and literature review. Case Report. 2011;29(2):180-183.

[57] Bhigjee AI, Rosemberg S. Neurology. Optimizing therapy of seizures in patients with HIV and cysticercosis. Neurology 2006;67(12 Suppl 4):19-22.

[58] Scholtz L, Mentis H. Pulmonary cysticercosis. SAMT1987; 72(1): 573.

[59] Bhigjee AI. Disseminated cysticercosis. J Neurol Neurosurg Psychiatry 1999;66(4):545

[60] Thomas MB, Thomas KM, Awotedu AA, Blanco-Blanco E, Anwary M. Cardiocysticercosis. South Africa Medical Journal. 2007; 97(7): 504-505

[61] Sobnach S, Khosa SA, Pather S, Longhurst S, Kahn D, Raubenheimer PJ. First case report of pharyngeal cysticercosis. Trans R Soc Trop Med Hyg. 2009;103(2):206-208.

[62] Foyaca-Sibat H, Ibañez-Valdés LdeF. "Pseudoseizures and Epilepsy in neurocysticercosis" Electron J Biomed 2003;2(2):20-29. http://www.uninet.edu/reb/2003/n2/2foyaca.html

[63] Ibañez-Valdés LdeF, Foyaca-Sibat H. Refractory epilepsy in neurocysticercosis. The Internet Journal of Neurology 2006;5(2):34-41. http://www.ispub.com/journal/the_internet_journal_of_neurology/volume_5_number_2_19/article/refractory_epilepsy_in_neurocysticercosis.html

[64] Foyaca-Sibat H. Ibañez-Valdés LdeF. Insular Neurocysticercosis: Our Finding and Review of the Medical Literature. The Internet Journal of Neurology 2006;5(2). http://www.ispub.com/journal/the_internet_journal_of_neurology/volume_5_number_2_19/article/insular_neurocysticercosis_our_findings_and_review_of_the_medical_literature.html

[65] Foyaca-Sibat H, Del Rio AR, Ibañez-Valdés LdeF, Vega-Novoa EC, Awotedu A. "Neuroepidemiological survey for Epilepsy and knowledge about neurocysticercosis at Sidwadweni location, South Africa" Electron J Biomed 2004;2(1):40-48. http://www.biomed.edu/2004/n1/foyaca.html

[66] Foyaca-Sibat H, Del Rio-Romero AH, Ibañez-Valdés LdeF, Vega-Novoa E. Neuroepidemiological Survey For Epilepsy And Knowledge About Neurocysticiercosis At Ngqwala Location, South Africa. The Internet Journal of Neurology 2005 3(2). http://www.ispub.com/journal/the_internet_journal_of_neurology/volume_3_number_2_31/article/neuroepidemiological_survey_for_epilepsy_and_knowledge_about_neurocysticiercosis_at_ngqwala_location_south_africa.html

[67] Foyaca-Sibat H, Del Rio-Romero A, Ibañez-Valdés LdeF Prevalence Of Epilepsy And General Knowledge About Neurocysticercosis At Ngangelizwe Location, South Africa . The Internet Journal of Neurology. 2005;4 (1). http://www.ispub.com/journal/the_internet_journal_of_neurology/volume_4_number_1_30/article/prevalence_of_epilepsy_and_general_knowledge_about_neurocysticercosis_at_ngangelizwe_location_south_africa.html

[68] Foyaca-Sibat H, Del Rio A: "Epilepsy, Neurocysticercosis and, Poverty at Mphumaze and Marhambeni Locations, in South Africa". The Internet Journal of Neurology (ISSN: 1531-295X). 2007;7(1):8-14. http://www.ispub.com/journal/the_internet_journal_of_neurology/volume_7_number_1_7/article/epilepsy_neurocysticercosis_and_poverty_at_mphumaze_and_marhambeni_locations_in_south_africa.html

[69] Foyaca-Sibat H, Ibañez-Valdés LdeF, Del Rio IA: "Prevalence of Epilepsy and General Knowledge about Neurocysticercosis at Ngangelizwe Location, South Africa". The Internet Journal of Neurology.(ISSN: 1531-295X). 2005; 4(1):23-37. http://www.ispub.com/journal/the_internet_journal_of_neurology/volume_4_number_1_30/article/prevalence_of_epilepsy_and_general_knowledge_about_neurocysticercosis_at_ngangelizwe_location_south_africa.html

[70] Foyaca-Sibat H, Del Rio- Romero AI: "Prevalence Of Epilepsy In An Endemic Area For Neurocysticercosis In South Africa". The Internet Journal of Neurology.(ISSN: 1531-295X). 2008;9(1):8-18. http://www.ispub.com/journal/the_internet_journal_of_neurology/volume_9_number_1_6/article/prevalence_of_epilepsy_in_an_endemic_area_for_neurocysticercosis_in_south_africa.html

[71] Del Rio- Romero A, Foyaca-Sibat H, Ibañez-Valdés LdeF: Neuroepidemiology Findings As Contributors For Epilepsy Due To Neurocysticercosis At Mngceleni Location, South Africa . *The Internet Journal of Neurology.* 2008 Volume 9 Number 1. http://www.ispub.com/journal/the_internet_journal_of_neurology/volume_9_number_1_6/article/neuroepidemiology_findings_as_contributors_for_epilepsy_due_to_neurocysticercosis_at_mngceleni_location_south_africa.html

[72] Kumar A, Goenka AH, Choudhary A, Sahu JK, Gulati S. Disseminated cysticercosisin a child: whole-body MR diagnosis with the use of parallel imaging. Pediatr Radiol. 2010;40(2):223-227.

[73] Del Brutto OH, Rajshekhar V, White AC jun., *et al.* Proposed diagnostic criteria fo neurocysticercosis. *Neurology* 2001; 57: 177-183.

[74] Hoberg EP, Alkire NL, de Queiroz A, and Jones A. Out of Africa: origins of the Taenia tapeworms in humans. Proc. R. Soc. Lond.B 2001;268:781–787.

[75] Heslip , S. 2001. Time-Space chart. ANP440. Hominid fossils. Spring Semester, 2001. http://www.msu.edu/~heslipst/contents/ANP440/index.htm (accessed 07 May, 2012).

[76] Critical Issues in Researching Hidden Communities. University of Glasgow, http://www.gla.ac.uk/departments/esharp/otherpublications/specialissues/hiddencommunities/

[77] Wikipedia, the free encyclopedia: Mbuti people. http://en.wikipedia.org/wiki/Mbuti_people. (accessed 08May, 2012).
[78] Wikipedia, the free encyclopedia: Indigenous peoples of the Americas. http://en.wikipedia.org/wiki/Indigenous_peoples_of_the_Americas. (accessed 08, May, 2012).
[79] Wikipedia, the free encyclopedia: Uncontacted peoples. http://en.wikipedia.org/wiki/Uncontacted_peoples.
[80] Survival International website - About Us/Work for Survival.
[81] Wikipedia, the free encyclopedia: Survival International. http://en.wikipedia.org/wiki/Survival_International
[82] Shanley JD, Jordan MC: Clinical aspects of CNS cysticercosis. *Arch Inter Med* 1980;140:1309-1315.
[83] Loo L, Braude A: Cerebral cysticercosis in San Diego: a report of 23 cases and review of the literature. *Medicine* (Baltimore) 1982;61:341-350.
[84] McComick G, Zec Chi-S, Heiden J. Cysticercosis Cerebri. Review of 127 cases. *Arch Neurol* 1982; 39:534-539.
[85] Schantz PM, Moore AC, Muñoz JL, et al.: Neurocysticercosis in an Orthodox Jewish community in New York City. *N England J Med* 1992;327:692-696.
[86] White AC Jr. Neurocysticercosis: a major cause of neurological disease worldwide. *Clin Infect Dis* 1997;24:101-106.
[87] White AC Jr. Neurocysticercosis: updates on epidemiology, pathogenesis, diagnosis and management. *Ann Rev Med* 2000;51:187-206.
[88] Rousseau MC, Guillotel B, Delmont J. Neurocysticercosis in the South-East of France1988-1998. *Presse Med* 1999;28(39):2141-2144.
[89] García HH, Del Brutto OH; Cysticercosis Working Group in Peru. Neurocysticercosis: updated concepts about an old disease. *Lancet Neurol*. 2005; 4:653-661.
[90] O'Neal S, Noh J, Wilkins P, Keene W, Lambert W, Anderson J, Compton Luman J, Townes J. Taenia solium Tapeworm Infection, Oregon, 2006-2009. *Emerg Infect Dis*. 2011;17(6): 1030-1036.
[91] Kelesidis T, Tsiodras S. Extraparenchymal neurocysticercosis in the United States: a case report. Journal of Medical Case Reports 2011;5:359 .
[92] Serpa JA, Gravis EA, Kas Js, White ACJr. Neurocysticercosis in Houston, Texas: an update. Medicine (Baltimore) 2011;90(1):81-86.
[93] Wallin M, Kurtzke J. Neurocysticercosis in the United States: review of an important emerging infection. *Neurology* 2004; 63: 1559-1564.
[94] Saxena H, Samuel KC, Singh B. Cysticercosis of the heart. *Indian Heart J* 1972;24: 313-315.
[95] Niakara A, Cisse R, Traore A, *et al*. Myocardial localization of a disseminated cisticercosis.
[96] Cutrone JA, Georgiou D, Gil-Gomez C, Burndage BH. Myocardial cysticercosis detected by ultrafast CT. *Chest* 1995; 108:1752-1754.

[97] Rahalkar MD, Shetty DD, Kelkar AB, Kelkar AA, Kinare AS, Ambardekar ST. The many faces of cysticercosis. *Clin Radiol* 2000; 55 (9): 668-674.

[98] Ibarra-Perez C, Fernandez-Diez J, Rodriguez-Trujillo F. Myocardial cysticercosis, report of two cases with coexisting heart disease. *South Med J* 1972; 65: 484-486;

[99] Deshpande VL, Patil SD. Silent myocardial cysticercosis. *Indian Heart J* 1976; 28(1): 58-60.

[100] Belagavi CS, Goravalingappa JP. Cysticercosis of the heart. A case report. *Indian Heart J* 1978;30: 118-119.)

[101] Wadia N, Deasi S, Bhat M. Disseminated cysticercosis; new observations, including CT scan finding and experience with treatment by praziquantel. *Brain* 1988; 111: 597-614;

[102] Hidron A, Vogenthaler N, Santos-Preciado JI, Rodriguez-Morales AJ, Franco-Paredes C, Rassi A. Cardiac Involvement with Parasitic Infections. Clin. Microbiol. Rev. 2010*; 23(2): 324-349.*

[103] Botero, D., H. B. Tanowitz, L. M. Weiss, and M. Wittner. 1993. *Taeniasis and cysticercosis.* Infect. Dis. Clin. North Am. 7:683-697.

[104] *Lino, R. D. S, Ribeiro PM, Antonelli EJ, Faleiros AC, Terra SA, dos Reis MA, Teixeira VDPA..* Developmental characteristics of Cysticercus cellulosae in the human brain and heart. *Rev. Soc. Bras. Med. Trop. 2002;35:617*-622. (In Portugese.)

[105] *Schantz, P. M., M. Cruz, E. Sarti, and Z. Pawlowski. 1993.* Potential eradicability of taeniasis and cysticercosis. *Bull. Pan Am. Health Organ. 27:397*-403.

[106] Cutrone JA, Georgiou D, Gil-Gomez C, Burndage BH. Myocardial cysticercosis detected by ultrafast CT. Chest 1995; 108:1752-1754.)

[107] Niakara A, Cisse R, Traore A, Niamba PA, Barro F, Kabore J. Myocardial localization of a disseminated cysticercosis. Echocardiography diagnosis of a case. Arch Mal Coer Vaiss 2002;95(6):606-608

[108] Asrani A, Morani A. Primary Sonographic Diagnosis of Disseminated Muscular Cysticercosis. J Ultrasound Med 2004; 23:1245–1248

[109] Takayanagui MO, Chimelli L. Disseminated muscular cysticercosis with myositis induced by praziquantel therapy. *Am J Trop Med Hyg* 1998; 56: 1002-1003.)

[110] Kirchhoff LV, Weiss LM, Wittner M, Tanowitz HB. Parasitic diseases of the heart. Front Biosci. 2004 Jan 1;9:706-23.

[111] Eberly MD, Soh EK, Bannister SP, Tavaf-Motamen H, Scott JS. Isolated cardiac cysticercosis in an adolescent. Pediatr Infect Dis J. 2008 Apr;27(4):369-71.

[112] Shogan PJ, Yasmer JF, Monson M. Cardiac Cysticercosis. AJR 2009;192(5): xxx

[113] Strawter C, Quiroga P, Zaidi S, Ardiles T. Pulmonary nodules with cutaneous manifestations: A case report and discussion. Southwest J Pulm Crit Care 2012;4:116-121.

[114] Bassermann FJ. Radiographic problems in pulmonary cysticercosis. *PTax Klin001 Pneumo. 1971;*11:669-676.

[115] Veliath AJ, Ratnalcar C, Thalcur Le. Cysticercosis in south India. *J TTop Med Hyg* 1985; 1: 25-29.

[116] Scholtz L, Mentis H. Pulmonary cysticercosis. SAMT1987; 72(1): 573.

[117] Walts AE, Nivatpumin T, Epstein A. Pulmonary cysticercus. Mod Pathol 1995;8:299-302.

[118] Choi JH, et al. A case of pulmonary cysticercosis. The Korean Journal of Internal Medicine.1991;6(1):38-43.

[119] Singh P, Saggar K, Kalia V, Sandhu P, Galhotra RD. Thoracic imaging findings in a case of disseminated cysticercosis. *Postgrad Med J.*2011;87:158-159.

[120] Iwatani K, KubotaI, Hirotsu I, Wakimoto J, Yoshioka M, Mori T, et al.Sparganum mansoni parasitic infection in the lung showing a nodule.Pathology International Pathology International 2006;56 (11):674-677.

[121] Mauad T, Battlehner CN, Bedrikow CL, Capelozzi VL, Nascimento Saldiva PH. Massive Cardiopulmonary Cysticercosis in a Leukemic Patient, Pathology Research and Practice.1997;193(7):527-529.

[122] Bastos AL, Marchiori E, Gasparetto EL, Andrade BH, Junior GC, Carvalho RC, Escuissato DL, Souza AS. Pulmonary and cardiac cysticercosis: helical CT findings. British Journal of Radiology .2007; 80(951):58-60.

[123] Jain BK, Sankhe SS, Agrawal MD, Naphade PS. Disseminated cysticercosis with pulmonary and cardiac involvement. Indian J Radiol Imaging. 2010; 20(4):310–313.

[124]] Cheung YY, Steinbaum S, Yuh WT, Chiu L. MR findings in extracranial cysticercosis. J Comput Assist Tomogr. 1987 Jan-Feb;11(1):179-81.

[125] Gupta S, Jain VK, Sen J, Gupta S, Arora B. Subcutaneous cysticercosis involving the eyelid: sonographic diagnosis. J Dermatol 2000; 27:35–39.

[126] Chadha V, Pandey PK, Chauhan D, Das S. Simultaneous intraocular and bilateral extraocular muscle involvement in a case of disseminated cysticercosis. Int Ophthalmol. 2005 Feb-Apr;26(1-2):35-7. Epub 2006 Jun 15.

[127] Pushker N, Bajaj MS, Balasubramanya R. Disseminated cysticercosis involving orbit, brain and subcutaneous tissue. J Infect. 2005;51(5):245-248.

[128] Nijjar I, Singh JP, Arora V, Abrol R, Sandhu PS, Chopra R, et al. MRI in intraocular cysticercosis - A case report. Indian J Radiol Imaging. 2005;15:309–10.

[129] Devi S, Singh B, Singh S, Singh B, Singh J, Chingsuingamba Y. A rare case of disseminated cysticercosis. *Neurology Asia 2007;12 :127 –130.*

[130] Kadhiravan T, Soneja M , Hari S , Sharma SK. Images in Clinical Tropical Medicine. Disseminated Cysticercosis. *Am. J. Trop. Med. Hyg.2009;* 80(5):699.

[131] Pushker N, Mehta M, Meel R, Bajaj MS. Disseminated cysticercosis with multiple bilateral orbital cysts. Ophthal Plast Reconstr Surg. 2009 Nov-Dec;25(6):499-501.

[132] Tamilarasu K, Manish S, Smriti H; Surendra SK. Images in clinical tropical medicine: disseminated cysticercosis The American Journal of Tropical Medicine and Hygiene, 2009;80 (5):699

[133] Pandey PK, Chaudhuri Z, Bhatia A. Extraocular muscle cysticercosis presenting as Brown syndrome. Am J Ophthalmol. 2001 Apr; 131(4):526-527.

[134] Sundaram PM, Jayakumar N, Noronha V. Extraocular muscle cysticercosis - a clinical challenge to the ophthalmologists. Orbit. 2004 Dec; 23(4):255-262.

[135] Review Extraocular muscle cysticercosis mimicking idiopathic orbital inflammation: case report. Angotti-Neto H, Gonçalves AC, Moura FC, Monteiro ML. Arq Bras Oftalmol. 2007 May-Jun; 70(3):537-9.

[136] Sharma A, Mahajan C, Rath GP, Mohapatra S, Padhy UP, Kumar L. Neurocysticercosis: Acute presentation and intensive care management of two cases. Indian J Crit Care Med. 2011 Jul; 15(3):185-7

[137] Gangadhar K, Santhosh D. An Uncommon Manifestation of a Common Tropical Disease: Disseminated Cysticercosis. Neuroradiology Journal 2012;25(2):200-205.

[138] Pandey PK, Bhatia A, Garg D, Singh R. Canine tooth syndrome due to superior oblique myocysticercosis J Pediatr Ophthalmol Strabismus. 2006 May-Jun; 43(3):185-187.

[139] Goenka AH, Garg A. Pseudomuscular male with seizures: disseminated cysticercosis. Int J Infect Dis. 2010;14(3):385-387.

[140] Thomas B, Krishnamoorthy T.Extensive brain and muscular cysticercosis. Neurology. 2006;66(3):13.

[141] Juhl ZK, Løgager VB. Subcutaneous cysticercosis and neurocysticercosis. Ugeskr Laeger. 2000 Dec 4;162(49):6691-6692.

[142] Chopra JS, Nand N, Jain K, Mittal R, Abrol L. Generalized muscular pseudohypertrophy in cysticercosis. Postgrad Med J 1986; 62:299–300.

[143] Kuruvilla A, Pandian J, Nair M, Joseph S. Neurocysticercosis: A clinical and radiological appraisal from Kerala State, South India. Singapore medical journal. 2001; 42(7): 297-303.

[144] Goenka AH, Garg A.Pseudomuscular male with seizures: disseminated cysticercosis. Int J Infect Dis. 2010 Sep;14 385-387.

[145] Satyanarayana S, Gorthi SP, Bhardwaj JR, Nath N, Sharma S. Disseminated Cysticercosis. J Assoc Physicians India 2002; 50:1180–1182.

[146] Saranya D, M Jawahar, K Bhanu. A case of disseminated neurocysticercosis. Images in Neurology.2011;14(1):56-57.

[147] Kadhiravan T, Soneja M , Hari S , Sharma SK. Images in Clinical Tropical Medicine. Disseminated Cysticercosis. *Am. J. Trop. Med. Hyg.2009;* 80(5):699.

[148] Saranya D, Jawahar M, Bhanu K. A case of disseminated neurocysticercosis. Images in Neurology 2011;14(1):56-57

[149] Hashmi MA, Sharma SK, Bera SP, Saha B. Disseminated cysticercus involving the vocal cords. Annals Tropical Medicine and Public Health. 2008;1(2):66-67.

[150] Gupta S, Sodhani P .Clinically Unsuspected Thyroid Involvement in Cysticercosis. A Case Report. Acta Cytologica 2010;54(5): 853-856.

[151] Verma R, Sharma P, Khurana N. Thousands of Lesions in Disseminated Cysticercosis. Am J Trop Med Hyg. 2011; 85(4): 583.

[152] Nakamura-Uchiyama F, Kobayash K, Ohnishi K. *An Imported Case of Disseminated Cysticercosis and Taeniasis.* Internal Medicine 2012; 51(3):347-348.

[153] CCD immnunocompromised patient.

[154] Goenka AH, Kumar A. Whole body MR and disseminated cysticercosis. Indian J Radiol Imaging. 2011; 21(2): 157–158.

[155] Kumar A, Goenka AH, Choudhary A, Sahu JK, Gulati S. Disseminated cysticercosis in a child: whole-body MR diagnosis with the use of parallel imaging. Pediatr Radiol. 2010;40(2):223-227.

Chapter 8

Uncommon Clinical Manifestations of Cysticercosis

Humberto Foyaca Sibat and Lourdes de Fátima Ibañez Valdés

Additional information is available at the end of the chapter

http://dx.doi.org/10.5772/53078

1. Introduction

Cysticercosis, a parasitic infection caused by the larval form of the pork tapeworm, *Taenia solium*, is increasingly recognized as a cause of epilepsy, headache, and neurological signs when it is located in the brain, optic nerve or spinal cord, known as neurocysticercosis (NCC). A high prevalence of cysticercosis/taeniosis has been reported from the developing countries because of the coexistence of poor sanitary conditions and domestic pig raising without veterinary control or surveillance systems. It occurs mainly in Eastern and Southern Africa, China, India, Mexico, Central America, Chile, Ecuador, Colombia, Venezuela, Peru, Brazil, Papua New Guinea, and non-Islamic South East Asia where human faces reach pigs and pork is eaten raw or undercooked.

An infection which leads to extra-intestinal disease (including NCC) usually occurs as a result of eating food or drinking water contaminated by human feces containing *T. solium* eggs. It is a preventable and potentially eradicable neurological disease which primarily affects people living in the developing world. The disease is endemic in Central and South America, Asia and Africa. There is a variable time interval between point of infection and the onset of symptoms: ranging from 1-30 years.

Seizures are widely reported to be the most common symptom, occurring in 70-90% of patients. Most patients respond to praziquantel if cystic lesions are located in the parenchyma tissue and albendazole when parasites are located in the ventricular system and subarachnoid space [1-16]. Seizure disorder is the most frequent clinical manifestation of the NCC observed in 50% to 80% of cases, in children and adults presenting intraparenchymal cystic lesions. [13-44]

Each day the cysticercosis is more and better known in the developed world or in developing countries, the immune diagnostic techniques are more reliable and neuroimaging studies are more accurate. The greatest success in the diagnosis of the disease

INTECH
open science | open minds

© 2013 Foyaca Sibat and de Fátima Ibañez Valdés, licensee InTech. This is a paper distributed under the terms of the Creative Commons Attribution License (http://creativecommons.org/licenses/by/3.0), which permits unrestricted use, distribution, and reproduction in any medium, provided the original work is properly cited.

control passes at the achievements attained by the agricultural sector, without which it is not possible try to sustain successful results. The knowledge that we have on the porcine cysticercosis today are much more certain and deep. In the epidemiological aspects, the African continent goes up to the head because it is the only basic information that has been made safe for almost all their countries, as can be seen in the chapter: "*Agricultural Impact of Porcine Cyisticercosis in Africa: A Review*" in this book written by Helena A Ngowi et al. This study included information from 54 African countries that were fully recognized by the United Nations as of 2012. The total population of pigs estimated in the study area in 2010 amounted 29,606,438. This was approximately 3.1% of the world pig population estimate (N = 965,855,414) of 2010. Out of the Africa regional pig population, approximately 0.2% was reared in the northern countries, while 6.1%, 43.3%, 16,4%, and 34.0% were reared in the southern, western, central, and eastern Africa, respectively. Overall, 19 (35.2%) of the 54 study countries reported prevalence of cysticercosis in pigs. While no data were available in the northern region, the remaining regions provided prevalence data, with more reporting frequency observed in the Eastern followed by Central Africa.

All these previous arguments together have favored the growing number of diagnosed uncommon presentations of cysticercosis that before passing unnoticed.

For purely didactic reasons we are going to aggregate all the uncommon forms of cysticercosis in accordance with the following classification:

- Uncommon cysticercosis in the head and neck
- Uncommon cysticercosis in the trunk
- Uncommon cysticercosis in the abdomen
- Uncommon cysticercosis in the limbs

2. Uncommon cysticercosis in the head and neck

2.1. Uncommon clinical presentations neurocysticercosis (UNCC)

Pseudoseizures and epilepsy in patients presenting neurocysticercosis

In our experience, the South African patients with NCC and fictitious attacks (pseudo-seizures) are more often in young women with a history of violations and/or sexual abuse and their attacks are usually characterized by absence of post ictal signs, irregular and asymmetrical stereotyped movements, and often accompanied by shouts or sounds in the middle of the "attack" that usually last for more than three minutes if the patients are not alone. We found that these manifestations contribute to characterize clinically patients with pseudo-crisis. These conclusions were the result of a study conducted some years ago. [4]

Refractory epilepsy in HIV/AIDS patients presenting NCC

At the present moment, more than 40 million people are living with HIV and more than 50 million people have neurocysticercosis (NCC) worldwide. About 5% of patients with HIV and most of the patients with NCC develop recurrent epileptic seizures. Although this comorbidity has not been reported as an additional public health problem, NCC and the HIV/AIDS infections are very common in the former Transkei (South Africa) and both cause recurrent epileptic seizures frequently. [3,5] Usually patients with NCC have partial seizures with or without secondary generalization. The epileptogenesis in patients with NCC can be attributed to several factors, such as: inflammation, gliosis and its frequent location in the frontal and temporal lobes. [47] While the basis for seizure production in HIV-positive patients include HIV itself, mass lesions, meningitis, encephalitis, ischemia, metabolic derangement, and drugs [48] In both conditions we recognize patients as epileptic when they present recurrent unprovoked epileptic seizures associated to a chronic brain disorder. [14]

We consider refractory epilepsy when seizures are so frequent that limit the patient's ability to live fully in line with their wishes and their physical and mental capabilities or when the antiepileptic drug (AED) does not control the crisis or their side effects are limited to a person's normal development. [6] Other authors have the same criteria. [49] Recently, The International League against Epilepsy has defined the patients with epilepsy resistant to drugs when there are no controls over the attacks with a combination of two AED well tolerated, and managed properly elected. BY understanding how the lack of control when the patients continue to have attacks with an interval of not less than one third of which presented before starting the antiepiileptic treatment [14]

Although this clinical presentation is not uncommon in our setting it may be very uncommon in other countries. Nevertheless, there is a novel presentation of motor partial simple seizures localized in the lower part of the hemiface in females at the stage IV of HIV/AIDS and CD4 below 100 x10^6. This type of seizures becomes secondarily generalized a few days or weeks of the beginning and are still uncommon in our region. At the present moment the mortality rate for these patients is 100%.

Managing seizures in HIV-positive patients present specific challenges, including the identification and treatment of the underlying cause, recognition that seizure production may be multifactorial, selection of the appropriate AED, and consideration of the effects of co-administered highly active antiretroviral therapy (HAART). Unfortunately, there has been little systematic study in these areas. The available information is confined to case reports, retrospective analyses, and small studies. [48] The cause of the seizures will depend on the stage of HIV infection. Since the causes are many and there may be more than one mechanism for seizure production, a meticulous clinical, laboratory, and neuroimaging survey must be undertaken. The older AEDs, phenobarbital, phenytoin, carbamazepine, and valproic acid are still widely used. [48] In our experience Valproic acid is the AED of choice for HIV/AIDS patients with epilepsy due to NCC and we did not find increased viral load in our series of these patients on HAART.

Finally we like to highlight that apart from NCC/HIV/AIDS sometimes other causes should be investigated for a better control of the seizures. [9]

Dementia is another uncommon presentation of NCC [50] and its prognosis is better if there is not an associated HIH/AIDS.

Massive neurocysticercosis

Massive brain infection with viable cysticerci, undetectable inflammatory reaction on CNS imaging, and an unexpectedly high (82%) prevalence of tapeworm infection represents a particular presentation of neurocysticercosis is different from the previously described syndromes of cysticercotic encephalitis and disseminated systemic cysticercosis according with Garcia et al. [51] In our series we did not find remarkable differences excepting a fatal prognosis when more than one thousand of cystic lesions are present [14,16] but without doubt it is another uncommon clinical presentation of NCC. (Figure 1)

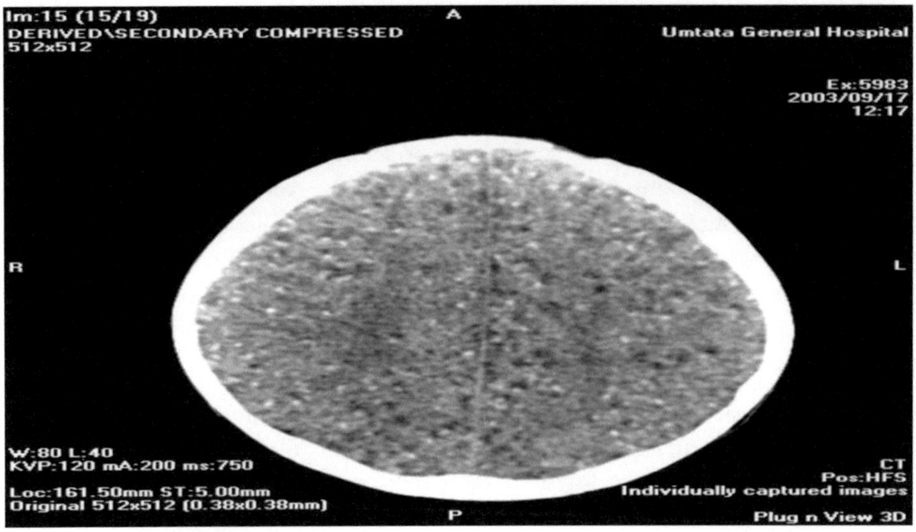

Figure 1. CT scan of the brain showing massive neurocysticercosis (more that 100 cysts)

Giant intraparenchymal/Giant subarachnoid neurocysticercosis

Parenchymal cysts usually involve the gray white matter junction, however giant cyst is usually located at the Sylvia fissure or deeper in the cerebral lobe.

Giant NCC is a rare condition defined by various authors as measuring more than five cm in its largest dimension [52] usually associated with intracranial hypertension but giant cysts may not always be associated with elevated intracranial pressure, probably due to slow growing of the cyst.

Almost all reported patients presenting intraparenchymal giant cyst had similar clinical manifestations at the beginning characterized by headache, altered mental status, hemiparesis mainly on the right side [9, 53-62] or uncontrolled epilepsy. [63] Between 1990 and 2006, only five patients have been reported in South Africa. All had associated epilepsy, one patient also presented visual hallucinations, dysnomia in blue and red, dyslexia and palinopsia, and the cyst (106mm) was located in the left occipital lobe. [9] (See figure 2)

All patients were treated with a 31-day course of praziquantel 50 mg/kg daily. Two patients had corticosteroids administered simultaneously. All five patients had anticonvulsant cover. In all cases there was rapid and complete resolution of the cysts. In three patients this occurred within 30 days. The computed tomographic features of giant cysticercal cysts in our series were: thin walled cystic lesions containing clear fluid, localized thickening of the wall with an eccentric scale in three patients, the absence of pericyst edema, and the presence of associated smaller and more typical cysticercal larval forms. Identification of a scolex in a cystic lesion with CSF intensity plays a key role in the diagnosis of NCC and the presence of internal septations is an atypical feature. [61]

Giant cysticercal cysts resolve remarkably rapidly on medical therapy. A therapeutic trial of praziquantel can, in suspected giant cysticercal cysts, obviate the need for exploratory craniotomy. [9, 56] Other authors [60] suggest repeating anthelmintic treatment to provide good response, when it is necessary, and we fully agree on that. However, surgical treatment may be required when it is associated with elevated intracranial pressure, [62] mainly if the pre-operatory diagnosis is not clear enough.

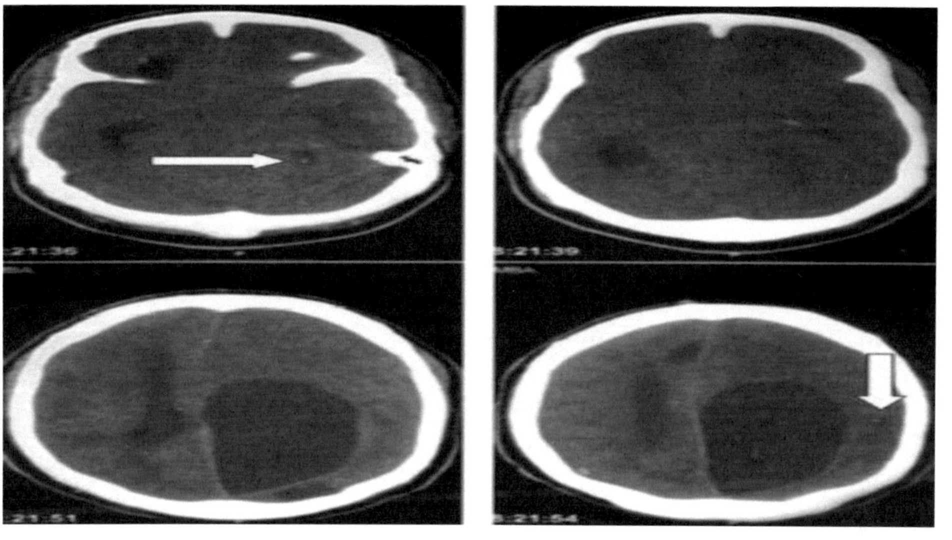

Figure 2. In upper right and lower left white arrow show identification of active viable cyst in vesicular stage with an eccentric scolex. Giant cyst measuring 106 mm on the left occipital lobe is seen.

Neurocysticercosis in the posterior cranial fossa

The posterior cranial fossa is part of the intracranial cavity, located between the foramen magnum and tentorium cerebelli. It contains the brainstem and cerebellum. This is the most inferior of the fossa. It houses the cerebellum, medulla and pons. Anteriorly it extends to the apex of the petrous temporal. Posteriorly it is enclosed by the occipital bone. Laterally portions of the squamous temporal and mastoid part of the temporal bone from its walls.

In the posterior fossa, NCC can involve the fourth ventricle, cerebellopontine angle cistern, cisterna magna and rarely, the cerebellum [64, 65] .Cysticercosis affecting one of the above-mentioned anatomical structures are grouped under the name of NCC of the posterior fossa (PFNCC).

One of the first articles about clinical manifestations was done by Bickerstaff et al., in 1956 [66] and about clinical and surgical management by Kla in 1964. [67] Other modalities of management including the diagnostic importance of laboratory and serological analysis of blood and cerebro-spinal fluid in cysticercosis of the posterior cranial fossa and description of the pseudotumoral form of Cysticercus cellulose to be remembered when one attempts to characterize the type of neoplasms of the posterior fossa as detected by brain scan in the infantile population were reported from 1971 and 1978. [68-71]

Anecdotal clinical presentations in patients with posterior fossa involvement may include signs of bilateral fourth nerve palsy, facial myokymia, upbeat nystagmus, periodic alternating nystagmus, and rhythmic oculopalatal myoclonus. [72] In patients presenting huge cystic lesions due to PFNCC then intermittent severe headache, epilepsy, and signs of raised intracranial pressure, cerebellar signs and cranial nerves signs can be seen. [63,73] Studies post-mortem have confirmed this correlation between signs of increased intracranial pressure, localizing cerebellar signs and even hearing loss in patients presenting PFNCC in the cerebellopontine cistern and obstructive hydrocephalus. [74,75]

Sang-Wook et al. [76] reported a case presenting headache, dizziness, drowsiness and ataxic gait. The magnetic resonance imaging showed hydrocephalus and an ill-defined, multicystic cerebellar mass with hypersignal on T2-weighted images, hyposignal on T1-weighted images and rim enhancement after gadolinium injection (the differential diagnoses of include abscess, tuberculosis, metastasis and other parasitic diseases). The patient underwent endoscopic third ventriculostomy and the cyst resection was done through a craniotomy. In surgical field, cysts were conglomerated in a dense collagen capsule that were severely adherent to surrounding cerebellar tissue, and transparent cysts contained white, milky fluid. Histological findings confirmed the diagnosis of cysticercosis. These authors concluded that racemose cysticercosis is rare in the cerebellar hemisphere but neurocysticercosis should be taken into consideration as a differential diagnosis of multiple cystic lesions in the cerebellum and we agree on that. As has been mentioned, T solium cysticercosis spread through the bloodstream and it may locate almost anywhere in the CNS, most frequently involves the cerebral hemispheres and sometimes ventricles, basal cisterns, subarachnoid space, and spinal cord. Cerebellar cysticercosis has been rarely reported [77-78]. Anecdotal presentations include multiple cranial nerve involvement (V, VI, VII, VIII) and cerebellar signs resembling anterior inferior cerebellar artery (AICA) syndrome. [79]

Other uncommon clinical locations of NCC (UNCC) are: intraventricular (IV), intra-spinal (IS), subarachnoid (SA) and others that we will explain below.

2.1.1. Neurocysticercosis intraventricular (IVNCC)

The ventricular system is a set of structures containing cerebro-spinal fluid in the brain. It is continuous with the central canal of the spinal cord. The ventricles are filled with cerebro-spinal fluid (CSF) which bathes and cushions the brain and spinal cord within their bony confines. Cerebro-spinal fluid is produced by modifying ependymal cells of the choroid plexus found in all components of the ventricular system except for the cerebral aqueduct and the posterior and anterior horns of the lateral ventricles. CSF flows from the lateral ventricles via the foramina of Monro into the third ventricle, and then the fourth ventricle via the cerebral aqueduct in the brainstem. From there it can pass into the central canal of the spinal cord or into the cisterns of the subarachnoid space via three small foramina: the central foramen of Magendie and the two lateral foramina of Luschka. The fluid then flows around the superior sagittal sinus to be reabsorbed via the arachnoid villi into the venous system. CSF within the spinal cord can flow all the way down to the lumbar cistern at the end of the cord around the cauda equina where lumbar punctures are performed.

The aqueduct between the third and fourth ventricles is very small, as are the foramina, which means that they can be easily blocked, causing high pressure in the lateral ventricles. This is a common cause of hydrocephalus (known colloquially as "water on the brain"), which is an extremely serious condition due to both the damage caused by the pressure as well as the nature of whatever caused the block (e.g. a tumour, cyst or inflammatory swelling). The cavities of the cerebral hemispheres are called lateral ventricles, or 1st & 2nd ventricles. These two ventricles open commonly into the 3rd ventricle by a common opening called the foramen of Monro.

The presence of T solium in the ventricular system may be seen in a 7-30% of patients with NCC [45] and although it has been reported less frequently (6 %) by other authors [46] everything seems to indicate that its frequency is much greater than had been thought previously. [45] Of all forms of presentation of the NCC, the IVNCC is sometimes associated with a fatal prognosis. The diagnosis of certainty is achieved by methods of neuroimaging, particularly the nuclear magnetic resonance imaging (MRI), which is also indispensable as prior checking to surgery, the choice of treatment and assessment of the response to the same. [80-82]

Some reports related to the clinical characteristics and the management of this entity confirm their increasing frequency in countries such as the Unite States of America. [83, 84] In 1906, Ludwig Bruns described a phenomenon characterized by sudden headache associated with acute vestibular syndrome, triggered by sudden movements of the head, or, at times, it could have a disastrous outcome, by leading to coma and even death. [85] A form of presentation of the NCCIv may be syndrome Bruns characterized by episodes of loss of consciousness to head movements and hydrocephalus due to a cyst in the IV ventricle their movement obstructs the exit of CSF through the holes of Luchka and Magendie, involuntary movements or intracranial hypertension. [86] Other clinical manifestations of the NCCIv have been reported according to the location of the cysticerci in the ventricular system [87] or when passing through the same. [88] The NCCIv of the lateral ventricles has not been reported that constitutes a diagnostic or therapeutic problem however the NCCIv of the III and IV ventricles constitute a major challenge to resolve. [80,89] The treatment of forms Iv is geared toward case by case, according to the pathogenic substrate. The first thing to define is the presence or risk of acute hydrocephalus, and, therefore, the option of a ventriculostomy emergency or making a ventriculoperitoneal shunt (DVP), with or without fenestration of the septum, according to the location of the Ct. To take the decision to remove the cysts must be taken into account: the number, location stage of cysticercus, general clinical conditions of the patient, abilities, and experience of the surgical team to perform open or endoscopic neurosurgical approach. [90, 91] Also add to the list other criteria such as: the mass effect, the ventricular obstruction, the dysfunction of the valve and the diagnostic doubt. [90] Some authors have argued that the confirmation of contrast in the wall cysticercus by MRI is a sign of a poor prognosis independent of the applied surgical treatment, as it translates the possibility of a process of ependimitis that will tend to chronicity with obstruction or entrapment, independent of the presence of the Ct. [90] The treatment of forms Iv includes not only surgical options, but also with anti-parasitic treatment (APT), corticosteroids [87, 90-93] and VPS when necessary. It is important to mention that the APT of the NCCIv should be indicated if there is a possibility to make an emergency-relief through a VPS in the case of acute obstruction. Variations in the number, volume and involution of the Ct, the secondary reactions, the eventual hydrocephalus, as well as the low number of patients who have this form of presentation, make it unlikely to carried out randomized clinical trials with an acceptable confidence. [94] On the other hand, Ramirez-Ceballos and Marquez [97] argue that the NCCIv requires an individualized treatment, medical, surgical, or a combination of both and in their experience Iv neuro-endoscopic has provided a good surgical approach allowing to explore properly the ventricular cavities with either the rigid or flexible endoscope. According to these authors, this treatment improves the prognosis and clinical course of patients, since in most of them it avoids the placement of derivatives systems and in those cases that require, decreases the risk of re-surgical interventions. In this regards, we did not find articles related to the NCCIv and infection by HIV/AIDS, its clinical features and treatment options therefore it will be another aspect to be discussed below from our results.

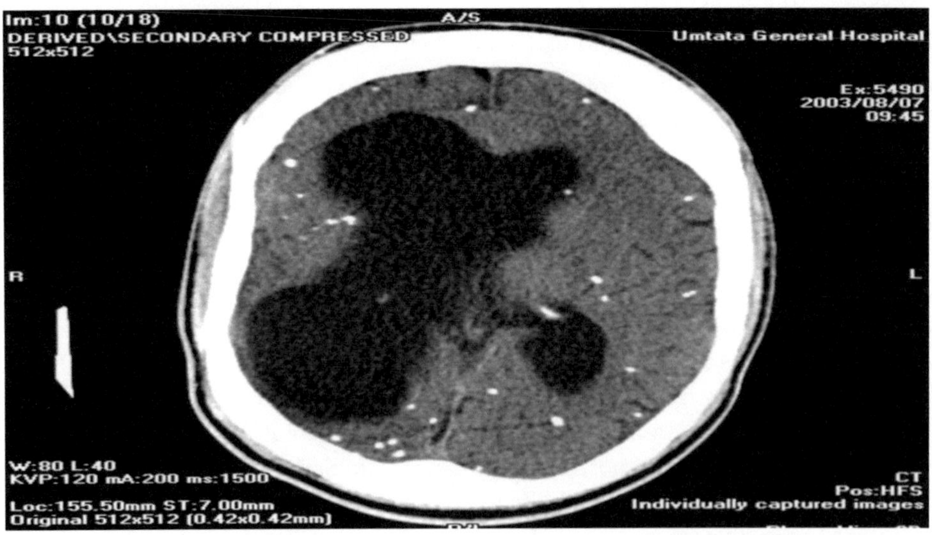

Figure 3. CT scan of the brain showing asymmetrical hydrocephalus due to intraventricular neurocysticercosis blocking foramen of Monro on the right side and calcified NCC.

Patients presenting intraventricular NCC (IvNCC) can have a different clinical presentation if they are HIV positive [2,3], although they have in common that the diagnosis must be confirmed by MRI as other have also pointed outr. [80, 97, 98] Should be emphasized that in HIV patients must be ruled out the presence an associated chronic meningitis by favoring the ventricular dilatation, (See figure 3) and in which case the serial lumbar punctures should be assessed carefully. The ABZ is the drug of choice, [2,3] if removal of the Ct by endoscopic is not possible. [15,16,90, 91]

Fourth ventricular neurocysticercosis (FVNCC)

Despite fourth ventricle is located in the posterior fossa, we decided to place apart here for didactic purposes, and because the fourth ventricle is the most frequent site of intraventricular infestation, a location that carries a higher risk of raise intracranial pressure due to cerebro-spinal fluid (CSF) blockage. We will comment a little bit more about this particular location of T solium cysticercosis.

The fourth ventricle is one of the four connected fluid-filled cavities within the human brain. These cavities, known collectively as the ventricular system, consist of the left and right lateral ventricles, the third ventricle, and the fourth ventricle. The fourth ventricle extends from the cerebral aqueduct (*aqueduct of Sylvius*) to the obex, and is filled with CSF. The fourth ventricle has a characteristic diamond shape in cross-sections of the human brain. It is located within the pons or in the upper part of the medulla. CSF entering the fourth ventricle through the cerebral aqueduct can exit to the subarachnoid space of the spinal cord through two lateral foramina of Luschka and a single, midline foramen of Magendie.

Clinical and imagenological aspects on FVNCC has been described in the medical literature [99- 108] and can be sumarized as follow: Symptoms and sings of intracraneal hypertension due to obstructive hydrocephalus [99,100-107] , blurred vision, loss of consciousness, [100] sudden death, [108] reversible parkinsonism following ventriculoperitoneal shunt, [109] Bruns syndrome, [110] positional vomiting [111] and comatose state [112]

From the point of view of imagenology, the magnetic resonance imaging (MRI) is the investigation of choice which can also show: cerebrospinal fluid (CSF) signal intensity (on all pulse sequences), intra fourth ventricular cyst with scolex, and wall enhancement. On T1-weighted and Fluid Attenuation Inversion Recovery images (FAIR), the cyst wall and scolex which are not seen in other routine sequences, and the CSF flow study can show the intraluminal nature of the cyst [113] and the even imagenological appearance of multicystic tumor. [114]

Most studies have been addressed to review the therapeutic approaches of IVNCC, as can be seen in our review. [99,110,115-127] and has been well established that available treatment options are: medical, external cerebro-spinal fluid diversion, microsurgical, or endoscopic removal alone or in combination. [122] Summarizing the reports in the medical literature we can conclude that the best choices for treatment of IVNCC are:

1. Albendazol (15 mg/kg/day for 2 weeks): A regimen of albendazole is the treatment of choice for IVNCC even after surgical procedures [122], although praziquantel may also be useful. [117]
2. Praziquantel (100 mg/kg/day for 2 weeks): Rapid regression of a large cyst of the fourth ventricle after oral praziquantel, avoiding the need for surgery has been reported. [116]

3. Direct surgical excision of the parasite after a shunt procedure is performed, [115] but the complication rate is high due to obstruction or material infection, which may justify other procedures such s endoscopic third ventriculostomy, [122] as you can read below. Resection of the fourth ventricle lesion through a sub occipital approach allowed for restoration of normal cerebro-spinal fluid (CSF) flow and relief of midbrain compression. [112]
4. If pericystic enhancement is present on MRI, shunt surgery should be performed, and craniotomy reserved for treatment of those patients with symptomatic lesions secondary to mass effect.[119]
5. Endoscopy approach: Neuroendoscopy provides a safe and effective management modality for the treatment of a variety of intracranial disorders, either temporal or non-tumoral, congenital, developmental, and degenerative, and its knowledge, indications, and limits are fundamental for the armamentarium of the modern neurosurgeon. [126] In patients presenting symptomatic obstructive hydrocephalus, aqueductal and foramen of Monro dilatations, endoscopic neurosurgery is a minimally invasive technique enabling removal of intraventricular cyticercal cysts from all locations, avoiding major craniotomies/posterior fossa explorations and shunts. The flexible fiberoptic scope is used for excising cysts in the fourth ventricle, through a transaqueductal route and patients should be treated with albendazole in the postoperative period. [118, 120, 122] Endoscopic third ventriculostomy for patients with ventricular outlet obstruction and a prior history of FVNCC has been reported as a successful management and no patient has required subsequent surgery. [121, 122] Endoscopic transaqueductal removal of fourth ventricular neurocysticercosis with an angiographic catheter has been used and there are good experiences from two series of 10 and 21 patients with IVNCC with obstructive hydrocephalus that underwent endoscopic removal along with endoscopic third ventriculostomy through a frontal precoronal burr hole. The author concluded that a 30-degree rigid telescope provide excellent image quality, with the ability to address intra-FVNCC through the dilated aqueduct with a curved-tip catheter without significant operative or postoperative complications. They concluded that neuro-endoscopic surgery is an effective treatment modality for patients with intraventricular NCC. It effectively restores CSF flow and is capable of removing cysts completely or partially from accessible locations causing mass effect. Partial removal or rupture of the cyst does not affect the clinical outcome of the patients. [123, 124] Other series of patients (n-13) presenting FVNCC with complete excised of cyst by using a transventricular, transaqueductal "scope-in-scope" endoscopic technique was reported and their author also concluded that endoscopic fourth ventricular cysticercal cyst excision along with internal cerebrospinal fluid diversion via endoscopic third ventriculostomy is an effective alternative to open microneurosurgical procedures and avoids shunt placement and its related complications [125] such as: Parkinsonism with evidence of midbrain dysfunction due to aqueductal stenosis after placement of ventriculoperitoneal shunt. [110]

2.1.2. Subarachnoid NCC (SANCC)

In the central nervous system, the subarachnoid space (SAE) is the interval between the arachnoid membrane and pia mater. It is occupied by spongy tissue consisting of trabeculae (delicate connective tissue filaments that extend from the arachnoid mater and blend into the pia mater) and intercommunicating channels in which the CSF is contained.

This cavity is small on the surface of the hemispheres of the brain. On the summit of each gyrus the pia mater and the arachnoid are in close contact, but in the sulci between the gyri, triangular spaces are left, in which the subarachnoid trabecular tissue is found. Whilst the pia mater closely follows the surface of the brain and dips into the sulci, the arachnoid bridges across them from gyrus to gyrus.

At certain parts of the base of the brain, the arachnoid is separated from the pia mater by wide intervals, which communicate freely with each other and are named subarachnoid cisternæ; in these the subarachnoid tissue is less abundant. The subarachnoid space is the location of the interface between the vascular tissue and the cerebro-spinal fluid and is active in the blood brain barrier.

The arachnoid mater continues down the spinal cord, and the subarachnoid layer with it. It serves a similar function in the spinal cord as it does in the brain.

Despite SANCC is an uncommon location compare with intraparenchymal NCC, the commonest location in the subarachnoid space is over the cerebral hemispheres.

In 2004, Wallin and col. [128] reported the prevalence of SANCC in 2% while other authors reported a higher prevalence (3.5 %) in patients with SANCC with visual and hormonal disturbances secondary to a direct compression of the pituitary stalk and the optic nerve, [129,130] in some studies it was not clear whether refers to the frequency of complications by compression of the optic nerve and the pituitary stalk within the group of patients with SANCC or within a group of patients with NCC in general. As in the above situations, the treatment of choice for the SANCC is individual. [94] There are numerous reports of cases and a series of cases treated with cesticidas and corticosteroids to repetition, but not compared with a control group, to confirm this hypothesis with the additional benefit of reducing the size of the cysts or of the inflammatory leptomeningeal process. [131,132] Despite the lack of evidence which originated in randomized clinical trials, there is consensus for this option [133] and other authors combine prolonged treatments (sometimes for several months) with cesticidas and corticosteroids. [134] According to some authors the reason why the clinical manifestations of ischemia with or without infarction, due to cerebral vasculitis infectious by NCC, were not detected in some patients is due to the age group with the highest incidence have no aggregated vascular risk factors. The cerebrovascular complications are predominantly associated with the prevalence of the CC especially in the basal cisterns and associated arachnoiditis of variable degree [133, 135-139] later we will discuss this aspect based on our experience and results. It is known that when cisticerci are confined to a small area with associated arachnoiditis and few changes in the CSF, these affect small blood vessels predominantly penetrating arterioles causing infarctions very similar to the lacunar infarctions of the basal ganglia which did not differ from those caused by arteriopatías or microateromas. [94] The most severe form of vasculopathy infectious for NCC is observed when the CC spreads through the SAE with major alterations of the LCR and a chronic evolution of the disease. The neurovascular syndrome (SNv) is usually the first manifestation of the focal SANCC that produces unique infarcts (90 %), which often have a good prognosis. [94] In contrast, many patients have non-vascular complications (including intracranial hypertension and a progressive neurological impairment) when the NCC is diffusely extended in the CNS, whereas the SNv occurs only late in the course of the disease and has a grim forecast. [94] We have not found in the reviewed medical literature references related to the SANCC (See figure 4) and cerebrovascular complications in patients with HIV/AIDS.

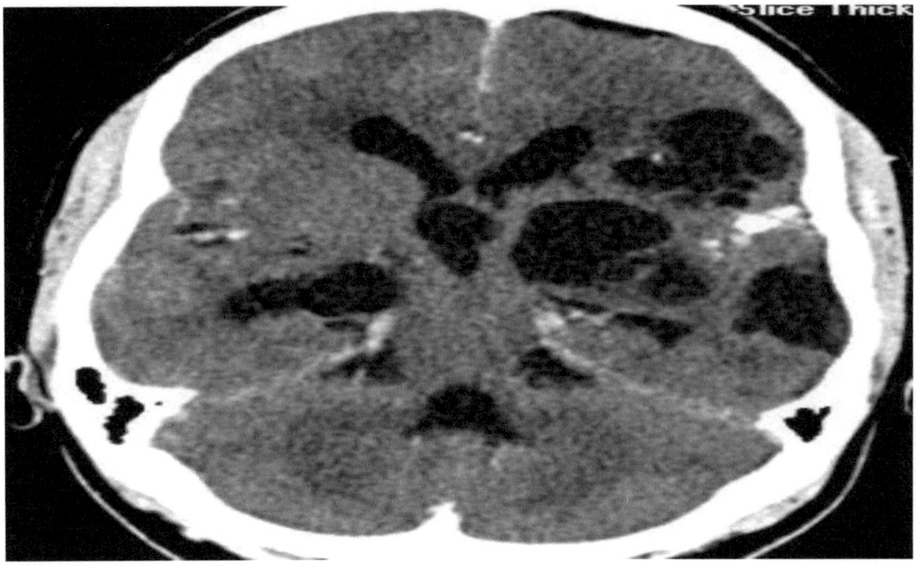

Figure 4. Racemose cystic lesions in left frontal and both temporal lobes. Intraventricular cyst causing obstructive hydrocephalus.

The SANCC also has some different features in the South African patient due to their frequent association with HIV infection. As is known, scattered Ct in the SAE cause the most severe forms of infectious vasculitis when evolve toward the chronicity [94], although no one knows the exact prevalence of this problem. [16] In our study we were able to determine that the risk to present an ischemic infarct is almost three times higher in patient with SANCC compared with the patient with intraparenchymal NCC and this risk increase more than seven times if the patient is HIV-positive. Therefore you have to exhaust all the possibilities of deworming to avoid cerebrovascular complications. [16]

2.1.3. Intraspinal NCC

The intra-spinal NCC (ISNCC) presentation include: Intra-medullary NCC (IMNCC) and extra-medullary NCC (EMNCC). The ISNCC is rare and there are only 45 cases reported in medical literature. Its frequency varies between 7 and 5.8 % and its incidence is very low but six times more on that in axial medullary. [140, 141] Other authors in 2002 reviewed of 95 published cases of medullary cysticercosis since 1856. [142]

Its clinical manifestations are the result of the presence of CC in the intra-spinal canal i.e. the space between the meninges of the spinal canal.[143] Other authors have found up to 200 cases reported in the international medical literature before the year 2001, [144] this low prevalence of the IMNCC is explained by the fact that the blood supply to the spinal cord is 100 times less than the blood flow to the brain [145, 146] and the Ct usually comes to the region's best irrigated. Most of the times the symptoms of the ISNCC are secondary to the mass effect or the secondary edema, and among the most common can be found: spastic paraplegia, bladder incontinence, radicular pain or sexual impotence; the degree of commitment depends on the site which locate the lesion. [147] When there is an associated arachnoiditis (EMNCC) dominate the radicular pain and muscle weakness and when it affects the axial medullary then the predominant clinical feature is similar to the transverse myelitis characterized by sphincter dysfunction with motor and sensory signs below the level of the lesion. [148]

In ISNCC the subarachnoid damage can be secondary to its spread through the SAE, and the more usual imaging presentation is the EMNCC and arachnoiditis. The IMNCC presentation has been associated with hematogenous spread or through the spinal canal; the latter is seen as expansive lesions with a ring enhancement after contrast injection. [141] This presentation is extremely rare, and the lesions may be single or multiple, or even with the appearance of clusters. [149] When there is a degenerative process of the cystic lesion can also be seen this thickening in the ring of the cystic wall after the administration of contrast during a CT scan of the thoracic spine. [141,143, 147,150-152] It is equally unusual the damage of the spinal canal and the most frequent space occupies lesion to level EM. As we before-mentioned, on very rare occasions IMNCC is confirmed. [153] The differential diagnosis for the IMNCC presentation includes the IM abscess [154], other parasitic diseases such as hydatid cysts, neoplasias (ependymomas), traumatic lesions, sarcoidosis [155], arachnoid cysts [156], ependymal cysts [157] and neuroenteric cysts. [158] In the presentation EM include congenital cystic lesions (dermoides cysts); infectious diseases, demyelinating disorders, inflammatory or granulomatous, such as tuberculosis and sarcoidosis, and neoplasms. The region of provenance of the patient and the characteristics of the MRI images help to establish the difference. [159,160] For this type of presentation there is a general consensus on the poor knowledge and limited experience of the problem. Surgical treatment is recommended alone or combined with APD and corticoids [133, 161], although others believe that surgery is the best treatment option for NCCIm counting with current techniques of microsurgery. [141] The recovery of patients with IMNCC with surgical treatment is fast, with ranges of a week with maximum recovery of 3 months after surgery. [162] Although they have also reported irreversible spinal injuries by NCCIm that logically do not recover with surgical intervention. [141] Finally, there are individual differences from the clinical point of view, imaging and of response to treatment according to the number and location of the lesions, that determine the characteristics of the presentations described [117,161] and which are by describing such as: medullary central cord syndrome, medullary conus and the horsetail, when this happens. In the meantime, report of isolated cases continues to unfold with more or less variations between the same. [162,163] We report a HIV patient presenting intraspinal calcified NCC and an associated tuberculosis of the spinal. [11] The clinical and imagenological features of NCC and TB of the spine in HIV-positive patients have not been previously reported. (See figure 5)

We have also seen patients with intramedullary granulomatous lesions and associated paravertebral calcified cysticercosis confirmed by biopsy and antigen/antibody cysticercosis serology test. (See figure 6)

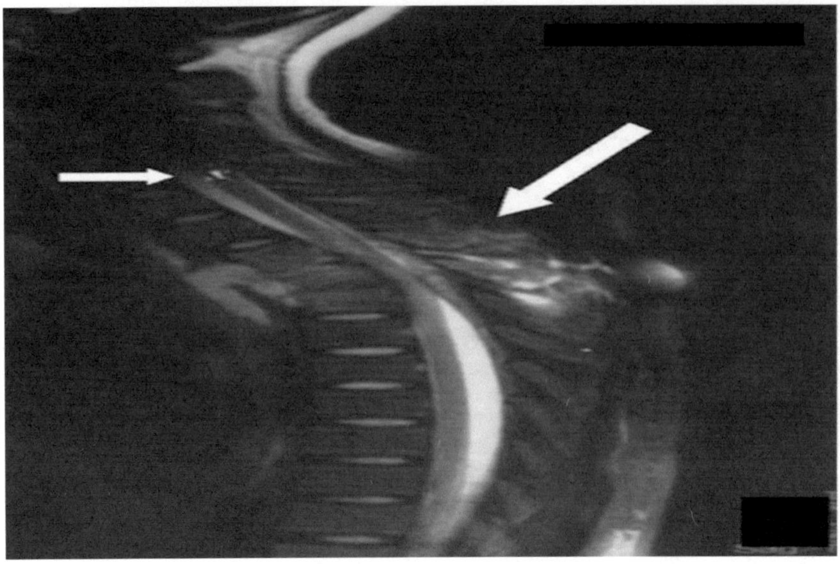

Figure 5. Shows calcified intramedullary calcified lesion and tuberculosis of the spine.

We will not discuss this observation in this chapter because we consider that this is just an anecdotal case that provides only casual interesting information. Some author thinks that EMNCC is explained by the downward migration of larvae from the brain to the spinal subarachnoid space and most larvae are expected to be stopped in the upper portions of the spinal canal due to peculiarities of the anatomy of the spinal cord; because it is hard to image cysticerci passing throughout foramen of Luscka and Magendie others authors support the hematogenous route. [11, 142, 163] Spinal intramedullary cysticercosis involving the conus medullaris is an extremelly uncommon clinical condition that may mimic an intramedullary tumor. It should be kept in mind in the differential diagnosis of intramedullary conus lesions and to rememeber that it can lead to irreversible neurological deficits if untreated.[164] Another clinical presentation is spastic paraplegia in patients presenting dorsal IMNCC but in some of them the neurological deficit may persist even after successful cyst excision. [165] Coexisting intramedullary schwannoma with intramedullary cysticercus has been reported. [166]

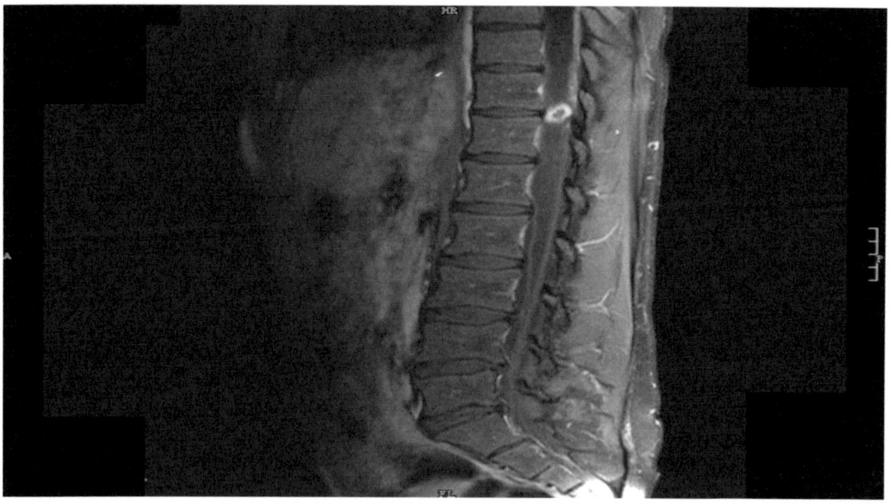

Figure 6. Multiplanar, multisequence MRI of the spine with IV contrast: Shows intramedullary ring enhancing lesion at the level of T11/T12 with enhancement of the meninges and nerve roots due to tuberculous radiculomyelitis, tuberculoma and calcified cysticercosis in the paravertebral muscles.

Disseminated cysticercosis

In the chapter entitled: "What is a low frequency of the disseminated cysticercosis suggests that neurocysticercosis is going to disappear?" Our readership will find detailed information about this uncommon presentation of cysticercosis. Therefore in this chapter we are going to mention only some remarkable issues.

Disseminated cysticercosis (DCC) was reported in 1912 by doctors of the English Navy stationed in India. An intensive search in PubMed revealed 22 cases reported by Wadia and collaborators in 1988 and only 16 additional cases were reported until 2006. [167] Two years later Bhalla et al., (2008) argued that fewer than 50 cases have been reported in the international medical literature most of them from India. [168] The characteristic features of the DCC is epilepsy, subcutaneous cysticercosis, the pseudo-hypertrophy in the four members and the allocation of any other organ or system. [164] However, a manifestation fairly typical of the DCC may be a subcutaneous cyst that occurs as an asymptomatic nodule. These subcutaneous nodules can be sliders in the muscle and measure up to 1.5 cm. (See figure 6) In the case of patients who have had for more than 5 years cysticerci, these cysts are calcified. [169] Finally, there are individual differences from the clinical point of view, imaging and of response to treatment according to the number and location of the lesions, that determine the characteristics of the described presentations. [117,160] Neurocysticercosis is always present in patients with DCC.

3. Other uncommon presentations of neurocysticercosis

The unusual location of the cysts may result in uncommon manifestations mimicking a host of neurological disorders. Thus, a high level of suspicion should be kept for NCC, especially in endemic zones and developing countries. Uncommon clinical presentations that demonstrate the spectrum of pleomorphism of NCC include extrapyramidal disease (parkinsonism and focal dystonia), Kluver-Bucy syndrome, Weber's syndrome, dementia and cortical blindness,[170] other authors include dorsal midbrain syndrome, isolated bilateral ptosis, papillitis, cerebral hemorrhage, painful cervical radiculopathy, progressive swelling of arm, paraplegia due to intramedullary cyst, third ventricular cyst, dystonia and nominal aphasia masquerading as transient ischaemic attacks, [171] and an associated pachymeningitis of the cervical spinal cord.[172]

3.1. Brainstem neurocysticercosis

3.1.1. Midbrain, pons and medulla oblongata NCC

In vertebrate anatomy the brainstem (or brain stem) is the posterior part of the brain, adjoining and structurally continuous with the spinal cord. The brain stem provides the main motor and sensory innervation to the face and neck via the cranial nerves. This is an extremely important part of the brain as the nerve connections of the motor and sensory systems from the main part of the brain to the rest of the body pass through the brain stem. This includes the corticospinal tract (motor), the posterior column-medial lemniscus pathway (fine touch, vibration sensation and proprioception) and the spinothalamic tract (pain, temperature, itch and crude touch). The brain stem also plays an important role in the regulation of cardiac and respiratory function. It also regulates the central nervous system, and is pivotal in maintaining consciousness and regulating the sleep cycle. The brain stem has many basic functions including heart rate, breathing, sleeping and eating. It is usually described as including the medulla oblongata (myelencephalon), pons (part of metencephalon), and midbrain (mesencephalon).Less frequently, parts of the diencephalon are included.

Isolated brainstem involvement in patients who have neurocysticercosis is rare, usually, it occurs in association with disseminated forms of cysticercosis and some patients can present acute midbrain syndrome responding well to corticosteroids [173,178-180] although tapering of corticosteroids should be performed very slowly in such cases [174] good response to albendazol therapy [175, 177, 178,179] and spontaneous resolution have been reported. The importance of recognizing this entity allows to avoid unnecessary surgical intervention, empirical anti-tuberculous chemotherapy, [176] and to recommend a conservative approach to case management, including observation. [175] The segment of the brainstem most frequently affected by the larval stage of the *T solium* is the midbrain, followed by the pons and in some anecdotal cases the medulla oblongata. We will comment a little bit more about this presentation.

3.1.2. Midbrain neurocysticercosis

The midbrain or mesencephalon is a portion of the central nervous system associated with vision, hearing, motor control, sleep/wake, arousal (alertness), and temperature regulation.

Anatomically, it comprises the tectum (or corpora quadrigemina), tegmentum and the cerebral peduncles, as well as several nuclei and fasciculi. Caudally the mesencephalon adjoins the pons (metencephalon) and rostrally it adjoins the diencephalon (Thalamus, hypothalamus, etc.). The midbrain is located below the cerebral cortex, and above the hindbrain placing it near the center of the brain. The clinical features of the midbrain neurocysticercosis (MIDNCC) could be summarized as follows:

1. *Pretectal syndrome*

The pretectal area, or pretectum, is a midbrain structure composed of seven nuclei and comprises part of the subcortical visual system. Through reciprocal bilateral projections to the retina, it is primarily involved in mediating pupillary light reflex, the optokinetic reflex, the accommodation reflex, and temporary changes to the circadian rhythm. In addition to the pretectum's role in the visual system, the anterior pretectal nucleus has been found to mediate somatosensory and nociceptive information. Parinaud's Syndrome, also known as a dorsal midbrain syndrome (Pretectal syndrome) is a group of abnormalities of eye movement and pupil dysfunction. It is caused by lesions of the upper brain stem and is named for Henri Parinaud (1844–1905), considered to be the father of French ophthalmology.

As before-mentioned, isolated brainstem involvement in patients who have neurocysticercosis is rare and symptoms and signs of MIDNCC can vary from one reported patient to another according to the exact location of *T solium* NCC. [174,175,181,182]

The symptoms of NCC of the pretectal area are nonspecific, but abnormal pupils, vertical gaze limitation, disjunctive horizontal and vertical eye position, lid retraction, and convergence-retraction nystagmus can be seen.[181]

2. *Weber syndrome*

Superior alternating hemiplegia is usually a form of stroke characterized by the presence of an oculomotor nerve palsy and contralateral hemiparesis or hemiplegia but cases secondary to MIDNCC (acute onset right 3rd nerve palsy with left hemiplegia) has been reported. [176]

3. *Third cranial nerve palsy*

Oculomotor nerve palsy is an eye condition resulting from damage to the third cranial nerve or a branch thereof. As the name suggests, the oculomotor nerve supplies the majority of the muscles controlling eye movements. Thus, damage to this nerve will result in the affected individual being unable to move their eyes normally. In addition, the nerve also supplies the upper eyelid muscle (Levator palpebrae superioris) and the muscles responsible for pupil constriction (sphincter pupillae). The limitations of eye movements resulting from the condition are generally so severe that the affected individual is unable to maintain normal alignment of their eyes when looking straight ahead, leading to strabismus and, as a consequence, double vision (diplopia). In the chapter entitled: "Orbital cysticercosis.A challenger for neurologists, ophthalmologists, neuro-ophthalmologists, and general practitioner" more detailed information about extraocular muscle palsy due to cysticercosis is available.

Isolated third cranial nerve palsy is usually due to vascular causes like posterior communicating artery aneurysm and it is rare in NCC and is usually caused by supratentorial or sub-arachnoid lesions with accompanying hydrocephalus or meningitis however patients presenting third cranial nerve palsy caused by neurocysticercosis involving the midbrain has been reported. [174, 183]

4. *Claude's syndrome*

Claude's syndrome is a distinctive brainstem syndrome characterized by ipsilateral third cranial nerve palsy with contralateral hemiataxia and is due to an intrinsic or extrinsic lesion in the midbrain. The most common cause of Claude's syndrome is ischemic stroke on the midbrain however one patient presenting Claude's syndrome secondary to MIDNCC is reported. Therefore, if we encounter Claude's syndrome, we should consider neurocysticercosis infection as one of the etiologic factors [179]

5. *Superior divisional oculomotor nerve palsy*

Superior divisional oculomotor nerve palsy caused by intrinsic brain stem disease occurs rarely. The first case of midbrain neurocysticercosis presenting as isolated superior divisional paresis of the oculomotor nerve was communicated by Chotmongkol et al,. in 2006. [177] They reported a 25-year-old woman presented with acute onset of headache and ptosis-upgaze palsy of the right eye. This is an anecdotal case but serve to keep in mind MIDNCC for the differential diagnosis in similar cases.

6. *Sudden-onset ptosis [184]*

Sudden onset of ptosis secondary to MIDNCC was identified in 2008 and the first two children were informed to the medical literature by Singhi et al. [184] Recently Naphade et al., [180] reported the case of a 45-year-old woman who presented with acute onset of bilateral symmetrical ptosis with no other neurological deficit. Her imaging revealed a single cystic ring-enhancing lesion with perilesional oedema in the midbrain suggestive of NCC.

3.1.3. Pontine neurocysticercosis

The pons is a structure located on the brain stem, named after the Latin word for "bridge" or the 16th-century Italian anatomist and surgeon Costanzo Varolio (Pons Varolii). It is cranial to the medulla oblongata, caudal to the midbrain, and ventral to the cerebellum. In humans and other bipeds this means it is above the medulla, below the midbrain, and anterior to the cerebellum. This white matter includes tracts that conduct signals from the cerebrum down to the cerebellum and medulla, and tracts that carry the sensory signals up into the thalamus. The pons measures about 2.5 cm in length. Most of it appears as a broad anterior bulge rostral to the medulla. Posteriorly, it consists mainly of two pairs of thick stalks called cerebellar peduncles which connect the cerebellum to the pons and midbrain. The pons contains nuclei that relay signals from the forebrain to the cerebellum, along with nuclei that deal primarily with sleep, respiration, swallowing, bladder control, hearing, equilibrium, taste, eye movement, facial expressions, facial sensation, and posture. The pons is implicated in sleep paralysis, and also plays a role in generating dreams.

Clinical features of pontine neurocyticercosis (PNCC) also depends of different locations of the T solium at the pontine level such as:

1. *Internuclear ophthalmoplegia*

Internuclear ophthalmoplegia (INO) is a disorder of conjugate lateral gaze in which the affected eye shows impairment of adduction. When an attempt is made to gaze contralaterally (relative to the affected eye), the affected eye adducts minimally, if at all. The contralateral eye abducts, however with nystagmus. Additionally, the divergence of the eyes leads to horizontal diplopia. That is, if the right eye is affected the patient will "see double" when looking to the left, seeing two images side-by-side. Convergence is generally preserved. Clinical presentations of INO can be divided into: unilateral INO, bilateral INO, and one-and-a-half syndrome in a similar descending frequency. [185] Perhaps the more difficult clinical diagnosis to perform is the One-and-a-half syndrome (OAHS). It is a neurological disorder of the extra ocular movements characterized by conjugate horizontal gaze palsy in one direction and internuclear ophthalmoplegia (INO) in the other. The commonest cause of the syndrome is a vascular lesion on the basilar territory followed by demyelinating lesions of the brainstem usually affecting the paramedian pontine reticular formation unilaterally or due to lesions on the abducens nucleus on one side, with interruption of internuclear fibbers of the ipsilateral medial longitudinal fasciculus after it has crossed the midline from its side of origin in the contra lateral abducens nucleus causing failure of adduction of the ipsilateral eye. [186]

In 2004, we proposed a new classification for OAHS based on our finding in patients with NCC and cerebrovascular diseases and we described the clinical features of One-and-a-half "plus" syndrome. We found patients with other combinations that can be called as: Five-and-a-half syndrome (1 ½ + 4-throclear nerve), Seven-and-a-half syndrome (1 ½ + 6-abducens) or Eleven-and-a-half syndrome (1 ½ + 7-facial nerve + 3-oculomotor nerve) due to racemose NCC, and midbrain lesions related to NCC. However we honestly considered at that time and even today that a generation of novel arithmetic combinations will bring more confusion than clarity to this problem and will increase unnecessarily the long list of different names of neuro-ophthalmological disorders, therefore we concluded that adding the term "plus" was good enough to distinguish these conditions from the typical OAHS. [186] Five years later Ranjith et al [178] studied an 18-year-old male presented with a history of sudden-onset diplopia of 1-week duration and blurring of vision. He had no history of headache, fever, seizures, walking difficulty, previous head injury, diabetes or hypertension. There was no history of a similar episode in the past. Diplopia was found to increase while looking to the left. Findings from general examination were normal. The left eye was deviated outward, and the right eye was central in primary gaze. There was a weakness of adduction in the left eye and paralysis of all conjugate horizontal eye movements in the right eye. The left eye also showed nystagmus while the patient attempted left lateral gaze. Vertical eye movements were normal, and no ocular bobbing was observed. There was no long tract sign, and the cerebellar system was normal. They confirmed OAHS secondary to PNCC.

2. *Simulating cystic tumor*

Characterized by focal neurological signs and clinical manifestation of intracranial hypertension including abducens palsy among other features. Cases have been reported [187]

3. *Hemifacial spasm*

Ipsilateral hemifacial spasm and associated bladder incontinence and confusional state secondary to PNCC has been reported [173]

4. *Isolated facial myokymia*

In patients presenting a history of continuous rippling and quivering movements of their hemiface suggestive of myokymia, a diagnosis of PNCC should be taking into account. The first well documented patient was reported in the medical literature by Bhatia et al in 2008 [188]

3.1.4. Medulla oblongata neurocysticercosis

The medulla oblongata is the lower half of the brainstem. In discussions of neurology and similar contexts where no ambiguity will result, it is often referred to as simply the medulla. The medulla contains the cardiac, respiratory, vomiting and vasomotor centers and deals with autonomic, involuntary functions, such as breathing, heart rate and blood pressure.

The medulla neurocysticercosis (MENCC) is an extremely rare presentation of NCC and the main affected area is the lateral aspect of the medulla leading to: Lateral medullary syndrome (also called Wallenberg syndrome and posterior inferior cerebellar artery syndrome) which is characterized by sensory deficits affecting the trunk and extremities on the opposite side of the MEDNCC and sensory deficits affecting the face and cranial nerves on the same side of the lesion. Specifically, there is a loss of pain and temperature sensation on the *contralateral* (opposite) side of the body due to damage of the spinothalamic tract and *ipsilateral* side of the face including an absence of corneal reflex due to lesion of the spinal trigeminal nucleus. Clinical symptoms include ataxia secondary to damage of the inferior cerebellar peduncle, facial pain, vertigo and nystagmus due to lesion of Deiters' nucleus and the inferior vestibular nucleus, and possibly palatal myoclonus may be observed due to disruption of the central tegmental tract. Damage to the hypothalamospinal fibers disrupts sympathetic nervous system relay and gives symptoms analogous to Horner syndrome. If patients also start vomiting then the extension of the damage toward the area postrema (dorsal vagal complex) should be considered. Remember that the area postrema is located outside of the blood–brain barrier and connects to the nucleus of the solitary tract and other autonomic control centers in the brainstem, which may serve as the beginning of the pathway triggering vomiting in response to various emetic inputs. The MEDNCC causing Wallenber syndrome has been communicated by Garg in 1999. [189]

Other uncommon presentations of NCC may include: Bilateral trigeminal neuralgia secondary to racemous cysticercus of the cerebellopontine angle, [190] and bradycardia due to right cerebellar peduncle neurocysticercosis, [191]

3.1.5. Insula lobe neurocysticercosis

In each hemisphere of the mammalian brain the insular cortex (often called insula, insulary cortex, *Island of Reil* or the insular lobe) is a portion of the cerebral cortex folded deep within the lateral sulcus between the temporal lobe and the frontal lobe. The insula is believed to be involved in consciousness and play a role in diverse functions usually linked to emotion or the regulation of the body's homeostasis. These functions include perception, motor control, self-awareness, cognitive functioning, and interpersonal experience. In relation to these it is involved in psychopathology.

The insular cortex is divided into two parts: the larger anterior insula and the smaller posterior insula in which more than a dozen field areas have been identified. The cortical area overlying the insula towards the lateral surface of the brain is the operculum (meaning "lid"). The Operculum, derived from Latin, meaning "little lid", refers to the cerebral cortex that covers the insula and is formed from parts of the enclosing frontal, temporal and parietal lobes. Operculum-insular cortex plays a role in the processing of nociceptive input. It has been convincingly established, over the past decade, that the human insular cortices are involved in processing both body feelings (such as pain) and feelings of emotion. Recently, however, an interpretation of this finding has emerged suggesting that the insular cortices are the necessary and sufficient platform for human feelings, in effect, the sole neural source of feeling experiences. [192]

Between the years 1999 and 2005 we studied a series of patients with NCC located in the lobe of the insula (INCC) confirmed by imagenology. All came from the epilepsy/NCC clinic and the neurology clinic of the Mthatha Hospital Complex. This study was designed for the screening of symptoms and clinical signs such as: dysphagia, dysarthria, attention deficit disorders, cardiovascular problems, and epileptic seizures.

All the patients underwent a CT scan of the brain and/or MRI, an ELISA test for the determination of antigens and antibodies of CC in serum and an electrocardiogram. For all patients a digital interictal EEG was performed based on, the 10-20 system and each study lasted about 20 minutes looking for focal or generalized alterations of the background rhythm or paroxysmal activity.

It was considered that the patient had difficulty swallowing liquids when they were choking or coughing after swallowing five cubic centimeters of water. In the first six month period of this study we explored the ability of the patients to differentiate between expressions of fear or disgust in photos or drawings that we show them for that purpose. Unfortunately many patients did not have the capacity to differentiate an expression of joy, fear or sadness; however we erroneously believe that this test did not work and it was eliminated from this study. In this research, special attention was given in the exclusion of patients with a history of other neurological diseases in addition to epilepsy, metabolic diseases of any type of ischemic heart disease or diseases causing difficulty in swallowing, the syndromes of Jervell-Lang -Nielsen, Romano-Ward and other causes of prolongation of the QT Segment.

Two patients died and in the postmortem studies *T solium* cystic lesions were confirmed in the insular cortex. (See figure 7) The problems most frequently encountered were functional dysphagia, the visual and somato-sensory inattention, ECG alterations such as ST-segment depression greater than 0.1 millivolts by more than 80 milliseconds and elongation of the QT Segment (greater than 0.44 seconds).

In our series, disturbances of the language due to the NCC are very uncommon excepting some patients presenting ischemic stroke due to cysticercotic /HIV/AIDS vasculitis. It is even rare in patients presenting T solium cystic lesions in the motor or sensory language cortical regions. In patients with lesions of the insula with involvement of the superior temporal gyrus and the inferior parietal region, conductive afasias have been reported, [193] but we have not been able to identify any single patient with isolated disorders of the speech or spoken languages without stroke.

The insula of the right cerebral hemisphere may play an important role in the autonomic control of the heart and the electrocardiographic abnormalities of the heart are often transient, but represent a diagnostic problem sometimes indistinguishable from a myocardial infarction. Some alterations of the T waves may be suggestive of cardiac pathology, but are not specific so it is important to consider this situation to avoid inappropriate treatment.

In the year 2004, Colivichi et al. [194] designed a study to establish the relationship between the vascular ischemic brain damage at the level of the right insular lobe and cardiac arrhythmias and they concluded that this area of the brain exerts a controlling function of the visceral autonomic activity on the heart with prognostic implications. However, the cardiac signs found in our series such as: asystole and bradycardia may also be suggestive of cardiac dysfunction secondary to left insula as has previously been reported in patients with temporal lobe epilepsy [195-198] and confirmed in 2009 by Koseoglu et al.[199] The epileptic activity spreads through the limbic system with the involvement of the amygdala, hypothalamus, and thalamus. These, in turn stimulate the autonomic system at medullar level including the nucleus tractus solitarius and the nucleus ambiguous which generate sympathetic and parasympathetic discharges.[200]

In our first study the ictal manifestations found were: laryngeal constriction, oppression of the chest, paresthesia of peri-oral region, the feeling of suspension or floating and some taste disorders. The characteristics of the epileptic seizures in these patients could not be defined convincingly at that time, therefore few years later, the realization of a methodological design addressed primarily to achieve that goal was made. However as noted earlier in this study could not arrive at confident conclusions. Later we concluded that the INCC is characterized by a functional dysphagia, ECG alterations such as: ST-segment depression and especially a prolongation of the QT segment, atypical epileptic seizures, a slight spastic dysarthria, sensory lapses and cardiovascular disorders. [7, 15]

Finally, we would like to highlight that even when the clinical features of the lesions in the insula are known mainly from neurophysiological studies and by electrical stimulation of the insular cortex, our clinical findings were not previously reported in the international medical literature although some of them were confirmed later by other authors. [201-203]

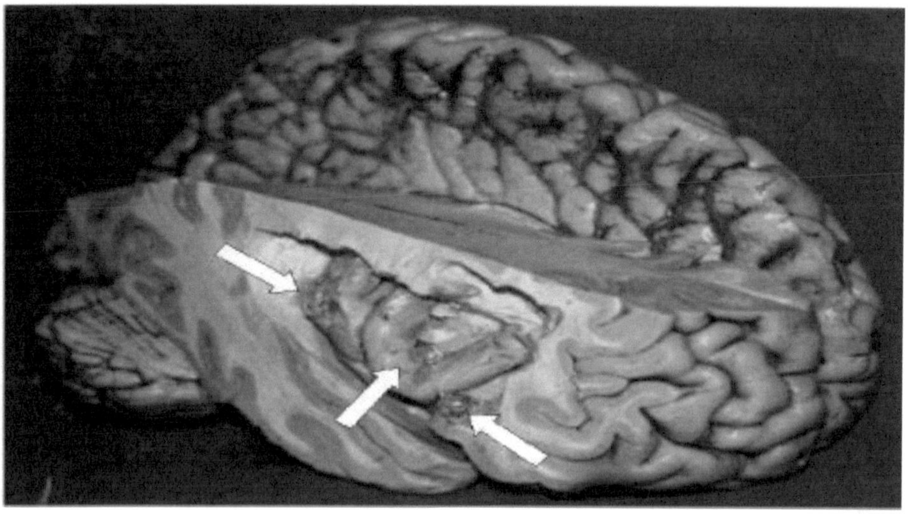

Figure 7. Right insular lobe with T solium cysticercosis in different stages. Unfortunately some cyst was damaged during disserting procedures.

In brief: patient with INCC may submit a functional dysphagia with visual and somatosensory inattention, signs of neurogenic heart and, ECG alterations such as ST-segment depression greater than 0.1 millivolts for longer than 80 milliseconds and elongation of the QT segment (greater than 0.44 seconds) and that special attention should be given to this mode of presentation by the serious complications that can be involved, including death.

The clinical features of epileptic seizures secondary to NCCI are characterized by paroxysmal feeling of laryngeal constriction, the functional dysphagia, and peribucal paresthesia. We must insist on the patient's interview about these symptoms if there is evidence of INCC in imagenology. Frequently, neither the patient nor the family or friends give importance to these symptoms and the situation is even worse when the patient is assisted by other doctor, another diagnosis is made and do not to pay too much attention is suggested especially if the seizures are sporadic and apparently banal. The diagnosis is based on the clinical confirmation of these manifestations as the conventional EEG with surface electrode is normal. [7,15]

3.1.6. Middle fossa neurocysticercosis

Apart from subarachnoid NCC, *T solium* can also affect directly or indirectly midline anatomical structures such as: optic quiasm, hypothalamus, pituitary gland, and sella turcica.

3.1.7. Optic quiasm NCC

The optic chiasm (OCh) is the part of the brain where the optic nerves partially cross. Several important structures are located adjacent to the OCh. The supraclinoid branches of the internal carotid artery flank the OCh. The cavernous sinuses are lateral and inferior to the OCh. The frontal lobe of the brain lies above. The pituitary gland sits below in the sella turcica. The sella turcica is bounded in front by the tuberculum sellae and behind of the dorsum sellae. Behind the chiasm lies the floor of the third ventricle. Chiasmal syndrome is the medical term used to describe the various signs and symptoms that are associated with lesions of the OCh, manifesting as various types of blindness or impairment in the sufferer's visual field according on the location of the lesions along the optic nerve.

Optic NCC has been well described in the past and all interested readers can find more information in the chapter entitled: "Orbital cysticercosis. A challenger for neurologists, ophthalmologists, neuro-ophthalmologists, and general practtioners" in this book. However optic chiasm NCC (OChNCC) caused by intra-chiasmatic cysticercosis has not been reported up to date. It's known that the clinical features of the OCh are caused by inflammatory processes secondary to cysticercotic vasculitis [204] or by released pro-inflammatory elements when close by cysticerci are dying. Neurocysticercosis may cause bitemporal hemianopsia due to chiasmatic compression secondary to obstructive hydrocephalus. [205]

3.1.8. Intra-Sellar turcica neurocysticercosis

The sella turcica is a midline depression in the sphenoid bone which contains the anterior and posterior lobes of the pituitary gland and the distal portion of the pituitary stalk. It is covered by a dural reflection, the diaphragm sellae. Above this lies the suprasellar cistern, which contains the supraclinoid carotid arteries and the optic tract, OCh, and nerves, and through which travels the pituitary stalk, Lateral to the sella turcica are the cavernous sinuses containing the carotid arteries, cranial nerves III, IV, and VI, and the first two divisions of the fifth cranial nerve. Anteriorly, the sella turcica is bound by the tuberculum sellae and anterolaterally by the anterior clinoid processes, Anteroinferiorly, the foramen rotundum conducts the maxillary branch of cranial nerve V. Posteriorly, there are the smaller posterior clinoid processes, the dorsum sellae, and the interpeduncular cistern containing cranial nerves III and IV. Inferiorly, the sella turcica has a thin floor of cortical bone, below which lies the air-containing sphenoid sinus. The sinus is extremely variable in size. Adjacent to the posteroinferior aspect of the cavernous sinus lies a Meckel's cave, containing the gasserian ganglion. Immediately below and lateral to the gasserian ganglion, the third branch of the fifth cranial nerve exits through the foramen ovale.

In 1915, Kufs described a woman in whom destruction of the pituitary by one of multiple basilar cysts was found at autopsy. The diagnosis was not suspected antemortem, and the patient had findings that may have been related to pituitary insufficiency. [206] In 1955, panhypopituitarism was diagnosed by Dickinson [207] in a British soldier who had served in India and developed epilepsy with X-ray evidence of cysticerci in the legs and a distorted pituitary phase CT scan of the brain was not available at that time. The case reported by Briceflo et al. (1961) was one of 97 cases of cysticercosis found among 2 ,767 routine autopsies over a 6-year period in a large Mexican hospital. Clinical data were not presented, and the authors did not record whether the patient had other lesions elsewhere in the CNS. [209] A fourth report describes a patient with cysticercosis masquerading as a pituitary tumor, but this probably represented enlargement and an erosion of the sella secondary to increased intra cranial pressure. [210] Therefore the fourth well documented patient with sella turcica neurocysticercosis (STNCC) was studied by Prosser et al in 1978. They reported *a* 42-year-old woman from El Salvador presented with arthralgias and headache. She was found to have an enlarged sella with an intrasellar mass. Transsphenoidal exploration of the sella revealed a cysticercus, the cyst was successfully removed and normal pituitary function was retained. These authors recommend that cysticercosis be considered in the differential diagnosis of any patient from an endemic area who presents with a mass lesion anywhere in the CNS, including intrasellar masses. [210] Few years later other authors reported cases presenting disturbances in both visual acuity and visual fields and other considerations were made. [211,212]

As a general rule, for patients from endemic areas presenting chiasmatic syndrome and hormonal disturbances to rule out STNCC is mandatory. Other authors have similar opinions. [210, 213-216]

Although NCC damages sellar structures with direct compression by large cysts, extension through the basal cisterns and third ventricle with focal arachnoiditis can result as an inflammatory response. Taking into consideration that the sellar region and the basal cisterns contain many vascular and CNS structures that are separated by only a few millimeters increasing the possibility that different pathologic entities could affect them simultaneously then analysis of imaging findings and knowledge of the varied clinical presentations of NCC are important to detect cases of sellar involvement in patients with unexplained visual loss or atypical cystic lesions in the sella, especially in endemic countries. [213] As in other locations in the brain, the parasite can affect the sellar structures through diverse mechanisms, ranging from direct or indirect invasion to a severe local inflammatory response [217-218] Although direct invasion of the sella turcica by the NCC vesicle affecting the hypophysis is the most commonly described form in the literature [206-212] and is often confused with the most common tumors of the area (eg, cystic adenoma and craniopharyngioma). The absence of clinical suspicion of STNCC usually results in surgical treatment of the lesions and postoperative diagnosis of the NCC with variable clinical results. [213]

A 7-year-old child presented with polyuria and polydipsia for 1 year due to a small cystic lesion in the proximal pituitary stalk was also reported in the medical literature. [214] And three patients presenting hypopituitarism secondary to the NCC have been reported as well. [216]

3.1.9. Hypothalamic neurocysticercosis

The hypothalamus is a portion of the brain that contains a number of small nuclei with a variety of functions. One of the most important functions of the hypothalamus is to link the nervous system to the endocrine system via the pituitary gland (hypophysis). The hypothalamus is located below the thalamus, just above the brain stem. In the terminology of neuroanatomy, it forms the ventral part of the diencephalon. All vertebrate brains contain a hypothalamus. In humans, it is roughly the size of an almond.

The hypothalamus is responsible for certain metabolic processes and other activities of the autonomic nervous system. It synthesizes and secretes certain neurohormones, often called hypothalamic-releasing hormones, and these in turn stimulate or inhibit the secretion of pituitary hormones. The hypothalamus controls body temperature, hunger, thirst, fatigue, sleep, and circadian cycles. In mammals, the axons of magnocellular neurosecretory cells of the paraventricular nucleus and the supraoptic nucleus, which contain oxytocin and vasopressin (also called antidiuretic hormone), comprise the posterior pituitary. Parvocellular neurons of the paraventricular nucleus contain neurons that release corticotropin-releasing hormone and other hormones into the hypophyseal portal system where these hormones diffuse to the anterior pituitary.

The hypothalamus is thus richly connected to many parts of the central nervous system, including the brainstem reticular formation and autonomic zones, the limbic forebrain (particularly the amygdala, septum, diagonal band of Broca, and the olfactory bulbs, and the cerebral cortex). The hypothalamic-pituitary-adrenal axis (HPA or HTPA axis), also known as the limbic-hypothalamic-pituitary-adrenal axis (LHPA axis) and, occasionally, as the hypothalamus-pituitary-adrenal-gonadotropic axis, is a complex set of direct influences and feedback interactions among the hypothalamus, the pituitary gland (a pea-shaped structure located below the hypothalamus), and the adrenal glands.

Hypothalamic neurocysticercosis (HTNCC) is another extremelly uncommon presentation of NCC and the most common clinical features of best documented patient are characterized by: obesity, galactorrhea and central diabetes insipidus (polyuria without solute diuresis), and panhypopituitarism due to an associated pituitary gland involvement can also be present.[207,217, 219-222, 224] It has been established that intracranial hypertension "per se" does not generate changes in the hypothalamopituitary axis function. [219]

At a Uberaba Teaching Hospital in Brazil, a total of 1.596 autopsies performed between 1974 and 1997 were studied. The study found a diagnosis of cysticercosis in 53 autopsies (3.3%) and in two obese patients with NCC the lesions were located in the ventromedial nucleus of the hypothalamus. [220]

Other authors also divided the unusual manifestations of neurocysticercosis into: intraventricular, subarachnoid, spinal, orbital, intraparenchymatous, and reactivation of previously calcified lesions and they reported frequencies of 15.69% of intraventricular presentations, subarachnoid: 11.63%; spinal: 3.49%; orbital: 0.58% and reactivated lesion: 0.58% and the frequencies for association of intraventricular and intraparenchymatous: 6.98%; association of subarachnoid and intraparenchymatous: 3.49; and association of subarachnoid and intraventricular: 2.32%. [225] but they did not include other presentations already mentioned in this chapter.

3.1.10. Solitary cysticercus granuloma

The solitary cysticercus granuloma (SCG) is considered the most frequent type of NCC in India and many other Southeast Asian countries and these lesions are the most frequent neuroimaging abnormality seen as: less than 20 mm ring-enhancing lesion in patients with new-onset epilepsy. [223] However, in our region SCG is not the most frequent presentation of NCC and compared with the prevalence of multiple active and the calcified intraparenchymal NCC which is highest, SCG is relatively uncommon probable related to unknown factors.

3.1.11. Sinus thrombosis

Only one patient presenting lateral sinus thrombosis secondary to NCC has been reported in the medical literature up to date. [226]

4. Extracraneal cysticercosis

Taenia solium cysticercosis can invade almost all extracraneal anatomical structures in the head excepting skin, nasal cavity, paranasal sinus, bone tissue and the periostium.

When a temporalis muscle is involved, clinical presentation can be a temporal headache. Two woman who complained of subacute onset of left temporal pain and another complaining headache due to cysticercosis of the temporalis muscle have been reported. [227, 228]

4.1. Ocular cysticercosis

Ocular cysts are mostly vitreous or may be found in subretinal locations. Cysts can impair vision by floating in the eye and can lead to blindness by causing retinal detachment. Visualization of cysts via fundoscopy may be diagnostic of the disease.

We dedicated a complete article for this issue and interested readers can find detailed information in the chapter entitled: "Orbital Cysticercosis. A challenger for neurologists, ophthalmologists, neurophthalmologists, and general practitioners"

4.2. Facial cysticercosis

We found facial cysticercosis in a patient presenting disseminate subcutaneous and muscular cysticercosis with cardiac involvement and NCC. [10] A cystic lesion on the right cheek and in the maxillofacial region have been also reported. [229, 230] A photo of patient showing a nodular lesion in the left hemiface at the zigomatic arch level that was removed by surgical procedures and histological examination confirmed T solium cysticercosis can be seen in a previous chapter.

4.3. Buco-lingua-pharyngeal cysticercosis

4.3.1. Oral cysticercosis

As other before-cited locations of cysticercosis this one, is also extremely uncommon. Patients presenting lesion in the lips, [231, 232] oral cavity, [233] oral mucosa, [232] and in the gums [232] due to cysticercosis have been well documented. In all cases clinical manifestations are related to the size of the nodule lesion and good response to antiparasitic medication is the rule.

Cysticercus in the tongue can be present up to 50% in porcine cysticercosis. However in human beings only anecdotal cases have been reported. [232, 234]

4.4. Parotid gland cysticercosis

Involvement of the parotid gland is manifest by a mass effect, masquerading as a salivary gland neoplasm or mild swelling with occasional aching sensation and headache, and features resembling acute parotitis [235-238] Parotid gland cysticercosis can be associated with NCC [237] or presenting as a solitary extracranial cysticercosis of the parotid gland. [238] In solitary lesions final diagnosis is based on fine needle aspiration cytology and immunological investigations and in patients with an associated NCC antigen/antibody tests for T solium cysticercosis can be useful.

4.5. Neck cysticercosis

Subcutaneous cysticercosis in the neck is usually part of the disseminated cysticercosis and it does not constitute an independent clinical entity by itself because its clinical features are similar to another subcutaneous location. [10] We studied one patient with this condition who is cited in the chapter entitled: "Orbital cysticercosis. A challenger for a neurologist, ophthalmologist, neurophthalmologists, and general practitioners". Other uncommon presentations of cysticercosis around the neck are: thyroid cysticercosis (one patient is from our region), [239, 240] cricothyroid muscle cysticercosis, [241] pharyngeal cysticercosis, first described in South Africa, [242] submandibular lymphadenopathy cysticercosis in a 7-y-old girl presented with seizures and a right submandibular lymph node enlargement confirmed by fine needle aspiration cytology [243] and cervical lymphadenopathy cysticercosis [244] cysticercosis of submandibular duct [245] and isolated cysticercosis of the sternocleidomastoid [246] were also reported.

5. Truncal cysticercosis

5.1. Thoracic cysticercosis

The thoracic cavity (or chest cavity) is the chamber of the human body (and other animal bodies) that is protected by the thoracic wall (thoracic cage and associated skin, muscle, and fascia) which can be infected by isolated T solium cysticercosis or disseminated cysticercosis as it has been reported in South African patients. [10, 240, 242, 247, 251] and others. [241, 252-255] Anatomical structures within the thoracic cavity include: structures of the cardiovascular system, including the heart where cardiac cysticercosis can be seen. [10,247,248, 256-267] Parasitic diseases may involve various anatomic structures of the heart which can be manifested clinically as myocarditis, cardiomyopathies, pericarditis, or pulmonary hypertension in many resource-constrained settings. [263] Other structures are:

great vessels and the trachea but up to date, tracheal cysticercosis is seen only in porcine cysticercosis. [265] Esophageal cysticercosis has not been described; T solium thymic cysticercosis has not been reported as yet. In the other hand; vagus nerves, the paired sympathetic chains, lymphatic and the thoracic duct cysticercosis have not been well documented in the medical literature neither. Finally we would like to emphasize that pericardial cysticercosis is also extremely uncommon and has been mentioned in the international medical literature occasionally. [264,266] Other intra-thoracic anatomical structures are: lungs where pulmonary cysticercosis has been communicated. [240, 249, 250] Pulmonary infiltration with eosinophilia is a disease entity characterized by lung disease and eosinophilia its commonest causes are tuberculosis, parasitic infestations, malignancy and connective tissue disorders. The first report about pleural effusion and subcutaneous cysticercosis in a 2 year old child is made by Salaria et al. in 2001. [268] In adults pleural effusion is the commonest presentation of pleural cysticercosis. [269, 270]

5.2. Breast cysticercosis

In women, the breasts overlay the pectoralis major muscles and usually extend from the level of the second rib to the level of the sixth rib in the front of the human rib cage; thus, the breasts cover much of the chest area and the chest walls. At the front of the chest, the breast tissue can extend from the clavicle (collarbone) to the middle of the sternum (breastbone). At the sides of the chest, the breast tissue can extend into the axilla (armpit), and can reach as far to the back as the latissimus dorsi muscle, extending from the lower back to the humerus bone (the longest bone of the upper arm). As a mammary gland, the breast is an homogeneous anatomic structure composed of layers of different types of tissue, among which predominate two types, adipose tissue and glandular tissue, which affects the lactation functions of the breasts. The blood supply to the breast is derived from 3 sources. The predominant supply of blood comes from the perforating branches of the internal mammary arteries, derived from the internal thoracic artery. The breast is supplied by the lateral thoracic and thoracoacromial arteries (branches of the axillary artery) as well as posterior intercostal arteries (branches of the thoracic aorta). Apart from breast pain, fibrocystic change, nipple discharge, tumor, bacterial and fungal infection and Paget's disease; breast can also be infected by T solium cysticercosis. Some patients can present from mastalgia, hyperprolactinaemia [271] and painless mobile swelling (lump) in the breast [272] to no clinical manifestations. [273]

In places where cysticercosis is frequent the before mentioned presentations are rare while in countries where cysticercosis had been exceedingly rare (i.e. Malaysia), with only one case of neurocysticercosis diagnosed during post-mortem in 1934 and another one diagnosed ante-mortem [274] any presentation is uncommon.

5.3. Limbs cysticercosis

Limbs cysticercosis may be isolated in the biceps brachii, deltoid, thigh, elbow, forearm, triceps, gluteal muscles [275-290] or as part of disseminated cysticercosis. [254, 291-296] The clinical features depend on the location of the cyst, the cyst burden, and the host reaction but most of patients' present painless, rubbery nodules around 2 cm in diameter, which do not carry any risk to the patient's health or can present pseudotumor, mass, pseudohypertrophy [295-298] and myalgias. [298] A positive diagnosis is established solely by incision and examination of the interior, where the parasite will be found. In the other hand , the role of ultrasonographic (USG) studies in the diagnosis of isolated soft tissue cysticercosis has been also confirmed. [295] The most common USG appearance is that of a cyst containing a scolex within and with surrounding abscess. The second most common appearance reported is that of a cyst containing a scolex within and with surrounding edema and the least common appearance is that of an irregular cyst with no scolex within and with surrounding edema. [295] Fine needle aspiration cytology [296] and even mitochondrial DNA analysis of extremely calcified cysts have demonstrated a good efficacy. [288]

We found a good response to 100 mg/kg of praziquantel for a day [292] but in most patients albendazole is the medication of choice.

Cysticercosis of the flexordigitorum profundus muscle producing flexion deformity of the fingers and cysticercosis of the tendon sheath of Tendoachilles have been reported. [300, 301]

Only one patient with cysticercosis presenting as an ulnar entrapment neuropathy due to a compressive mass in the flexor digitorum profundus has been reported. In this case magnetic resonance imaging suggested an inflammatory mass compressing the neurovascular bundle and the final diagnosis was confirmed by histologic examination. [302]

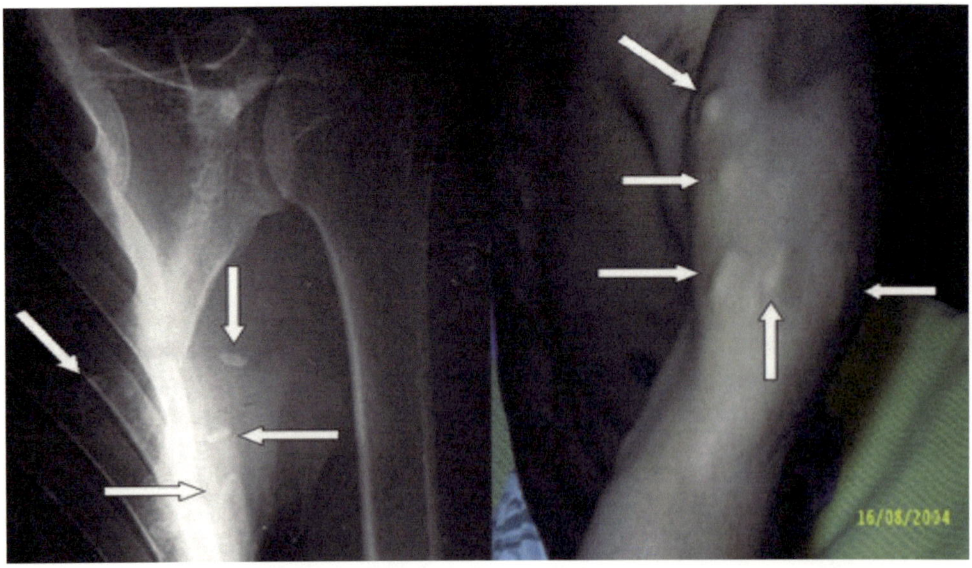

Figure 8. Subcutaneous and intramuscular cysticercosis in the proximal region of the limbs predominantly

The most common location for soft tissue cysticercosis is in the skeletal muscles of the upper extremities (33. %) as we show in the next figure. , and the least common sites for isolated muscular cysticercosis are the back, buttock and cheek, which accounted for 3% each [287].

5.4. Monoarticular cysticercosis

A joint is the location at which two or more bones make contact. They are constructed to allow movement (except for skull bones) and provide mechanical support to the body. A joint disorder is termed an arthropathy, and when involving inflammation of one or more joints the disorder is called: arthritis.

Arthropathies are called *polyarticular* when involving many joints and *monoarticular* when involving only one single joint how can happens cysticercotic arthropathy. Fortunately it is another very rare condition. Kurrein and Vickers [303] reported a former regular soldier who had served in India before the Second World War. He was in 1953-1955 diagnosed as suffering from cysticercosis affecting the brain and spinal cord as well as the muscles. Twenty years later he was found to have sustained severe damage to the lumbar spine, eventually proved due to cysticercosis involving the bones, **joints** and psoas muscles. The problem of why and how the disease remained active 40 years after the initial exposure remains unexplained. Searches of the literature and enquiries from appropriate specialists have failed to produce any record of similar cases. Kumar e al., [304] studied a 62-years old man presented with complaints of pain in the large peripheral joints with limitation of movement for two months. Fine needle aspiration cytology of the nodular eruptions over joints demonstrated negatively birefringent needle shaped crystals while that of calcific lesion in soft tissue demonstrated *cysticercus cellulose* with scolex. However the majority of the researchers that we have consulted, agree that the diagnosis of joint cysticercosis in this patient demonstrates some doubts though cannot be rejected.

The last report is made by Banu and Veen. [305] They studied an immunocompetent patient with disseminated cysticercosis who had involvement of the brain, subcutaneous tissues, lungs and skeletal muscles and presented with arthritis. This patient was otherwise asymptomatic in spite of the extensive involvement of multiple organs.

6. Abdominopelvic cysticercosis

Unfortunately we have come to the final part of this chapter faced severe space restrictions by what we have to reduce the content of each paragraph without sacrificing the quality of this chapter.

The abdominopelvic cavity (APC) is the cavity of the human body that holds the bulk of the viscera including include the stomach, liver, gallbladder, spleen, pancreas, small intestine, kidneys, large intestine and reproductive organs, the urinary bladder, the pelvic colon, and the rectum. The APC is lined with a protective membrane termed the peritoneum. The kidneys are located in the abdominal cavity behind the peritoneum, in the retroperitoneum. The viscera are also covered, in the front, with a layer of peritoneum called the greater omentum. The peritoneal cavity is a potential space between the parietal peritoneum and visceral peritoneum, that is, the two membranes that separate the organs in the abdominal cavity from the abdominal wall. The peritoneal cavity is the largest serosa sac in the body and secretes approximately 50 ml of fluid per day. This fluid acts as a lubricant and has anti-inflammatory properties.

Cysticercosis of the whole APC is another preventable faeco-oral transmitted T solium infection but for didactic purposes we will divide this topic in extra-abdominal and intra-abdominal cysticercosis.

6.1. Extra-abdominal cysticercosis

In the abdominal, wall *T solium* cysticercosis can be found involving the anterior abdominal wall musculature [306-308] and diagnosis can be done by sonography which can reveal a well-defined cystic lesion with an eccentric hyperechoic area within it and an eccentric, echogenic, pedunculated structure is seen within the cystic area of the lesion without calcification but inflammation and hypervascularity in the surrounding muscle also can be noted or can be confirmed by histopathology. Clinical manifestations include vague abdominal discomfort, tender or painless nodules. This presentation is more commonly seen in patients presenting disseminated cysticercosis [283, 292, 293, 296-298, 300-303] rather than isolated cysticercosis. [277-282, 286-289, 294]

6.2. Intra-Abdominal cysticercosis

In some anecdotal cases intra-abdominal cysticercosis is presenting as abdominal pain secondary to acute abdomen and reported cases have shown psoas muscle cysticercosis mimicking appendicitis [309] and mesenteric lymph node enlargement cysticercosis and associated appendicitis. [310] In this case is postulated that the larvae, after evagination in the small intestine, penetrated the mesenteric lymphatic, burrowing through the bowel wall, hence reaching the mesenteric lymph node. The before-cited case is the second case of isolated lymph node enlargement due to cysticercus infestation reported in the medical literature.

One study made by Vianna et al., [311] shows the frequency of cutaneous, muscular and visceral forms of cysticercosis in anatomopathological examinations and necropsies in the Federal District of Sao Paulo. In 64.911 protocols of anatomopathological examinations they found that 30 (0.05%) had the diagnosis of cysticercosis, 90% had cysticerci in the subcutaneous tissue, skeletal muscle or mucous membrane, 3.3% in lymph node and 6.7% in the central nervous system and two (7.4%) patients had cysticerci in the tongue. In 1520 autopsy protocols reviewed, 25 (1.6%) autopsies with cysticercosis were found. 96% had cysticerci in the central nervous system, 8% in the heart, 8% in the skeletal muscle and 4% in the liver, either isolated or associated with cysticerci in other viscera. A total of 1122 people were also examined and the muscular cysticercosis was found in 42.4%, subcutaneous cysticercosis was present in 20.3% and the visceral cysticercosis was found in 3.4% of cases.

In this series patient with visceral cysticercosis, the cysts were localized in the heart, pleura, kidney and ovary without clinical manifestations of importance.

6.3. Hepatic cysticercosis

Cysticercosis of the liver by T solium or other tapeworms has been reported in the animal population since long time ago, [312] and the first human being patient with hepatic cysticercosis and clinical manifestations of liver damage and not associated to disseminate cysticercosis was reported in the international medical literature in 1995. [313] Up to date only four patients with hepatic cysticercosis have been well documented.[313-316] Solitary nodular lesion remains asymptomatic while multinodular lesions may manifest as acute or chronic hepatitis. The experience of the last report highlights the need to use high resolution ultrasonography of abdomen in patients with a high index of suspicion. [314]

6.4. Pancreatic cysticercosis

In one of the previous chapter we mentioned that DCC is a rare form of cysticercosis caused by dissemination of the larval form of the pork tapeworm *T. solium* and fewer than 50 cases have been reported worldwide. Involvement of the pancreas and spleen is even rarer. The best of our knowledge, the first patient presenting splenic and pancreatic involvement by cysticercosis leading to pancreatitis was born and grew up at the former rural Transkei in South Africa (where we are living) and was reported in 1987 by Scholtz and Mentis [240] the second case is reported by Jain et al., [317] and their patient presented a history of headache and vomiting and was found to have DCC with pulmonary, cardiac , pancreatic, intraocular, and extradural spinal canal involvement. The third (last one) patient presented a disseminated cysticercosis involving the brain, orbit, myocardium, muscle, subcutaneous tissues, spleen and pancreas but without clinical or biochemical evidence of pancreatitis due to infection by cysticerci. [318]

6.5. Spleen and Kidney cysticercosis

Cysticercosis of the spleen [318,319] and the kidneys [240, 311,319] have been reported in two and three occasions respectively, always as part of a disseminate cysticercosis. Clinical manifestations secondary to the spleen or renal damage caused by *T solium* are uncertain up to date. The first reported patient presenting renal cysticercosis came from our region.

6.6. Pelvic cysticercosis

Tenia solium cysticercosis can infect ovary and one anecdotal case has been without remarkable clinical manifestation has been reported. [311]

6.7. Peritoneal cysticercosis

There are several types of tapeworms such as *T pisiformis, T hydatigena, T saginata, Taenia crassiceps* and other parasites that can be found in the peritoneal cavity in several types of animals, [320-324] but we are not aware of patients with peritoneal cysticercosis caused by T solium cysticercosis up to date.

6.8. Adrenal gland cysticercosis

The adrenal glands (also known as suprarenal glands) are endocrine glands that sit atop the kidneys; in humans, the right adrenal gland is triangular shaped, while the left adrenal gland is semilunar shaped. On CT scan, the average measurements for the right adrenal gland were: maximum width 0.61 cm (S.D. 0.2), the width of the medial limb 0.28 cm (S.D. 0.08), and width of the lateral limb 0.28 cm (S.D. 0.06). The average measurements for the left adrenal gland were: maximum width 0.79 cm (S.D. 0.21), width of the medial limb 0.33 cm (S.D. 0.09), and width of the lateral limb 0.30 cm (S.D. 0.10), [325] typically, they are less than 4 cm in length and less than 1 cm in width.

Although variations of the blood supply to the adrenal glands are common, there are usually three arteries that supply each adrenal gland such as: the superior suprarenal artery, the middle suprarenal artery and the inferior suprarenal artery which represent three paths for cysticercosis to reach the adrenal glands. However due to the size of the adrenal glands the cysticerci cannot be accommodated there; therefore, the adrenal cistticercosis does not exist. Nevertheless, there are clinical manifestations of adrenal dysfunction related to T solium cysticercosis (even simulating pheocromocytoma) but secondary to NCC [326-328] when it is affecting the limbic-hypothalamic-pituitary-adrenal axis.

7. Conclusion

After an extensive review of the medical literature and from our database, we concluded that the uncommon clinical manifestations of cysticercosis are related to the immune status of the patient, the location and numbers or cisticercus in any organ or tissue able to accommodate cysticerci depending of its size, consistency of the tissue, and the characteristics of its blood supply.

From the before-mentioned postulate is that there will never be cysticercosis in the skin, hair, nails, bones, and or organs, tissues and membranes with dimensions less than one centimeter. Outside of this rule, the cysticerci can be viewed in any organ of the human body causing direct or indirect damage with or without clinical manifestations. So any patient from an endemic area or not presenting clinical manifestation of unknown causes deserves an investigation in search of cysticercosis.

Author details

Humberto Foyaca Sibat and Lourdes de Fátima Ibañez Valdés

Department of Neurology, Stroke Unit, Epilepsy and neurocysticercosis Clinic in Nelson Mandela Academic Hospital, Faculty of Health Sciences,
Walter Sisulu University, Mthatha, South Africa

Acknowledgement

We wish to mention our eternal and deepest gratitude to Lorna María Foyaca García, Fátima Susana Foyaca Ibañez and Thabo Humberto Foyaca Ibañez for their delight support.

Hereby, we acknowledge financial support from the Directorate of Research Development, Walter Sisulu University in South Africa, South African Medical Research Council and NRF. The founder had no role in study design, data collection and analysis, decision to publish, or preparation of the manuscript.

8. References

[1] Foyaca-Sibat H, Ibañez-Valdés LdeF."Clinical trial of praziquantel and prednisone in rural patients with neurocysticercosis presenting recurrent epileptic attacks" The Internet Journal of Neurology 2002;2):41-50. http://www.ispub.com/journal/the_internet_journal_of_neurology/volume_1_number_2_39/article/clinical_trial_of_praziquantel_and_prednisone_in_rural_patients_with_neurocysticercosis_presenting_with_recurrent_epileptic_attacks.html

[2] Foyaca-Sibat H, Ibañez-Valdés LdeF."Intraventricular neurocysticercosis in HIV patients. Should be approaching surgically?" II International Congress of Neurosurgery on Internet. 2003 Conference Proceeding http://www.neuroc.sld.cu/paper/TL-neurocys.htm

[3] Foyaca-Sibat H, Ibañez-Valdés LdeF "Intraventricular neurocysticercosis in HIV patients" The Internet Journal of Neurology 2003;2(1):23-31. http://www.ispub.com/journal/the_internet_journal_of_neurology/volume_2_number_1_37/article/intraventricular_neurocysticercosis_in_hiv_positive_patients.html

[4] Foyaca-Sibat H, Ibañez-Valdés LdeF."Pseudoseizures and Epilepsy in neurocysticercosis" Electron J Biomed 2003;2(2):20-29. http://www.uninet.edu/reb/2003/n2/2foyaca.html

[5] Foyaca-Sibat H, Ibañez-Valdés LdeF "Neurocysticercosis in HIV-positive patients" The Internet Journal of Infectious Diseases 2003:2(2):15-23. http://www.ispub.com/ostia/index.php?xmlFilePath=journals/ijn/current.xml

[6] Ibañez-Valdés LdeF, Foyaca-Sibat H. Refractory epilepsy in neurocysticercosis. The Internet Journal of Neurology 2006;5(2):34-41. http://www.ispub.com/journal/the_internet_journal_of_neurology/volume_5_number_2_19/article/refractory_epilepsy_in_neurocysticercosis.html

[7] Foyaca-Sibat H. Ibañez-Valdés LdeF. Insular Neurocysticercosis: Our Finding and Review of the Medical Literature. The Internet Journal of Neurology 2006 vol 5 Number 2. http://www.ispub.com/journal/the_internet_journal_of_neurology/volume_5_number_2_19/article/insular_neurocysticercosis_our_findings_and_review_of_the_medical_literature.html

[8] Carabin H, Krecek RC, Cowan LD, Michael L, Foyaca-Sibat H, Nash T, Willingham AL "Estimation of the monetary burden of Taenia solium cysticercosis in the Eastern Cape, South Africa". Trop. Med. Int. Health.(ISSN: 1360-2276). 2006;11: 906-916.

[9] Foyaca-Sibat H, Ibañez-Valdés LdeF : Occipital Lobe Syndrome Due To Giant Intraparenchymal Neurocysticercosis . The Internet Journal of Neurology. 2006 Volume 5 Number 2. http://www.ispub.com/journal/the_internet_journal_of_neurology/volume_5_number_2_19/article/occipital_lobe_syndrome_due_to_giant_intraparenchymal_neurocysticercosis.html

[10] Foyaca-Sibat H, Ibañez-Valdés LdeF: "Generalized Cysticercosis With Cardiac Involvement". The Internet Journal of Neurology.(ISSN: 1531-295X). 2007;7(2):6-11 http://www.ispub.com/journal/the_internet_journal_of_neurology/volume_7_number_2_5/article/generalized_cysticercosis_with_cardiac_involvement.html

[11] Foyaca-Sibat H, Ibañez-Valdés LdeF: "Co-morbidity of Spinal Cord Neurocysticercosis And Tuberculosis In A HIV-Positive Patient". The Internet Journal of Neurology. (ISSN: 1531-295X). 2007;7(3):5-10 http://www.ispub.com/journal/the_internet_journal_of_neurology/volume_7_number_2_5/article/comorbidity_of_spinal_cord_neurocysticercosis_and_tuberculosis_in_a_hiv_positive_patient.html

[12] Foyaca-Sibat H Cowan LD, Carabin H, Serrano-Ocaña G, , Krecek RC, Willingham A. "Accuracy of serological exam for the diagnosis of neurocysticercosis in outpatients with epilepsy, Eastern Cape Province, South Africa" PLOS Negleted Trop.Dis.Dec.2009;3(3):1-7.

[13] Foyaca-Sibat H, Ibañez-Valdés LdeF & J. Moré-Rodríguez: Parasitic Zoonoses Of The Brain: Another Challenger?. The Internet Journal of Neurology. 2010 Volume 12 Number 2 http://www.ispub.com/journal/the_internet_journal_of_neurology/volume_12_number_2_4/article/parasitic-zoonoses-of-the-brain-another-challenger.html

[14] Humberto Foyaca-Sibat and Lourdes de Fátima Ibañez-Valdés (2011). Treatment of Epilepsy Secondary to Neurocysticercosis, Novel Treatment of Epilepsy, Humberto Foyaca-Sibat (Ed.), ISBN: 978-953-307-667-6, InTech, Rijeka

[15] Humberto Foyaca-Sibat and Lourdes de Fátima Ibañez Valdés (2011). Clinical Features of Epilepsy Secondary to Neurocysticercosis at the Insular Lobe, Novel Aspects on Epilepsy, Humberto Foyaca-Sibat (Ed.), ISBN: 978-953-307-678-2, InTech, Rijeka

[16] Humberto Foyaca-Sibat (2011). Epilepsy Secondary to Parasitic Zoonoses of the Brain, Novel Aspects on Epilepsy, Humberto Foyaca-Sibat (Ed.), ISBN: 978-953-307-678-2, InTech, Rijeka

[17] Takayanagui OM, Jardim E. Clinical aspects of nerocysticercosis: analysis of 500 cases. Arq Neuropsiquiatr 1983; 41(1):50-63.

[18] Takayanagui OM. Neurocysticercosis: I.Clinical and laboratory course of 151 cases. *Arq Neuropsiquiatr* 1990; 48(1):1-10.

[19] Takayanagui OM, Leite JP. Neurocysticercosis. *Rev Soc Bras Med Trop* 2001;34(3):283-290.

[20] Sarti E. La taeniasis y cisticercosis en México (revisión bibliográfica). *Salud Pública Mex* 1986; 28:556-563.

[21] McComick G, Zec Chi-S, Heiden J. Cysticercosis Cerebri. Review of 127 cases. *Arch Neurol* 1982; 39:534-539.

[22] Lopez-Hernández A, Garaizar C. Childhood Cerebral Cysticercosis: clinical features and computed tomographic findings in 98 Mexican children. *Can J Neurol SC* 1982;9:401-407.

[23] Kalra V, Paul VK, Marwah RK, Kichhar Gs, Bhargava S. Neurocysticercosis in childhood. *Trans R Soc Trop Med Hyg* 1987;81(3):371-373.

[24] Scharf D. Neurocysticercosis. Two hundred thirty-eight cases from a California Hospital. *Arch Neurol* 1988; 45:777-780.

[25] Sotelo J, Penagos P, Escobedo F, Del Brutto OH: Short course of albendazole therapy for neurocysticercosis. *Arch Neurol* 45:1130-1133, 1988.

[26] Villa AM, Monteverde DA, Rodríguez W, Boero A, Sica RE. Neurocysticercosis in a hospital of the city of Buenos Aires: study of 11 cases. *Arq Neuropsiquiatr* 1993;51(3):336-336.

[27] Pitella JEH. Neuro schistosomiasis. *Brain Pathol* 1997;7:649-662.

[28] Singh G. Neurocystycercosis in South-Central America and the Indian subcontinent. A comparative evaluation. *Arq Neuropsiquatr* 1997; 55(3A):349-356.

[29] Singhi P, Ray M, Singhi S, Khandelwal N. Clinical spectrum of 500 children with neurocysticercosis and response to albendazole therapy. *J Child Neurol* 2000;15(4):207-213.

[30] Del Bruto OH, Santibáñez R, Rubio CA, Aguirre R, Diez E, Alarcón TA. Epilepsy due to neurocysticercosis: analysis of 203 patients. *Neurology* 1992; 42:389-392.

[31] Del Brutto OH. Neurocysticercosis in children: clinical and radiological analysis and prognostic factor in 54 patients. *Rev Neurol* 1997; 25(147):1681-1484.

[32] Del Brutto OH. Neurocysticercosis. *Rev Neurol* 1999; 29(5):4456-4466.

[33] Del Bruto OH, Rajshekhar V, White AC Jr, Tsang VC, et al. Proposed diagnostic criteria for Neurocysticercosis. *Neurology* 2001; 57(2):177-183.

[34] Rousseau MC, Guillotel B, Delmont J. Neurocysticercosis in the South-East of France 1988-1998. *Presse Med* 1999;28(39):2141-2144.

[35] Sanchez AL, Ljungstrom I, Medina MT. Diagnosis of human neurocysticercosis in endemic countries: clinical study in Honduras. *Parasitol Int* 1999;48(1):81-89.

[36] Turkulov V, madle-Samardzija N, Canak G, Vukadinov J, Aleksic-Dordevic M. Clinical and diagnostic approaches to neurocysticercosis. *Med Pregl* 2001; 54(7-8):353-356.

[37] Varma A, Gaur KJ. The clinical spectrum of Neurocysticercosis in the Uttraranchal region.*Assoc Physicians India* 2002;50:1398-1400.

[38] Carpio A. Neurocysticercosis: an update. *Lancet Infect Dis* 2002;2:751-62.

[39] Carpio A, Hauser WA. Prognosis for seizure recurrence in patients with newly diagnosed neurocysticercosis. *Neurology* 2002;59:1730–1734.

[40] García HH, del Brutto OH. *Taenia solium* cysticercosis. *Infect Dis Clin North Am* 2000; 14(1):97-119.

[41] García HH, Evans CA, Nash TE, Takayanagui OM, White AC jret al., Current Consensus Guidelines for Treatment of Neurocysticercosis. *Clin Microbiol Rev* 2002; 15(4)747-756.

[42] White AC Jr. Neurocysticercosis: a major cause of neurological disease worldwide. *Clin Infect Dis* 1997;24:101-106.

[43] White AC Jr. Neurocysticercosis: updates on epidemiology, pathogenesis, diagnosis and management. *Ann Rev Med* 2000;51:187-206.

[44] Uddin J, Garcia HH, Gilman RH, Gonzalez AE, Friedland JS. Monocyte-astrocyte networks and the regulation of chemokine secretion in neurocysticercosis. *J Immunol.* 2005 Sep 1;175(5):3273-3281.

[45] Figueroa JJ, Davis LE, Magalhaes A. Extraparenchymal neurocysticercosis in Albuquerque, New México. *J Neuroimaging.* 2011;21(1):38–43.

[46] Wallin M, Kurtzke J. Neurocysticercosis in the United States: review of an important emerging infection. *Neurology* 2004; 63: 1559-1564.

[47] De Giorgio CM, Medina MT, Duron R, Zee C,. Escueta SP: Neurocysticercosis. Epilepsy Curr: 2004;4(3):107-111.

[48] Bhigjee AI, Rosemberg S Optimizing therapy of seizures in patients with HIV and cysticercosis. NEUROLOGY 2006;67(Suppl 4):S19–S22.

[49] Devinsky O. Patients with refractory seizures. *N Engl J Med* 1999; 340: 1.565-1.570.

[50] Ramirez-Bermudez J, Higuera J, Sosa AL,et al. Is dementia reversible in patients with neurocysticercosis? *J Neurol Neurosurg Psychiatry* 2005; 76:1164-1166.

[51] García HH, Del Brutto OH,The Cysticercosis Working Group in Perú. Heavy nonencephalitic cerebral cysticercosis in tapeworm carriers. Neurology *1999;* 53(7):1582.

[52] Colli BO, Martelli N, Assirati JA Jr, et al. Surgical treatment of cysticercosis of the central nervous system. Neurosurgery Quarterly 1995:5;34-35.

[53] Umredkar A, Singla N, Mohindra S, Bal A, Gupta SK. Giant intraparenchymal neurocysticercosis: Report of surgical aspects two cases. Neurol India 2009;57:800-802.

[54] Agarwal PP, Gaikwad SB, Garg A, Gupta V, Mishra NK, Mehta VS. Giant intraparenchymal neurocysticercosis: Unusual MRI findings. Neurol India 2004;52:259-260.

[55] Prachi P. Agarwal, Shailesh B. Gaikwad, Ajay Garg, Vipul Gupta, N. K. Mishra, V. S. Mehta. Giant intraparenchymal neurocysticercosis: Unusual MRI Findings.Neurology India 2004;52(2):259-260.

[56] Joubert J, Van As AD. Rapid and complete resolution of giant cysticercal cysts after administration of praziquantel. A report of 4 cases. S Afr Med J. 1990;77(3):154-157.

[57] Berman JD, Beaver PC, Cheever AW, Quindlen EA. Cysticercus of 60-milliliter volume in human brain. Am J Trop Med Hyg 1981;30:616-619.

[58] Castellanos F, Montes I, Porras LF, Peragallo E, Ampuero J, Rueda R. Quistes subarachnoideos gigantes por neurocisticercosis: a propósito de dos casos observados en un área rural de Extremadura. Rev Neurol 2000;30:433-435.

[59] Ramesh VG, Parthiban A. Giant parenchymal cysticercosis with unusual imaging features. J Clin Neurosci 2008;15:1404-1406.
[60] Proaño JV, Madrazo I, Avelar F, López-Félix B, Díaz G, Grijalva I. Medical treatment for neurocysticercosis characterized by giant subarachnoid cysts. N Engl J Med 2001;345:879-85.
[61] Agarwal PP, Gaikwad SB, Garg A, Gupta V, Mishra NK, Mehta VS. Giant intraparenchymal neurocysticercosis: unusual MRI findings. Neurol India. 2004 Jun;52(2):259-260.
[62] Umredkar A, Singla N, Mohindra S, Bal A, Gupta SK. Giant intraparenchymal neurocysticercosis: Report of surgical aspects two cases. Neurology India 2009;57(6):800-802.
[63] Takeshita I, Li HZ, Imamoto N, Cao YP, Gou CF, Liu DQ, Piao HZ, Fukui M.Unusual manifestation of cerebral cysticercosis. Fukuoka Igaku Zasshi. 1994;85(1):29-34.
[64] Amaral L, Maschietto M, Maschietto R, Cury R, Ferreira NF, Mendonça R, et al. Unusual manifestations of neurocysticercosis in MR imaging : analysis of 172 cases. Arq Neuropsiquiatr. 2003;61:533–541.
[65] Rocca U, Rosell A, Alvarez C. Surgical options in neurocysticercosis therapy. Neurosurg Q. 2005;15:5–13.
[66] Bickerstaff Er, Small JM, Woolf AL. Cysticercosis of the posterior fossa. Brain 1956;79:622-634.
[67] Kla O. The clinical aspects and surgical treatment of racemose cysticercosis of the posterior cranial fossa. Vopr Neirokhir. 1961;25:30-34.
[68] Lopes PG.Surgical treatment of cysticercosis of the posterior cranial fossa. Arq Neuropsiquiatr. 1971;29(1):76-92.
[69] Filizzolo F, Nastasi G, Morello A. Cysticercosis of the posterior cranial fossa. Acta Neurol (Napoli). 1972;27(6):632-638.
[70] Lushchenko AI. Diagnostic importance of laboratory and serological analysis of blood and cerebrospinal fluid in cysticercosis of the posterior cranial fossa. Lab Delo. 1975;(7):409-411.
[71] de Morais-Rêgo SF, Latuf NL. Cysticercosis of the fourth ventricle simulating a posterior fossa neoplasm in cerebral scintillography. Report of a case. Arq Neuropsiquiatr. 1978 Dec;36(4):371-374.
[72] Keane JR.Cysticercosis: unusual neuro-ophthalmologic signs. J Clin Neuroophthalmol. 1993 Sep;13(3):194-199.
[73] Kim JH, Suh SI, Kim JH, Kwon TH, Chung HS. Giant neurocysticercosis cyst in the cerebellar hemisphere. Neurol Med Chir (Tokyo) 2006; 46:412-4.Neurol India. 2004 Jun;52(2):259-60.
[74] Cheepsattayakorn R, Tantachamroon T. Cysticercosis in the posterior cranial fossa. J Med Assoc Thai 1994;77:544-548.
[75] Chang JH, Chang JW, Park YG, Kim TS.Cysticercosis of cerebellopontine cistern: differential diagnosis using MRI. Acta Neurochir (Wien). 2004 Apr;146(4):325-328.

[76] Sang-Wook K, Moon-Kyu K, Sae-Moon O, Se-Hyuck P. Racemose Cysticercosis in the Cerebellar Hemisphere. J Korean Neurosurg Soc. 2010;48(1):59–61.

[77] Zhu L, Shi Y, Pan X, Mo L, Weng X. Successful treatment of isolated cerebellar cysticercosis with albendazole. Chin Med J (Engl) 2003;116:637–638.

[78] Kim JH, Suh SI, Kim JH, Kwon TH, Chung HS. Giant neurocysticercosis cyst in the cerebellar hemisphere. Neurol Med Chir (Tokyo) 2006;46:412–414.

[79] Lalla RS, IyerVV, Asgaonkar DS. Neurocysticercosis as Anterior Inferior Cerebellar Artery syndrome. *Bombay Hospital Journal.* 2011;*53(3): 643-645.*

[80] Zee CS, et al. MRI of intraventricular cysticercosis: Surgical implications. *J Comput Assist Tomogr* 1993;17(6):932-939.

[81] Govindappa SS, et al. Improved detection of intraventricular cysticercal cyst with the use of three-dimensional constructive interference in steady state MR sequences. *Am J Neuroradiol* 2000;21(4):679- 684.

[82] Sánchez L, Abad L, Lozano E, Maldonado G. Neurocisticercosis intraventricular. Presentación de un caso localizado en el tercer ventriculo. *Radiologia.* 2002;44:309-313.

[83] Earnest MP, Reller LB, Filley CM, Grek AJ. Neurocysticercosis in the United States: 35 cases and a review. *Rev Infect Dis.* 1987;9(5):961-979.

[84] Kelesidis T, Tsiodras S. Extraparenchymal neurocysticercosis in the United States: a case report. *Journal of Medical Case Reports* 2011;5:359 .

[85] Aguilar-Amat M, Martínez-Sánchez J, Medina P, et al. Síndrome de Bruns causado por neurocisticercosis intraventricular. *Med Clin* (Barc). 2011;137(1):45-46.

[86] Carod-Artal FJ, et al. Neurocisticercosis intraparenquimatosa diseminada. *Rev Neurol* 2000;30(5):498-499.

[87] Cuetter AC, et al. Neurocisticercosis: Focus of intraventricular disease. *Clinical Infectious Disease* 1997;24:157-164.

[88] Kramer J, et al. Transaqueductal migration of a neurocysticercus cyst. *J Neurosurgery* 1992;77:956-958.

[89] Neal JH. An endoscopic approach to cysticercosis cysts of the posterior third ventricle. *Neurosurgery* 1995;36(5):1040-1043.

[90] Madrazo I, Proaño J. Tratamiento quirúrgico de la neurocisticercosis. En: Arriagada C, Nogales-Gaete J, Apta W, eds. *Neurocisticercosis.* Santiago: ARRYNOG 1997; 299-321.

[91] García HH, Gonzalez AE, Evans CA, Gilman RH; Cysticercosis Working Group in Peru. Taenia solium cysticercosis. *Lancet.* 2003; 362: 547-556.

[92] Proaño JV, Madrazo I, García L, García-Torres E, Correa D. Albendazole and praziquantel treatment in neurocysticercosis of the fourth ventricle. *J Neurosurg* 1997; 87: 29-33.

[93] Kelley R, Duong D, Locke G. Characteristics of Ventricular Shunt Malfunctions among patients with Neurocysticercosis. *Neurosurgery* 2002; 50:757-762.

[94] Nogales-Gaete J, Arriagada RC, Rodrigo SR. Tratamiento de la neurocisticercosis: Revisión crítica. *Rev Méd Chile* 2006; 134: 789-796.

[95] Ramírez-Ceballos JA, Marquéz RMC.Tratamiento endoscópico de la neurocisticercosis intraventricular. *Rev Neurocir* 2007;9(4):107-113.

[96] Govindappa SS, et al. Improved detection of intraventricular cysticercal cyst with the use of three-dimensional constructive interference in steady state MR sequences. *Am J Neuroradiol* 2000;21(4):679- 684.

[97] Sánchez L, Abad L, Lozano E, Maldonado G. Neurocisticercosis intraventricular. Presentación de un caso localizado en el tercer ventriculo. *Radiologia*. 2002;44:309-313.

[98] Gallonel L, Bedushi A, D'Andrea F. Clinical aspects and therapeutic possibilities in cysticercosis of the fourth ventricle. Riv Patol Nerv Ment. 1957;78(3):1183-1186.

[99] Patharangkura P, Jariya P, Tandhavadhana. Cysticercus racemosus in the fourth ventricle: report of two cases. Southeast Asian J Trop Med Public Health. 1980;11(4):532-534.

[100] Palmer J, Poulgrain P. Cysticercosis of the fourth ventricle: a report of two cases. Aust N Z J Surg. 1980 Feb;50(1):60-63.

[101] Elliott EM, Fried RA. Cerebral cysticercosis of the fourth ventricle: a problem in primary care diagnosis. J Fam Pract. 1984;19(4):553-557.

[102] Gupta RK, Jain VK, Kumar S, Gupta S, Haque I, Gujral RB. Unusual MRI appearances of cysticercus within the fourth ventricle. Neuroradiology. 1993;35(6):457-458.

[103] Flisser A, Madrazo I. Evagination of Taenia solium in the fourth ventricle. N Engl J Med. 1996;335(10):753-754.

[104] Govindappa SS, Narayanan JP, Krishnamoorthy VM, Shastry CH, Balasubramaniam A, Krishna SS. Improved detection of intraventricular cysticercal cysts with the use of three-dimensional constructive interference in steady state MR sequences. AJNR Am J Neuroradiol. 2000;21(4):679-684.

[105] Savindra TL et al. Neurocysticercosis in Asia. The Internet Journal of Infectious Diseases 2002:1(2):21-23.

[106] Singh S, Gibikote SV, Shyamkumar NK. Isolated fourth ventricular cysticercus cyst: MR imaging in 4 cases with short literature review. Neurol India. 2003;51(3):394-396.

[107] Hortobágyi T, Alhakim A, Biedrzycki O, Djurovic V, Rawal J, Al-Sarraj S. Cysticercosis of the fourth ventricle causing sudden death: a case report and review of the literature. Pathol Oncol Res. 2009;15(1):143-146.

[108] Prashantha DK, Netravathi M, Ravishankar S, Panda S, Pal PK. Reversible parkinsonism following ventriculoperitoneal shunt in a patient with obstructive hydrocephalus secondary to intraventricular neurocysticercosis. Clin Neurol Neurosurg. 2008;110(7):718-721.

[109] Das A, Kesavadas C, Radhakrishnan VV, Nair NS. Teaching NeuroImages: Bruns syndrome caused by intraventricular neurocysticercosis. Neurology. 2009 Aug 18;73(7):e34.

[110] Roongpiboonsopit D, Shuangshoti S, Phanthumchinda K, Bhidayasiri R. Positional vomiting as the initial manifestation of Bruns syndrome due to cysticercosis in the fourth ventricle: a symptom reminiscent of an old disease. Eur Neurol. 2012;67(3):184-185.

[111] Hanak BW, Walcott BP, Codd PJ, Jones PS, Nahed BV, Butler WE, Asaad WF. Fourth ventricular neurocystercercosis presenting with acute hydrocephalus. J Clin Neurosci. 2011;18(6):867-869.

[112] Singh S, Gibikote SV, Shyamkumar NK. Isolated fourth ventricular cysticercus cyst: MR imaging in 4 cases with short literature review. Neurol India. 2003;51(3):394-396.

[113] Costa CU, von Einsiedel HG, Disko R, Berthele A. Multicystic tumor in the fourth ventricle: consider neurocysticercosis. J Neurol. 2006;253(8):1092-1093.

[114] Loyo M, Kleriga E, Estañol B. Fourth ventricular cysticercosis. Neurosurgery. 1980;7(5):456-458.

[115] Allcut DA, Coulthard A. Neurocysticercosis: regression of a fourth ventricular cyst with praziquantel. J Neurol Neurosurg Psychiatry. 1991;54(5):461-462.

[116] Proaño JV, Madrazo I, García L, García-Torres E, Correa D.Albendazole and praziquantel treatment in neurocysticercosis of the fourth ventricle. J Neurosurg. 1997;87(1):29-33.

[117] Anandh B, Mohanty A, Sampath S, Praharaj SS, Kolluri S. Endoscopic approach to intraventricular cysticercal lesions. Minim Invasive Neurosurg. 2001;44(4):194-196.

[118] Citow JS, Johnson JP, McBride DQ, Ammirati M. Imaging features and surgery-related outcomes in intraventricular neurocysticercosis. Neurosurg Focus. 2002 Jun 15;12(6):e6.

[119] Zymberg ST, Paiva Neto MA, Gorgulho AA, Cavalheiro S. Endoscopic approach to fourth ventricle cysticercosis. Arq Neuropsiquiatr. 2003;61(2A):204-207.

[120] Psarros TG, Coimbra C. Endoscopic third ventriculostomy for patients with hydrocephalus and fourth ventricular cysticercosis: a review of five cases. Minim Invasive Neurosurg. 2004;47(6):346-349.

[121] Lapergue B, Hosseini H, Liance M, Rosso C, Decq P. Hydrocephalus and racemose cysticercosis: surgical alternative by endoscopic third ventriculostomy. Neurochirurgie. 2005;51(5):481-488.

[122] Husain M, Rastogi M, Jha DK, Husain N, Gupta RK.Endoscopic transaqueductal removal of fourth ventricular neurocysticercosis with an angiographic catheter. Neurosurgery. 2007;60(Suppl 2):249-253.

[123] Husain M, Jha DK, Rastogi M, Husain N, Gupta RK. Neuro-endoscopic management of intraventricular neurocysticercosis (NCC). Acta Neurochir (Wien). 2007;149(4):341-346.

[124] Suri A, Goel RK, Ahmad FU, Vellimana AK, Sharma BS, Mahapatra AK. Transventricular, transaqueductal scope-in-scope endoscopic excision of fourth ventricular neurocysticercosis: a series of 13 cases and a review. J Neurosurg Pediatr. 2008;1(1):35-39.

[125] Cappabianca P, Cinalli G, Gangemi M, Brunori A, Cavallo LM, de Divitiis E, Decq P, et.al. Application of neuroendoscopy to intraventricular lesions. Neurosurgery. 2008; 62(2):575-597.

[126] Hanak BW, Walcott BP, Codd PJ, Jones PS, Nahed BV, Butler WE, Asaad WF. Fourth ventricular neurocystercercosis presenting with acute hydrocephalus. J Clin Neurosci. 2011;18(6):867-869.

[127] Wallin M, Kurtzke J. Neurocysticercosis in the United States: review of an important emerging infection. *Neurology* 2004; 63: 1559-1564.

[128] Del Brutto O, Sotelo J. Neurocysticercosis Up date. *Rev. Inf. Dis.*1988;10(6):1075-1087.

[129] Del Bruto OH, Rajshekhar V, White AC Jr, Tsang VC, et al. Proposed diagnostic criteria for Neurocysticercosis. *Neurology* 2001; 57(2):177-183.

[130] Del Brutto O, Sotelo J. Albendazole therapy for subarachnoid and ventricular cysticerciosis. *J Neurosurgery* 1990; 62: 816-817.

[131] Proaño JV, Madrazo I, Avelar F, López-Félix B, Díaz G, Grijalva I. Medical treatment for neurocysticercosis characterized by giant subarachnoid cysts. *N Engl J Med.* 2001;345:879–885.

[132] García HH, Evans CA, Nash TE, Takayanagui OM, White AC jret al., Current Consensus Guidelines for Treatment of Neurocysticercosis. *Clin Microbiol Rev* 2002; 15(4)747-756.

[133] Cruz-Ultreras I, Cruz M. Tratamiento médico de la neurocisticercosis. En: Arriagada C, Nogales-Gaete J, Apta W, eds. *Neurocisticercosis.* Santiago: ARRYNOG 1997; 287-98.

[134] Hatano S. Experience from a multicentre stroke registry: a preliminary report Bull World Health Organ. 1976;54:541–553.

[135] Portenog RK, Abissi CJ, Lipton RB. Headache in acute cerebrovascular disease. *Stroke* 1985;15:1009–1012.

[136] Chodosh EH, Foulkes MA, Kase CS. Silent stroke in NINCDS stroke data bank. *Neurology* 1988;38: 1674–1679.

[137] Cárdenas F, Quiroz H, Plancarte A. Taenia solium ocular cysticercosis: findings in 30 cases. *Ann Ophthalmol* 1992; 24:25–28.

[138] Alarcon F, Vanormelingen K, Moncayo J, Vinan I. Cerebral cysticercosis as a risk factor for stroke in young and middle–age people. *Stroke* 1992;23:1563–1565.

[139] Dantas FL. Fagundes-Pereyra WJ, De Souza CT, Vega MG, De Souza AA. Intramedullary cysticercosis: *case report Arq Neuropsiquiatr* 1999;57(2A):301-305.

[140] Musumdar D, Nadkarni T, Desai K, Dindorkar K, Goel A. Thoracic intramedullary cysticercosis. *Neurol Med Chir* (Tokyo)2002; 42 :575-579.

[141] Gallani NR, Zambelli HJ, Roth-Vargas AA, Limoli Júnior C.Spinal cord cysticercosis: report of 2 cases, review of the literature, and comments on its pathogeny. Arq Neuropsiquiatr. 1992 Sep;50(3):343-350.

[142] Mohanty A, Venkatrama SK, Das S. Spinal intramedullary cysticercosis. *Neurosurgery.* 1997;40(1):82–87.

[143] Chang GY, Keane JR. Visual loss in cysticercosis: analysis of 23 patients. Neurology. 2001;57:545–548.

[144] Kishore LT, Gayatri K, Naidu MR, Mateen MA, Dinakar I, Ratnakar KS. Intramedullary spinal cord cysticercosis-a case report and literature review. *Indian J Pathol Microbiol.* 1991;34:219–221.

[145] Isidro-Llorens A, Dachs F, Vidal J, Sarrias M. Spinal cysticercosis. Case report and review. *Paraplegia.* 1993;31:128–130.

[146] Parmar H, Shah J, Patwardhan V. et al. MR imaging in intramedullary cysticercosis. *Neuroradiology*. 2001;43(11):961–967.

[147] David J. Neurocysticercosis. "Dr. House Series" .Tuesday, February 22, 2011.(Last review on September 22, 2011) Full article is free available at the URL: http://mentiraomedicina.blogspot.com/2011/02/neurocisticercosis.html

[148] Amaya MA, Roa JL. Neurocisticercosis raquídea: Reporte de caso. *Rev Colomb Radiol.* 2011;22(1):3134-3137.

[149] Mathuriya SN, Khosla VK, Vasishta RK et al. Intramedullary cysticercosis: MRI diagnosis. *Neurol India*. 2001;49(1):71–74.

[150] Ahmad FU, Sharma BS. Treatment of intramedullary spinal cysticercosis: report of 2 cases and review of literature. *Surg Neurol*. 2007;67(1):74–77.

[151] Agrawal R, Chauhan SP, Misra V. et al. Focal spinal intramedullary cysticercosis. *Acta Biomed*. 2008;79(1):39–41.

[152] Leite CC, Jinkins JR, Escobar BE, et al. MR imaging of intramedullary and intradural-extra medullary spinal cysticercosis. *AJR* 1997;169:1713-1717.

[153] Tacconi L, Arulampalam T, Johnston FG. et al. Intramedullary spinal cord abscess: case report. *Neurosurgery*. 1995;37(4):817–819.

[154] Clifton AG, Stevens JM, Kapoor R. et al. Spinal cord sarcoidosis with intramedullary cyst formation. *Br J Radiol*. 1990;63(754):805–808.

[155] Lamejjati M, Aniba K, Haddi M. et al. Spinal Intramedullary arachnoid cyst in children. *Pediatr Neurosurg*. 2008;44(3):243–246.

[156] Iwahashi H, Kawai S, Watabe Y. et al. Spinal Intramedullary ependymal cyst: a case report. *Surg Neurol*. 1999;52(4):357–361.

[157] Riviérez M, Buisson G, Kujas M. et al. Intramedullary neurenteric cyst without any associated malformation. One case evaluated by RMI and electron microscopic study. *Acta Neurochir*. 1997;139(9):887–890.

[158] Rahalkar MD, Shetty DD, Kelkar AB, et al. The many faces of cysticercosis. *Clin Radiol.* 2000;55:668-674.

[159] Thurnher MM, Cartes-Zumelzu F, Mueller-Mang C, et al. Demyelinating and infectious diseases of the spinal cord. *Neuroimaging Clin N Am*. 2007;17:37-55.

[160] Colli B, Morales M, Carlotti C, Rubens H, Assirati J. Spinal cord cysticercosis: neurosurgical aspects. *Neurosurg Focus (e-journal)* 2002; 12 (6): available at the URL http://www.medscape.com/viewpublication/65_toc?vol=12 & iss=6. (Last review on August 09, 2012)

[161] Villanueva M, Alcocer JL, Martinez J, Horna A. Cisticercosis intramedular. Reporte de un caso. *Arch Neurocien* 2004;9(2):110-113.

[162] Ichiro A. Tetsuji F, Hitoshi M, Hideo M, Masakuni K. Intramedullary spinal cysticercosis. *Neurology* 1979; 29: 1531-1534.

[163] Alsina GA, Johnson JP, Mc Bride DQ, *et al*. Spinal neurocysticercosis. *Neurosurg Focus* 2002: 12(6):e8.

[164] Izci Y, Moftakhar R, Salamat MS, Baskaya MK.Spinal intramedullary cysticercosis of the conus medullaris.WMJ 2008;107(1):37-39.

[165] Mathuriya SN, Khosla VK, Vasishta RK, Tewari MK, Pathak A, Prabhakar S.Intramedullary cysticercosis : MRI diagnosis. Neurol India. 2001;49(1):71-74.
[166] Vij M, Jaiswal S, Jaiswal AK, Behari S.Coexisting intramedullary schwannoma with intramedullary cysticercus: report of an unusual collision. Indian J Pathol Microbiol. 2011;54(4):866-867.
[167] Wadia N, Desai S, Bhatt M: Disseminated cysticercosis. New observations, including CT scan findings and experience with treatment by praziquantel. *Brain* 1988, 111:597-614.
[168] Bhalla A, Sood A, Sachdev A, Varma V. Disseminated cysticercosis: a case report and review of the literature *Medical Case Reports* 2008; 2:137-140. Full article is available at the URL: http://www.jmedicalcasereports.com/content/2/1/137 (Last access on August 10, 2012)
[169] Flisser A. Cisticercosis subcutáneo. *Ciencias,* UNAM 2011. Available at the URL: http://hydra.fciencias.unam.mx:8080/xmlui/handle/123456789/62343?show=full (last accessed on August 11, 2012)
[170] Patel R, Jha S, Yadav RK.Pleomorphism of the clinical manifestations of neurocysticercosis. Trans R Soc Trop Med Hyg. 2006;100(2):134-141.
[171] Sawhney IM, Singh G, Lekhra OP, Mathuriya SN, Parihar PS, Prabhakar S. Uncommon presentations of neurocysticercosis. J Neurol Sci. 1998;154(1):94-100.
[172] Kahn P. Cysticercosis of the central nervous system with amyotrophic lateral sclerosis: case report and review of the literature. J Neurol Neurosurg Psychiatry. 1972;35(1):81-87.
[173] Revuelta Gutierrez R, Soto-Hernández JL, Suastegui-Roman R, Ramos-Peek J. Transient hemifacial spasm associated with subarachnoid brainstem cysticercosis: a case report. Neurosurg Rev.1998;21(2-3):167-170.
[174] Kim JS, Jeong SM, Moon SY, Park SH. Third cranial nerve palsy from midbrain neurocysticercosis: repeated exacerbation on tapering corticosteroids. J Neuroophthalmol. 2004 Sep;24(3):217-220.
[175] Lath R, Rajshekhar V. Solitary cysticercus granuloma of the brainstem. Report of four cases. J Neurosurg. 1998;89(6):1047-1051.
[176] Singh NN, Verma R, Pankaj BK, Misra S. Neurocysticercosis presenting as Weber's syndrome. Neurol India. 2003;51(4):551-552.
[177] Chotmongkol V, Sawanyawisuth K, Limpawattana P, Phuphatham A, Chotmongkol R, Intapan PM. Superior divisional oculomotor nerve palsy caused by midbrain neurocysticercosis. Parasitol Int. 2006;55(3):223-225.
[178] Ranjith MP, Divya R, Sahni A. Isolated one and a half syndrome: An atypical presentation of neurocysticercosis. Indian J Med Sci [serial online] 2009 [cited 2012 Aug 13];63:119-120. Available from: http://www.indianjmedsci.org/text.asp?2009/63/3/119/49291
[179] Song TJ, Suh SH, Cho H, Lee KY.Claude's syndrome associated with neurocysticercosis. Yonsei Med J. 2010;51(6):978-979.

[180] Naphade PU, Singh MK, Garg RK, Rai D. Bilateral ptosis: an atypical presentation of neurocysticercosis. *BMJ Case Reports.*2012; doi:10.1136/bcr-2012-006195 http://casereports.bmj.com/content/2012/bcr-2012-006195.abstract

[181] Keane JR. The Pretectal Syndrome: 206 Patients. Neurol 1990;40:684-690

[182] Garg RK, Karak B. Neurocysticercosis presenting as midbrain syndrome. J Assoc Physicians India. 2000;48(5):533-535.

[183] Ranjith MP, Divya R, Sahni A.Isolated third cranial nerve palsy: a rare presentation of neurocysticercosis. Ir J Med Sci. 2011;180(4):905-907.

[184] Singhi P, Mahajan V, Khandelwal NK. Sudden-onset ptosis caused by midbrain neurocysticercosis in 2 children. J Child Neurol. 2008 Mar;23(3):334-337.

[185] Bolaños I, Lozano D, Cantú C. Internuclear ophthalmoplegia: causes and long-term follow-up in 65 patients. Acta Neurol Scand. 2004;110(3):161-165.

[186] Foyaca-Sibat H, Ibanez-Valdes LdeF.One-and-a half syndrome. Clinical Classification. / Electron J Biomed 2004;3:15-21. http://biomed.uninet.edu/2004/n3/foyaca.html

[187] Arruda WO, Ramina R, Pedrozo AA, et al. Brainstem cysticercosis simulating cystic tumor lesion. A case report. Arq Neuropsiquiatr 1994;52:431- 434.

[188] Bhatia R, Desai S, Garg A, Padma MV, Prasad K, Tripathi M. Isolated facial myokymia as a presenting feature of pontine neurocysticercosis. Mov Disord. 2008;23(1):135-137.

[189] Garg RK. Wallenberg's lateral medullary syndrome: a new non-vascular cause. J Assoc Physicians India. 1999;47(11):1110-1111.

[190] Aguiar PH, Miura FK, Napoli PR, Sendenski M, Rotta JM, Cescato VN, Teixeira MJ, Marino Junior R. Unusual cause for bilateral trigeminal neuralgia: unilateral racemous cysticercus of cerebellopontine angle. Case report. Arq Neuropsiquiatr. 2000;58(4):1138-1141.

[191] Nadkarni T, Kansal R, Goel A. Right cerebellar peduncle neurocysticercosis presenting with bradycardia. Acta Neurochir (Wien). 2010;152(4):731-732.

[192] Damasio A, Damasio H, Tranel D.Persistence of Feelings and Sentience after Bilateral Damage of the Insula. Cereb. Cortex (2012) doi: 10.1093/cercor/bhs077 First published online: April 3, 2012. http://cercor.oxfordjournals.org/content/early/2012/04/03/cercor.bhs077.short

[193] Marshall R, Lazar R, Mohr JP, Van Heertum R, Mast H. "Semantic" conduction aphasia from a posterior insular cortex infarction. J Neuroimaging. 1996;6:189-191.

[194] Colivicchi F, Bassi A, Santini M, Caltagirone C. Cardia autonomic derangement and arrhythmias in right sided stroke with insular involvement. Stroke 2004;35:2094-2098.

[195] Massetani R, Strata G, Galli R, Gori S, Gneri C, et al., Alteration of Cardiac Function in Patients with Temporal Lobe Epilepsy: Different Roles of EEG-ECG Monitoring and Spectral Analysis of RR Variability. Epilepsia 1997;38(3):363-369.

[196] Locatelli ER, Varghese J, Shuaib A, Potolicchio SJ. Cardiac Asystole and bradycardia as a manifestation of left temporal lobe complex partial seizure. Ann Intern Med 1999;130:581-583.

[197] Druschky A, Hilz MJ, Hopp P, Platsch G, et al. Interictal cardiac autonomic dysfunction in temporal lobe epilepsy demonstrated by [^{123}I]metaiodobenzylguanidine-SPECT. Brain 2001;124(12):2372-2382.

[198] Ansakorpi H, Korpelainen JT, Huikuri HV, Tolonen U, Myllylä VV, Isojärvi JIT. Heart rate dynamics in refractory and well controlled temporal lobe epilepsy. J Neurol Neurosurg Psychiatry 2002;72:26–30.

[199] Koseoglu E, Kucuk E, Arman F, Ersoy AO. Factors that affect interictal cardiovascular autonomic dysfunction in temporal lobe epilepsy: Role of hippocampal sclerosis. Epilepsy & Behavior 2009;16(4): 617–621.

[200] Nouri S. Epilepsy and the Autonomic Nervous System. (2010) Full article is availale at the URL: http://emedicine.medscape.com/article/1186872-overview.

[201] Park YS, Lee YH, Shim KW, Lee YL, Kim HD, Lee J-S, Kim D-S. Insular epilepsy surgery under neuronavigation guidance using depth electrode. Childs Nerv Syst ((2009) 25:591–597.

[202] Von Lehe M, Wellmer J, Urbach H, Schramm J, Elger CE and H. Clusmann. Insular lesionectomy for refractory epilepsy: management and outcome. Brain 2009: 132; 1048–1056.

[203] Meng H, Yudan LV, Cui l, Wang Z, Kin W, et al. Hypothalamus mediates the cardiovascular changes induced by insular epilepsy. Human Health and Biomedical Engineering (HHBE), 2011 International Conference on 19-22 Aug. 2011. Available at the URL:
http://ieeexplore.ieee.org/xpl/login.jsp?tp=&arnumber=6027962&url=http%3A%2F%2Fieeexplore.ieee.org%2Fxpls%2Fabs_all.jsp%3Farnumber%3D6027962

[204] Enríquez Coronel E, Santos Marcial E, Cabrera Aldana EE. Cerebral cycticercosis vasculitis and optic neuropathy. Case report. Arch. Neurocien (Mex., D.F.) 2004;9(3):

[205] Salcedo-Villanueva G, Rueda-Villa A, Hernández-Ábrego MP. Hemianopsia bitemporal secundaria a hidrocefalia por neurocisticercosis. *Archivos de la Sociedad Española de Oftalmología.* Full article is free available at the URL:
http://linkinghub.elsevier.com/retrieve/pii/S0365669112003401?via=sd&cc=y

[206] Kufs T, von basaler F. Cysticerkenmeningitis mit Cysticercus der Hypophhysis und schwerer depressiver Psychose. Z. Ges.*Neurol. Psych.,* 1915;*30:286-304.(Cited by* Prosser PR)

[207] Dickinson, C. J. Cysticercosis and panhypopituitarism. Proc. R. Soc. Med., 1955; 48:892.

[208] Argenta, G., 1956. Su di un caso di cisticercosis generalizata con sindrome di adenoma ipofisario. Riv. Neurol. (Napoli). 1956;26:197-204.

[209] Briceflo, C. E., Biagi, F., and Martinez, B.,.Cysticercosis. Observaciones sobre 97 casos de autopsia. Prensa Med. Mex., 1961;26:193-197.

[210] Prosser PR, Wilson CB, Forsham PH. Intrasellar cysticercosis presenting as a pituitary tumor: successfully transphenoidal cystectomy with preservation of pituitary function. J Trop Med Hyg.1978;27(5):976-979.

[211] Gómez-Llata *RH.* Intrasellar cysticercosis. *J Neurosurg 1985;63:*975*–976.*

[212] Del Brutto OH, Guevara J, Sotelo J. Intrasellar cisticercosis. J Neurosurg 1988;69:58–60.

[213] Arriada-Mendicoa N, Celis-López MA, Higuera-Calleja J, Corona-Vázquez T. Imaging features of sellar cysticercosis. Am J Neuroradiol. 2003;24(7):1386-1389.

[214] Rohilla S, Rawal M, Yadac RK, Ahula A, Nanda S, Dhaulakhandi DB. Neurocysticercosis-presenting-as-central-diabetes-insipidus-in-a-boy J Pediat Neurol 2009;7(3):307-310. Full article is available at the URL: http://www.docstoc.com/docs/44022185/Neurocysticercosis-presenting-as-central-diabetes-insipidus-in-a-boy

[215] Jin Hwan Cheong, M.D., Jae Min Kim, M.D., Choong Hyun Kim, M.D. Neurocysticercosis Involving the Pituitary Stalk :Case Report and Literature Review. J Korean Neurosurg Soc 2010;48:91-93.

[216] Kelesidis T, Tsiodras S. Hypopituitarism caused by neurocysticercosis. Am J Med Sci. 2011;341(5):414-416.

[217] *Del Brutto OH, Sotelo J, Román GC. Neurocysticercosis: A Clinical Handbook. Lisse, the Netherlands: Swets & Zeitlinger;1998.*

[218] *Del Brutto OH, Sotelo J.* Some unusual manifestations of neurocysticercosis. *Rev Neurol* Neurosurg Psychiatry (Mexico) 1989;29:23–26.

[219] Madrazo I, Sandoval M, González D. Evaluation of the hypothalamic-hypophyseal axis in patients with hypertensive hydrocephalus due to neurocysticercosis. Arch Invest Med (Mex). 1991 Apr-Jun;22(2):113-115.

[220] Lino RS Jr, Reis MA, Teixeira VP. Occurrence of encephalic and cardiac cysticercosis (Cysticercus cellulosae) in necropsy. Rev Saude Publica. 1999;33(5):495-498.

[221] Júnior Lino RS, Reis LC, Reis MA, Gobbi H, Teixeira VP. Hypothalamic neurocysticercosis as a possible cause of obesity. Trans R Soc Trop Med Hyg. 2000 ;94(3):294.

[222] Prajej R, Thananat B, · Pasiri S, Yupin B, Warin ·Ch, Suchinta U, Thanom S. Hypothalamic neurocysticercosis presenting. with polyuria: a first report of an unusual manifestation. Nephrol Dial Transplant. 2006;21:2308–2310.

[223] Garg RK, Malhotra HS. Solitary cysticercus granuloma. Expert Review of Anti-infective Therapy. 2012;10(5):597-612.

[224] Maguire JH, Tierney MR. Case records of the Massachusetts General Hospital. Weekly clinicopathological exercises. Case 8-1993. A 62-year-old Cape Verdean woman with blurred vision, diplopia, a suprasellar mass, and lymphocytic meningitis. N Engl J Med 1993; 328: 566–573.

[225] Amaral L, Maschietto M, Maschietto R, Cury R, Ferreira NF, Mendonça R, Lima SS. Ununsual manifestations of neurocysticercosis in MR imaging: analysis of 172 cases. Arq Neuropsiquiatr. 2003;61(3A):533-541.

[226] Prasad R, Singh R, Joshi B. Lateral sinus thrombosis in neurocysticercosis. Trop Doct. 2005;35(3):182-183.

[227] Sethi PK, Sethi NK, Torgovnick J, Arsura E. Cysticercosis of temporalis muscle: an unusual cause of temporal headaches. A case report. J Headache Pain. 2007;8(5):315-317.

[228] Kumar V, Gulati A, Mehra B. Cysticercosis of the temporalis muscle causing temporal headache in a pregnant woman.Int J Gynaecol Obstet. 2011;114(1):79.

[229] Sarma DP, Omaha MD. Biopsy of a 1.5-cm cystic lesion on the right cheek of a 28-year-old man. Available at URL: http://www.scribd.com/doc/93186763/Cutaneous-Cysticercosis.

[230] Sidhu R, Nada R, Palta A, Mohan H, Suri S. Maxillofacial cysticercosis: uncommon appearance of a common disease. J Ultrasound Med 2002; 21:199–202.

[231] Pinswasdi P, Charoensiri DJ. Cysticercosis in labial tissue. Case report. Aust Dent J. 1997;42(5):319-321.

[232] Mazhari NJ; Kumar N; Jain S. Cysticercosis of the oral mucosa: aspiration cytologic diagnosis. J Oral Pathol Med 2001; 30:187-189.

[233] de Souza PEA, Barreto DC, da Silva Fonseca LM, Batista de Paula AM, Silva EC, Gomez RS. Cysticercosis of the oral cavity: report of seven cases. Oral Diseases. 2000;6(4): 253–255.

[234] Bhandary S, Sury R, Karki P, Sinha AK: Cysticercosis of Tongue-diagnostic dilemma; Pac Health Dialog. 2004;11(1): 87-88.

[235] Corona S, Apt W. Multiple hydatid cysts and generalized cysticercosis. Rev Med Chil 1989;117:311-314.

[236] Natarajan A, Rameshkumar K, D'Souza RE. Cysticercosis masquerading as a salivary gland neoplasm. Trop Doct 2002;32:120-121.

[237] Chakraborty PP , Bhattacharjee R, Chatterjee K. Parotid Gland Cysticercosis. 2007;55:

[238] Veena G, Shon GM, Usha K, NayarRC. Extracranial cysticercosis of the parotid gland: a case report with a review of the literature. The Journal of Laryngology & Otology 2008;122(9):1008-1011.

[239] Leelachaikul, Chuahirun S. Cysticercosis of thyroid gland in severe cerebral cysticercosis: report of a case. J Med Assoc Thai 1977;60:405–10.

[240] Scholtz L, Mentis H. Pulmonary cysticercosis. SAMT1987; 72(1): 573.

[241] Smiti S, Sripathi H, Naik L. Cricothyroid muscle cysticercosis. Muscoloskeletal 2003: 13(2):157-158.

[242] Sobnach S, Khosa SA, Pather S, Longhurst S, Kahn D, Raubenheimer PJ. First case report of pharyngeal cysticercosis. Trans R Soc Trop Med Hyg. 2009;103(2):206-208.

[243] Sodhi PK, Ratan SK. Submandibular lymph node enlargement due to cysticercosis infestation. Scandinavian journal of infectious diseases. 2004;36: 227-229.

[244] Geeta V, Devi P, Sirisha A, Devi R, Bai J, Kumar S. Unusual location of Cysticercosis lesion presentation. JEMDS 2012;42. Article is fully available at the URL: http://www.jemds.com/latest-articles.php?at_id=42 (Last checked on August 27, 2012)

[245] Vikas Sinha V, Raizada RM, Jain SKT, Chaturvedi VN. Cysticercosis of Submandibular Duct. Indian Journal of Otolaryngology and Head & Neck Surgery. 1999;51(4):51-52.

[246] Sharma R, Gautam P, Kumar S, Elhence P, Bansal R, et al. Isolated Cysticercosis Cellulosae of Sternocleidomastoid Muscle: A Case Report with Review of Literature. Indian Journal of Otolaryngology and Head & Neck Surgery 2011;24:127-130.

[247] *Thomas MB, Thomas KM, Awotedu AA, Blanco-Blanco E, Anwary M. Cardiocysticercosis.*S Afr Med J *2007;*97(7):504-505.

[248] Eberly MD, Soh EK, Bannister SP, Taraf-Motamen H, Scott JS: Isolated Cardiac Cysticercosis in an adolescent; Pediatr Infect Dis J. 2008; 27(4); 369-71.

[249] Jain BK, Sankhe SS, Agrawal MD, Naphade PS. Disseminated cysticercosis with pulmonary and cardiac involvement. Indian J Radiol Imaging 2010;20:310-313.

[250] Mamere AE, Muglia VF, Simao GN, Belucci AD, Carlos dos Santos A, Trad CS, et al. Disseminated cysticercosis with pulmonary involvement. J Thorac Imaging 2004;19:109–111.

[251] Bhigjee AI. Disseminated cysticercosis. *J Neurol Neurosurg Psychiatry* 1999;66(4):545

[252] Banu A, Veena N. A rare case of disseminated cysticercosis: Case report and literature review. Case Report. 2011;29(2):180-183.

[253] Kumar A, Goenka AH, Choudhary A, Kumar Sahu JK, Gulati S.Disseminated cysticercosis in a child: whole-body MR diagnosis with the use of parallel imaging. Pediatric Radiology 2110;45:223-227.

[254] Smiti S, Sripathi H, Naik L. Pectoralis Major muscle cysticercosis. MUSCULOSKELETAL 2003;13(2):157-158.

[255] Wadia N, Deasi S, Bhat M. Disseminated cysticercosis; new observations, including CT scan finding and experience with treatment by praziquantel. *Brain* 1988; 111: 597-614.

[256] Saxena H, Samuel KC, Singh B. Cysticercosis of the heart. *Indian Heart J* 1972;24: 313-315.

[257] Niakara A, Cisse R, Traore A, *et al.* Myocardial localization of a disseminated cisticercosis.

[258] Cutrone JA, Georgiou D, Gil-Gomez C, Burndage BH. Myocardial cysticercosis detected by ultrafast CT. *Chest* 1995; 108:1752-1754.

[259] Rahalkar MD, Shetty DD, Kelkar AB, Kelkar AA, Kinare AS, Ambardekar ST. The many faces of cysticercosis. *Clin Radiol* 2000; 55 (9): 668-674.

[260] Ibarra-Perez C, Fernandez-Diez J, Rodriguez-Trujillo F. Myocardial cysticercosis, report of two cases with coexisting heart disease. *South Med J* 1972; 65: 484-486.

[261] Deshpande VL, Patil SD. Silent myocardial cysticercosis. *Indian Heart J* 1976; 28(1): 58-60.

[262] Belagavi CS, Goravalingappa JP. Cysticercosis of the heart. A case report. *Indian Heart J* 1978;30: 118-119.)

[263] Kirchhoff LV, Weiss LM, Wittner M, Tanowitz HB. Parasitic diseases of the heart. Front Biosci. 2004;9:706-723.

[264] Fan PC, Chung WC, Guo JX, Ma YX, Xu ZJ. Experimental studies on physiological and morphological aspects of Cysticercus cellulosae in pigs. J Microbiol Immunol Infect. 2001;34(4):252-258.

[265] Franco-Paredes C, Rouphael N, Méndez J, Folch E, Rodríguez-Morales AJ, Santos JI, Hurst JW. Cardiac manifestations of parasitic infections part 3: pericardial and miscellaneous cardiopulmonary manifestations. Clin Cardiol. 2007;30(6):277-280.

[266] Franco-Paredes C, Rouphael N, Méndez J, Folch E, Rodríguez-Morales AJ, Santos JI, Hurst JW. Cardiac manifestations of parasitic infections part 1: overview and immunopathogenesis. Clin Cardiol. 2007;30(4):195-199.

[267] Hidron A, Vogenthaler N, Santos-Preciado JI, Rodriguez-Morales AJ, Franco-Paredes C, Rassi A Jr. Cardiac involvement with parasitic infections. Clin Microbiol Rev. 2010 ;23(2):324-349.

[268] Salaria M, Parmar V, Kochar S, Mehta S. Eosinophilia, Pleural Effusion and Cysticercosis - Unknown Association? Indian Pediatrics 2001; 38: 671-674.

[269] Mayo F, Baier H. Cysticercotic cyst involving the pleura. An unusual case of an abnormal chest roentgenogram. Arch Intern Med. 1979;139(1):115-116. http://www.scielo.br/scielo.php?pid=S0036-46651991000200007&script=sci_abstract

[270] Yaqoob N, Haq EU,Thomali K, Kamran A, Zaharani A. Cysticercosis of Soft Tissue (BREAST). Journal of Pakistan Medical Association.2009;59(2):108-110.

[271] Agnihotri S, Talwar OP, Pudasaini S, Baral R. Cysticercosis of breast - a case report. Pol J Pathol 2006; 57:53-54.

[272] Lucarelli AP, Martins MM, Marques de Oliveira V, Rinaldi JF, Roveda Jr D., Longo Galvão MA, et al. Cysticercosis of the Breast, a Rare Imaging Finding. *Am. J. Trop. Med. Hyg.,2008;*79(6):864–865.

[273] Chew NK, TAN CT, GOH KJ, Kamarulzaman A, Paul G, Ramli N, Anuar K. The first case of neurocysticercosis diagnosed ante-mortem in Malaysia. *Neurol J Southeast Asia 2001;7:135–138.*

[274] Mani NB, Kalra N, Jain M, Sidhu R. Sonographic diagnosis of a solitary intramuscular cysticercal cyst. J Clin Ultrasound 2001; 29:472-475.

[275] Inamadar AC, Yelikar BR. Cysticercosis cellulose cutis. Indian J Dermatol Venereol Leprol. 2001 Jul-Aug;67(4):198-189.

[276] Abdelwahab IF, Klein MJ, Hermann G, Abdul-Quader M. Solitary cysticercosis of the biceps brachii in a vegetarian: a rare and unusual pseudotumor. Skeletal Radiol 2003; 32:424-428.

[277] Yamasaki H, Nagase T, Kiyoshige Y, Suzuki M, Nakaya K, Itoh Y, et al. A case of intramuscular cysticercosis diagnosed definitively by mitochondrial DNA analysis of extremely calcified cysts. Parasitol Int 2006; 55:127-30.

[278] Nagaray C, Singh S, Joshi A, Trikha V: Cysticercosis of biceps brachii: a rare cause of Posterior Interosseous nerve syndrome; Joint Bone Spine. 2008;75(2):219-221.

[279] Jankharia B, Chavan G, Krishnan, Jankharia B: MRI and Ultrasound in solitary muscular and soft tissue cysticercosis; Skeletal Radiol.2005; 34: 722-726.

[280] Mani NBS , Kalra N et al Sonographic diagnosis of solitary intramuscular Cysticercal cyst. J clin ultrasound. 2001;29:472-475.

[281] Tripathy SK, Sen RK, Sudes P, Dhatt S. Solitary cysticercosis of deltoid muscle in a child: The diagnostic dilemma and case report. J of Orthopaedics 2009;6:e11.

[282] Asrani A, Morani A. Primary sonographic diagnosis of disseminated muscular cysticercosis. J Ultrasound Med 2004;23:1245-1248.

[283] Jhankaria BG, Chavhan GB, Krishnan P, Jhankaria B. MRI and ultrasound in solitary muscular and soft tissue cysticercosis. Skeletal Radiol 2005;34:722-726.

[284] Sirikulchayanonta V, Jaovisidha S. Correlation of Magnetic Resonance Imaging and Histopathology. *J Med Assoc Thai 2007;90(6):1248-1252.*

[285] Smiti S, Sripathi H, Naik L.Cysticercosis in the right thigh. MUSCULOSKELETAL 2003;13(2):157-158.

[286] Sirikulchayanonta V, Sirikulchayanonta Ch, Leopairat J.A Descriptive study of 36 cases of solitary soft tissue cysticercosis at Ramathibodi Hospital. Southeast Asian J Trop Med Public Health. 2007;38(3): 407.

[287] Yamasaki H, Nagase T, Kiyoshige Y, Suzuki M, Nakaya K, Itoh Y, et al. A case of intramuscular cysticercosis diagnosed definitively by mitochondrial DNA analysis of extremely calcified cysts. Parasitol Int. 2006;55:127-130.

[288] Inamadar AC, BR Yelikar BR. Cysticercosis cellulose cutis. Indian J Dermatol Venereol Leprol 2001;67(4):198-199.

[289] Ogilvie CM, Kasten P, Rovinsky D, Workman KL, Johnston JO. Cysticercosis of the triceps: an unusual pseudotumor. Clin Orthop 2001; 382:217–221.

[290] Akhtar MN, Sharat Agarwal S.Disseminated cysticercosis incidentally diagnosed in a patient of low backache: a case report and concise review of literature. *Asian Pac J Trop Med* Jul 2012.

[291] Foyaca-Sibat H, Ibanez-Valdes LdeF, Mashiyi MK. Disseminated cysticercosis. One day treatment in a case. Electron J Biomed 2004;3:39-43. http://www.biomed.edu/2004/n1/foyaca.html

[292] Park SY, Min HK, Jung HK, Kwan YS. Disseminated cysticercosis. *Journal of Korean Neurosurgical Society*. 2011;49(3):190-193.

[293] Sirikulchayanonta V, Jaovisidha S: An intramuscular cysticercosis, a case report with correlation of magnetic resonance imaging and histology; J Med Assoc Thai. 2007;90(6):1248-1252.

[294] Jacob JC, Mathew NT, 1968. Pseudohypertrophic myopathy in cysticercosis. *Neurology 18:* 767–771.

[295] Gill M, Dua S, Gill P, Gupta V, Gupta S, Sen R . Cytomorphological spectrum of subcutaneous and intramuscular cysticercosis: A study of 22 cases. *J Cytol 2010; 27(4):123-126.*

[296] Sawhney BB, Chopra JS, Banerji AK, Wahi PL, 1976. Pseudohypertrophic myopathy in cysticercosis. *Neurology 1976;26:*270–272.

[297] Armbrust-Figueiredo J, Speciali JG, Lison MP, 1970. Forma miopatica da cisticercose. *Arq Neuropsiquiatr 28:* 385–390.

[298] Naik D, Srinath MG, Kumar A.Soft tissue cysticercosis - Ultrasonographic spectrum of the disease. *Indian Journal of Radiology and Imaging. 2011;21(1):60-62.*

[299] GA Anderson, SM Chandi: Cysticercosis of the Flexordigitorum profundus muscle producing flexion deformity of the fingers; J of Hand Surgery (British & European Volume), 1993; Vol.18, No.3; 360-36.

[300] Sharat Agarwal, Paragjyoti Gogoi: An unusual case of Cysticercosis of the tendon sheath of Tendoachilles – A case report; Electronic Physician. 2010; 2: 45-48.

[301] Ray M, Kothur K. Entrapment ulnar neuropathy caused by cysticercosis. Journal of Pediatric Neurology. 2006;4(3):203-206.

[302] Kurrein F, Vickers AA. Cysticercosis of the spine. Ann Trop Med Parasitol. 1977 ;71(2):213-217.

[303] *Kumar P,AnsariJA, Dwivedi S, Sinha AK.* Peripheral Joint Pain, Hypertension, Multiple Skeletal and CNS Calcific Lesions. *JIACM 2002; 3(2):148-152.*

[304] Banu A, Veena N A rare case of disseminated cysticercosis: case report and literature review. Indian J Med Microbiol 2011 Apr-Jun; 29(2):180-1833.

[305] Mani NB, Kalra N, Jain M, Sidhu R. Sonographic diagnosis of a solitary intramuscular cysticercal cyst. J Clin Ultrasound 2001; 29:472-475.

[306] Bangal V , Kwatra A, Garg S. Rare case of cysticercosis of rectus abdominis muscle presenting as pelvi abdominal lump during puerperium. *Pravara Med Rev 2010; 5(2):21-24.*

[307] Khan RA, Wahab S, Chana RS A. Rare Cause of Solitary Abdominal Wall Lesion. *Iran J Pediatr. 2008;18(3):291-292.*

[308] Mittal A, Sharma NS 2008 Sep : Psoas muscle cysticercosis presenting as Acute Appendicitis; J Clin Ultrasound. 2008 Sep; 36(7): 430-431.

[309] Mohan H, Bal A, Aulakh R. Multiple cysticerci as an unusual cause of mesenteric lymph node enlargement: a case report. *Journal of Medical Case Reports* 2008,2:196.

[310] Vianna LG, Macedo V, Costa JM. Cutaneous, muscular and visceral cysticercosis - a rare disease? *Rev. Inst. Med. trop. S. Paulo* 1991;33(2):129-136.

[311] G Everett, de Gruchy PH. Hepatic cysticercosis Veterinary Record 1982;111:24 565.

[312] Fultz PJ, Penwarden B, Laczin J.Hepatic cysticercosis. Report of an unusual case. J Clin Gastroenterol. 1995;20(2):160-163.

[313] Figurnov VA, Churin AN, Lenshin AV, Grigorenko AA, Churina SA, Figurnova EV, Soldatkin PK. .A case of isolated hepatic cysticercosis in a nine-year-old girl. Med Parazitol (Mosk). 2002 ;(1):56-57.

[314] Vishwanath S, Charudutt S, Kavitha S, Abdul R, Ashwin P, Rao SN. (2011) *A rare case of hepatic cysticercosis.* Asian Pacific Journal of Tropical Biomedicine 2011;1(1)139-140.

[315] Bal MS, Suri A, Kumar R, Vijay M. Disseminated cysticercosis in a post mortem case. J Punjab Acad Forensic Med Toxicol 2012;12(1):40.

[316] Jain BK, Sankhe SS, Agrawal MD, Naphade PS.Disseminated cysticercosis with pulmonary and cardiac involvement. Indian J Radiol Imaging. 2010; 20(4):310–313.

[317] Jakhere SG, Chemburkar VC, Yeragi BS, Bharambay HVImaging findings of disseminated cysticercosis with unusual involvement of spleen and pancreas. J Glob Infect Dis 2011;3(3):306-308.

[318] Bal MS, Suri A, Kumar R, Vijay M. Disseminated cysticercosis in a post mortem case. J Punjab Acad Forensic Med Toxicol 2012;12(1):40.

[319] Norman RJ. Tetraphyllidean cysticerci in the peritoneal cavity of the common dolphin. J Wildl Dis. 1997;33(4):891-895.

[320] Chung WC, Lin CY, Fan PC. Ectopic locations of Taenia saginata asiatica cysticerci in the abdominal cavity of domestic pig and monkey. J Parasitol. 1996;82(6):1032-1034.

[321] Dyer NW, Greve JH. Severe Cysticercus Longicollis Cysticercosis in a Black Lemur (Eulemur Macaco Macaco. J VET Diagn Invest 1998;10:362.

[322] Fraga CM, Costa TL, Bezerra JC, de Souza Lino Junior R, Vinaud MC.Fatty acids oxidation and alternative energy sources detected in Taenia crassiceps cysticerci after host treatment with antihelminthic drugs. Exp Parasitol. 2012;131(1):111-115.

[323] Stringer JL, Marks LM, White AC Jr, Robinson P. Epileptogenic activity of granulomas associated with murine cysticercosis. Exp Neurol. 2003;183(2):532-536.

[324] Vincent JM, Morrison ID, Armstrong P, Reznek RH.The size of normal adrenal glands on computed tomography. Clin Radiol. 1994;49(7):453-455.

[325] Rajatanavin R, Dheandhanoo D, Siridej N, Somburanasin R. Cerebral cysticercosis simulating pheochromocytoma: a case report. J Med Assoc Thai. 1981;64(7):351-355.

[326] Liu Y, Wang L. Telemedicine in border area of China. Telemed J. 1998;4(1):39-41.

[327] Kelesidis T, Tsiodras S. Hypopituitarism caused by neurocysticercosis. Am J Med Sci. 2011;341(5):414-416.

Section 2

Neurocysticercosis

Chapter 9

Epidemiology of Neurocysticercosis in Mexico: From a Public Health Problem to Its Control

Ana Flisser

Additional information is available at the end of the chapter

http://dx.doi.org/10.5772/53839

1. Introduction

Cysticercosis is a parasitic disease of humans caused by the establishment of the larval stage of the cestode *Taenia solium* in several organs (Figure 1).

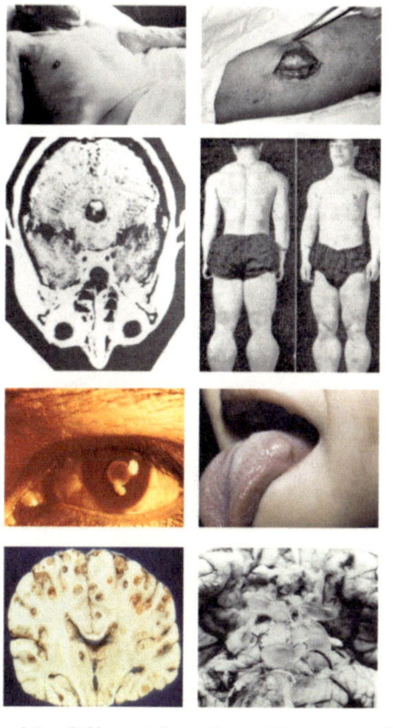

Figure 1. Images of cysticerci lodged in different locations. From top (left) to the bottom (right): diseminated sbcutaneous cysticercosis, confirmed by biopsy, lingual cysticercosis, intramuscular (pseudohypertrophy), intraocular (anterior chamber), intraventricular (IV ventricle), multiple locations of cellulosae type and subarachnoid (racemose) neurocysticercosis.

INTECH
open science | open minds

© 2013 Flisser, licensee InTech. This is a paper distributed under the terms of the Creative Commons Attribution License (http://creativecommons.org/licenses/by/3.0), which permits unrestricted use, distribution, and reproduction in any medium, provided the original work is properly cited.

The main clinical presentation is neurocysticercosis (NCC); it is due to the establishment of cysticerci in the Central Nervous System, where, depending on the specific location, can cause different symptoms, the main being epilepsy and hydrocephalus. Cysticercosis is a disease associated to poverty, lack of health education, inadequate hygienic habits and insufficient sanitary infrastructure; therefore it is common in underdeveloped countries. The life cycle of the parasite includes the human being, which is the only definitive host and, thus, lodges the adult tapeworm, which measures 1-4 meters long and is formed by a scolex, a neck and a long chain of proglottids that, as they are farther away from the neck, they develop into sexual maturity and, afterwards, gravidity.

Each gravid proglottid contains around 60,000 microscopic eggs; these segments are periodically released with feces. When outdoor defecation or improper latrines are found, pigs ingest feces; if contaminated with tapeworm eggs or proglottids, the embryos transform into the larval stage or cysticercus in the musculature and the central nervous system.

If humans eat insufficiently cooked or raw pork that is contaminated with cysticerci, the scolex evaginates, and with its doble row of hooks and four suckers in the rostellum, anchors to the intestinal mucosa and, after a few months, a new gravid tapeworm initiates the life cycle (Figure 2) [1].

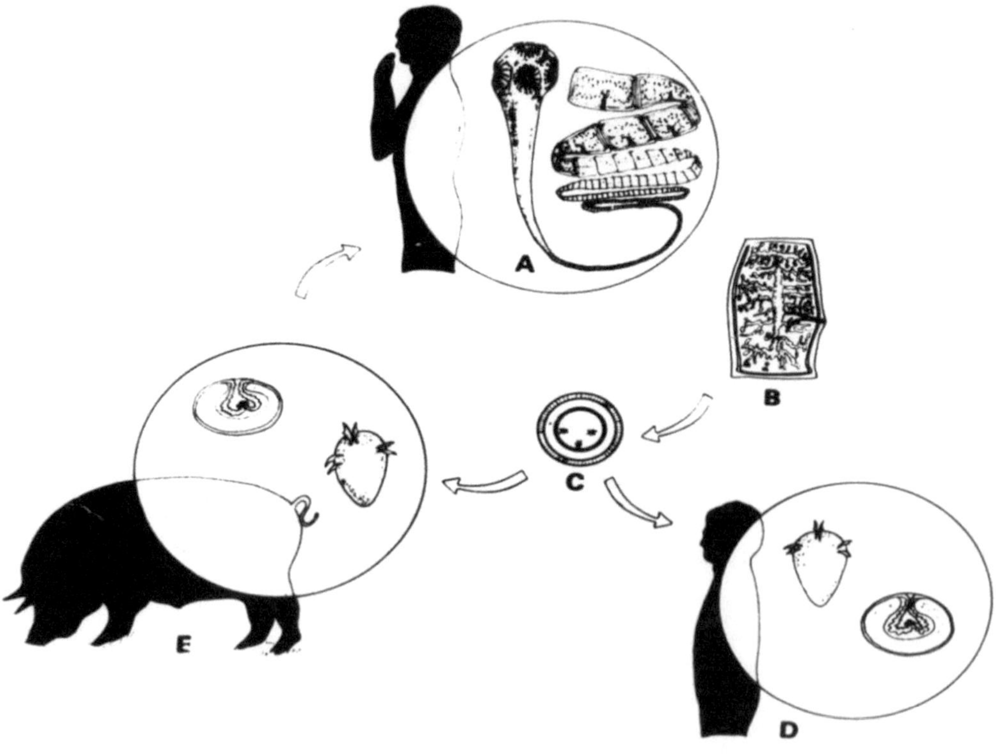

Figure 2. Life cycle of *T solium*. A- Adult in the small intestine. B- gravid proglotid. C- infective egg containing an oncosphere. D- Human cysticercosis. E- Porcine cysticercosis an hexacanth oncosphere and an invaginated cysticercus are drawn.

Cysticercosis has been known since ancient times; it was detected in an Egyptian mummy by paleoparasitologists [2]. In a popular Greek theater play "The Knights" by Aristophanes, the slave Demosthenes says "We will set his mouth open with a wooden stick as the cooks do with pigs; we will tear out his tongue, and, looking down his gaping throat, will see whether his inside has any pimples" [3]. Egyptian and Greek cultures also distinguished tapeworms, but the relation between both developmental stages was not known. Probably Egiptians had *Taenia saginata* because they did not eat pork meat; Hipocrates, Aristoteles y Teofrastus called the worms "flatworms" while the Romans, Celsus, Galenus and Pliny the elder, called them "lumbricus latus" that meant "wideworm". At the beggining of the Christian era, some Arab authors such as Serapio, considered that each proglottid was a different worm and were named "cucurbitinum" not only because of their resemblance to pumpkin seeds, but also because these seeds were used to release tapeworms, and, interestingly, are still in use nowadays [4].

The species T. solium was described by Villanovani in 1585 and reflects the common finding of a solitary tapeworm, *T. solium* was differentiated from *T. saginata* and *Diphyllobothrium latum* by Tyson in 1683 who discovered and described the different types of heads or scolices of tapeworms; Redi published the following year illustrations of the scolex of dog and cat tapeworms. Van Beneden 170 years later stated that a tapeworm was an animal formed by multiple individuals and that cysticerci in pigs develop after ingesting *T. solium* segments. At that time Kuchenmeister, in spte of severe ethical criticisms, identified that humans are the hosts of the adult stage of *T. solium*. In two occasions (1854 and 1859) he fed death convicts with 63 and 40 cysticerci each, and found developing tapeworms in the small intestine after necropsy. Interestingly the number of tapeworms found was 10 and 20 respectively and, since the second prisoner ingested the bladder worms much before death than the first convict (four months vs 4 days) 11 worms had mature proglottids and the largest reached five feet (1.5 meters) in length. This finding further demonstrates that *T. solium* is not necessarily a solitary parasite. He stated that the sheer number of tapeworms produced ought to convince even the most skeptical that they were derived from the cysticerci that the convicts ingested. Nevertheless he recommended that the experiment of bladder worm feeding should be allowed to be repetead on criminals under death sentences and, in the case of subsequent pardon, the tapeworms could be easily expelled, calming anxious souls and serving science at the same time [4]. Figure 3 shows pictures of some of the scientists that made outstanding contributions to the understanding of the life cycle of T. solium: Malpighi, Tyson, van Beneden and Kuchenmeister. Not until last century the precise knowledge of the complete anatomy of a tapeworm, as well as its organization and individuality were defined, considering it a single animal.

Rumler was the first clinician that described a case of human cysticercosis in 1558 but considered it to be a tumor in the dura matter of a person with epilepsy. Panarolus, one hundred years later, reported similar cysts in the corpus callosum of the brain of an epileptic priest and Wharton found many cysticerci, that he considered to be glands in the adipose and muscle tissues of a soldier. The disease was not clearly identified as parasitic until

Malpighi in 1698 discovered the animal nature of these cysts and described their scolex. Goeze, not knowing this study, examined swine cysticerci and described their helminthic nature. The taxonomic clasification of "Cysticercus cellulosae" was given by Zeder and Rudoplphi [4]. The use of a scientific name for this parasite was abolished when it was demonstrated that cysticerci are larval stages of *T. solium*. Therefore, when mentioning cysticerci it should only be stated "celluosae type of *T. solium* cysticerci" or simply "*T. solium* cysticerci". Yoshino published detailed histological descriptions of the development of cysticerci, including the formation of the scolex and the size and appearance of its hooks, after he fed proglottids to pigs, released by him because he ingested cysticerci [5-8] and Rabiela demonstrated that there are intermediate forms between a cellulose and a recemose type cysticercus and that cysticerci evaginate through a pore. (Figure 4) [9, 10].

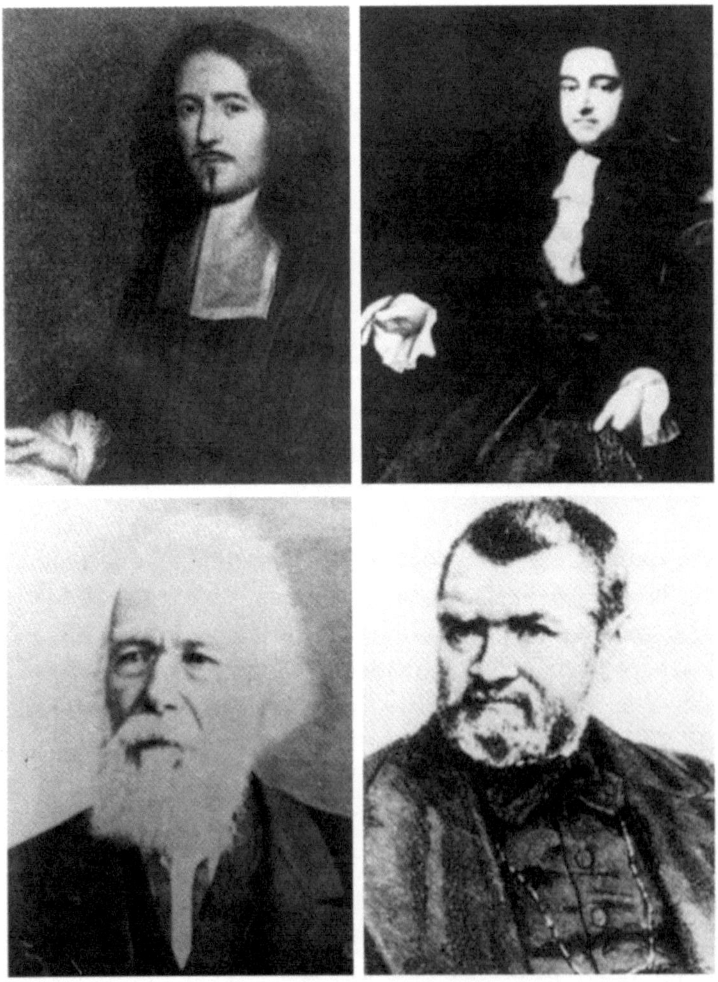

Figure 3. Photograps of M. Malpighi, E. Tyson, PJ van Beneden and F Kuchenmeister

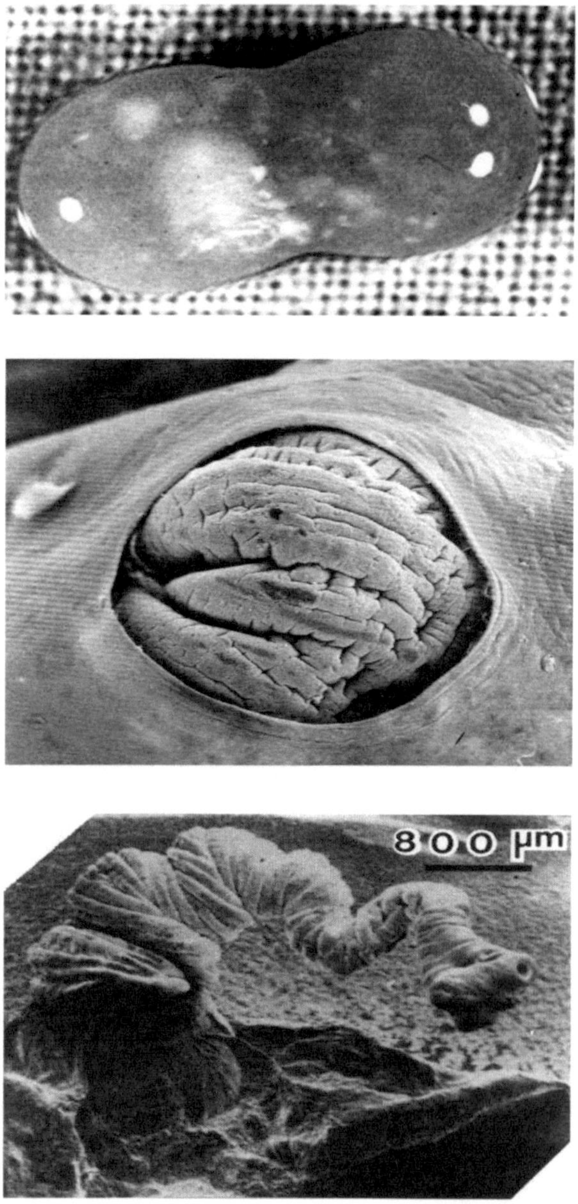

Figure 4. Micrographs of the evagination pore of a cysticercus and an evaginated cysticercus as well as a photograph of a bilobulated cysticercus; its appearance suggests the beginning of transformation from a cellulosae to a racemos type cysticercus. Kindly donated by Dr. Maria Teresa Rabiela (RIP)

The first report regarding NCC in Mexico, probably lost in the old Mexican literature, was published in 1901; the author, Dr. Ignacio Gómez-Izquierdo, described a patient from Cuba who died in a psichiatric asylum with diagnosis of alcoholism or tuberculosis. During necropsy multiple cysticerci were found. The author stated his doubts regarding the diease: "Diagnosis is almost impossible, because, with the exception of those cases in which cysticerci are found in superficial tissues or in the eye, symptomatology by itself does not provide enough information in order to establish its diagnosis, and, if diagnosis could have been done with precision, would prognosis stop to be fatal? Are there medical or surgical treatments to successfully fight this disease? Our answer, sadly to say, is negative" [11]. The questions posed by Dr. Gómez-Izquierdo 110 years ago have illuminated the path of knowledge and reflect major advances in the last 30 years because NCC is diagnosed and treated with high efficiency and its fatality rate has dramatically diminished [12,13].

2. Epidemiology

Human cysticercosis was considered in the past to be less frequent than taeniosis due to the possibility of finding a tapeworm in feces, while muscle cysticerci mostly do not cause clinical signs and neurocysticercosis generally could not be identified due to its pleomorphic symtomatology [14,15]. Interest in NCC arouse after Dixon and Lipscomb identified soldiers that acquired NCC when they were were stated in India [16]. This study is the only one that allowed identifying the duration of the disease and of the appearance of clinical manifestations, since it became clear when soldiers acquired NCC while stationed in India. Figure 5 shows a histogram of the time when soldiers presented the first convulsive crisis and/or subcutaneous nodules; as it can be seen in around 50% symptoms appeared two to four years after being in India, and cases were also identified as far as 30 years afterwards. MacArthur suggested that symptomatology was due to the death of parasites and suggested that the biological objetive of cysticerci, while in the tissues of the intermediate host, is to remain silent in order to be able to continue their life cycle. He also suggested that parasite death could be associated to toxin release that increases irritation [17].

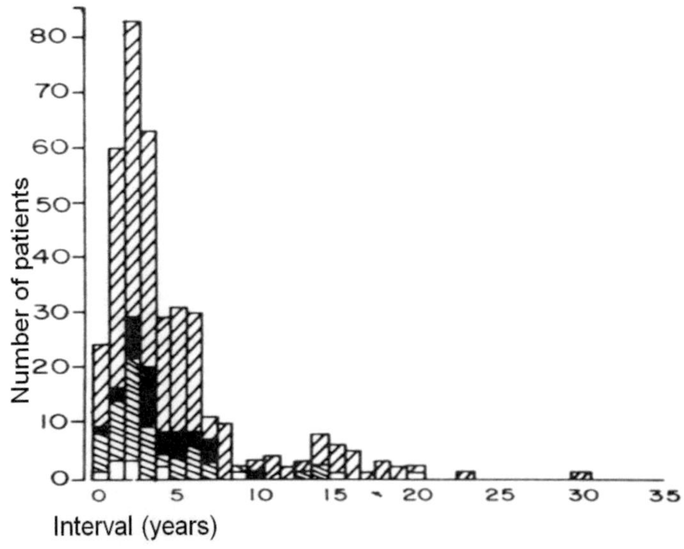

Figure 5. Histogram showing the interval in years in which signs and symptoms related to cysticercosis appearaed in 450 soldiers after they returned from being stationed in India. Convulsive crisis (///), subcutaneous nodules (\\\\\\), both (black) or other data (white), reproduced from [16].

Because human cysticercosis is a disease related to underdevelopment, it is present in countries that lack proper sanitary infrastructure and hygiene as well as insufficient health education [15,18,19]. An outstanding example is the emergence of neurocysticercosis in West New Guinea among the Ekari population, to whom the disease was unknown prior to the entrance of cysticercotic pigs as official gifts. Some 18-20% of the population acquired cysticercosis. The disease was detected by an epidemic of severe burns resulting from convulsions manifested while the people were sleeping around house fires; individuals also had subcutaneous nodules [20]. Between the 1940's and 1970's several reports of human necropsies performed in Latin America revealed the presence of cysticerci in the brain with different frequencies, so high that NCC is considered a public health problem in some countries [15,21,22]. As it can be seen in table 1, necropsies performed in Mexico reported an average of 2% of NCC. In addition, hospital-based reports provided data on the magnitude of cysticercosis in patients; the National Institute of Neurology and Neurosurgery reported a prevalence of 6% among its neurological patients [23]. This prompted the development and standardization of immunodiagnostic assays, and the detection of specific serum antibodies facilitated the shift to epidemiological information instead of that coming from autopsies, because these do not strictly represent the Mexican population since they were performed in people dying in public government hospitals, while seroepidemiological surveys are performed in open populations including both rural and urban settings [24].

Country	Years reported	%
Peru	1961-1974	5.9
Mexico	1947-1957	2.8
Brazil	1960-1979	2.4
Brazil	1965-1970	2.2
Mexico	1963-1974	2.2
Brazil	1992-1997	1.5
Mexico	1963-1973	1.5
Mexico	1953-1970	1.3
Peru	1961-1974	0.99
Colombia	1944-1964	0.78
Chile	1939-1966	0.70
Venezuela	1967	0.49
Ecuador	1947-1968	0.47
Costa Rica	1967	0.45
Colombia	1955-1970	0.40
El Salvador	1961	0.40
Chile	1947-1979	0.09
Honduras	1951-1966	0.02

Table 1. Frequency of neurocysticercosis in necropsies

For the first seroepidemiologic studies reported in Mexico, immunoelectrophoresis was used, initially in communities in the state of Chiapas: 1610 samples obtained from 9 communities, mostly rural, were analyzed. Interestingly, in spite of the low sensitivity of immunoelectrophoresis (50%), its high specificity (100% because practically no echinococcosis is found in Mexico) allowed to identify a clear correlation: communities with less than 4000 inhabitants had 1-8% seropositivity, while populations with more inhabitants (35,000 was the biggest) had 1% or less antibody frequency; indicating that the parasite was more prevalent in small, an thus less developed, towns [25]. Afterwards, using 20,000 samples from a national survey, a central area in Mexico, in which people had between 0.6 and 1% of anti-cysticercus antibodies, was identified; remarkably this geographic area, called "El Bajio", is the most important pig breeding area for national consumption of pork meat [26]. A few years later, in El Sotano, a small community in the state of Hidalgo, 6% of the 124 inhabitants had antibodies detected by ELISA, 25% of their pigs had cysticerci that were palpated in their tongues and 3% of the people had *Taenia* eggs. *Ascaris, Trichuris* and *Toxocara* eggs were found in soil samples but no *Taenia* eggs were identified in soil. The clustered distribution of infected pigs, tapeworm carriers and people with serologic or clinical evidence of cysticercosis suggested intra-household transmission. Furthermore, although the correlation of seropositivity and clinical history suggestive of NCC in individual residents was poor, there was an apparent spatial association between tapeworm carriers and persons with serologic or clinical histories associated to NCC [27]. This information was very interesting because it identified, for the first time ever, the main risk factor for NCC: the presence of a person infected with an adult tapeworm at home (which I consider my most important contribution to the control of NCC), instead of egg transmission through strawberries, lettuce, coriander and any other vegetable grown at floor level, eaten unpeeled, uncooked and probably unwashed, that could have been irrigated with sewage.

In a study undertaken in order to determine markers of *T. solium* transmission and risk factors in an urban community, 1000 soldiers from a military camp in Mexico City and their families were studied. Serum samples were used to detect cysticercus antigens and antibodies and fecal specimens were examined for *Taenia* coproantigens (CpAgs) and eggs. Antibodies were detected in 12.2% of soldiers and 5.8% and 10% of relatives of positive and negative soldiers, respectively. Antigens in serum were detected in 2.8% of the soldiers and in 4.2% of the relatives of antibody-positive soldiers. CpAgs were found in 0.5% and *Taenia* eggs in 0.1% of soldiers but were not found in their families. Interestingly, 12% of the family members of positive soldiers had had a history of proglottid release, compared to only 3.7% of the family members of negative soldiers. Lastly, 86% of the family members of positive soldiers had eaten in street food stores, compared to only 62.5% of those of negative soldiers. Both risk factors identified were statistically significant, indicating again, that the main risk factor was an association with the presence of a tapeworm carrier at home confirming its importance for the transmission of *T. solium* [28]. Therefore, a clinical history of taeniosis in a family member, defined as elimination of proglottids in feces, should be taken into account by health personnel in order to be treated in spite of being asymptomatic, and to prevent other members of the family from becoming infected. Likewise, public health authorities should control street food vendors to reduce new cases of *T. solium* infections by means of hygienic and sanitary measures. The results obtained support that the prevalence of human cysticercosis in Mexico was, as indicated by previous necropsy findings, around 2%, while the prevalence of antibodies was much higher, suggesting exposure to the parasite but not current infection. In another national survey, using indirect hemaglutination, a similar antibody prevalence was found (15% of the 11,611 homes analyzed), and 2.2% had two or more seropositive members, pointing to the presence of an intestinal tapeworm carrier [29].

Many epidemiological surveys were performed with ELISA in the 1980′s, supported by direct detection of cysticerci in pigs' tongue and tapeworm eggs in human feces [27, 28, 30-34] and, in the 1990's, by western blot (WB) [27, 30, 35-41] using an enriched fraction of glycoproteins as antigen source [42] allowing the demonstration of the presence of all the components of the life cycle (Tables 2 and 3), [24]). Table 3 also shows that swine cysticercosis is higher in Peru, suggesting that Peruvian pigs have easier access to human feces. Furthermore, one survey was performed in two rural communities of Mexico in order to compare the performance of both assays; 2524 individuals were studied, 7.5% were positive by WB, 2.1% by ELISA and only 3.1% in both assays [43]. Reports of predictive values indicate that for screening purposes, WB would be the test of choice, and for diagnosis, performing WB and CT tests would yield the best results, although with clinical data suggestive of NCC even ELISA is useful to support diagnosis [24].

Community studied, state	Year	Number of samples	% pigs with tongue cysticerci	% people with eggs in feces	% people positive in ELISA
El Sótano, Hidalgo	1984	124	24	3.1	6
San Pedro Martir, DF	1985	928	0	0	0
El Salado, Sinaloa	1986	432	Present	1.2	12
Los Sauces, Guerrero	1987	440	6.6	3.0	2.3
La Curva, Sinaloa	1989	549	1.4	1.3	11

Table 2. Epidemiologic studies performed with ELISA for detection of people with anti-cysticercus antibodies

When data from table 1 are compared to those of tables 2 and 3, it is evident that the prevalence of anti-cysticercus antibodies in humans (2.3-24%) is much higher than the finding of the parasite in pathology studies (0.02-5.9%), indicating that antibodies reflect exposure and not necessary the presence of the parasite; its serologic confirmation can be obtained by detecting cysticercal antigens. One survey used monoclonal antibodies in a capture ELISA [44,45] in 900 inhabitants of the community of Cerritos, San Luis Potosí, 1% positive samples for antigens and 4.2% for antibodies were found, only one sample was positive in both tests. Interestingly, although antigen detection was lower, two of the three positive cases that accepted undergoing computed tomography (CT) had images compatible with cysticerci, while only two of the seven antibody positive individuals had CT images resembling cysticerci [46]. These data point to a higher correlation with the disease in open populations when parasite antigens are being searched than when antibodies are detected.

Another field study showed and association between the presence of antigens and that of late onset epilepsy, while antibodies were associated to the presence of subcutaneous nodules; furthermore specificity and positive predictive values for the antigen capture ELISA was high with samples of epileptic people [47]. It has also been demostrated that this capture ELISA is useful to evaluate symtomaticos patients, who can benefit with immediate treatment [48]. Similar studies have been implemenented in the last decade in Asia and Africa.

Community studied, state	Year	Number of samples	% pigs with tongue cysticerci	% people with eggs in feces	% people positive in WB
Xoxocotla, México	1988	13227	4	0.3	11
Angahuan, México	1988	3065	6.5	0.5	5
Churusapa, Perú	1988	279	49	1	7
Maceda, Perú	1988	421	43	1	8
Haparquilla, Perú	1990	365	46	ND	13
Jocote, Guatemala	1991	1161	14	3	17
Quesada, Guatemala	1991	1204	4	1	10
Saylla, Perú	1990-3	501	36	3	24
San Pablo, Ecuador	1992	2723	ND	ND	10
Tegucigalpa, Honduras	1998	404	ND	0.6	16
Salama, Honduras	1999	480	ND	2.5	17
Cd. de México, México	1999	1000	ND	0.5	12

Table 3. Epidemiologic studies performed with western blot for detection of people with anti-cysticercus antibodies

3. Risk factors and intervention trials

It has been considered for a long time in Mexico that fruits, such as strawberries, and vegetables, such as lettuce, that are eaten unpeeled and uncooked and that grow at ground level, are the main sources of *Taenia* eggs that cause human NCC. But in a study carried out in the counties of Irapuato in the state of Guanajuato and Zamora, Michoacan, which are important locations for the production of strawberries, no *Taenia* eggs were identified in large amounts of homogenized strawberries collected throughout one year but low numbers of protozoan cysts and one *Ascaris* egg were found [49]. This indicated that, although there was contamination with human feces, strawberries did not carry tapeworm eggs. Also, the absence of *Taenia* eggs in domestic flies was demonstrated in the community of Tianquizolco, where over one thousand flies were caught in homes and assessed for their role in the transmission of *Taenia solium* [50]. On the other hand, multiple studies have demonstrated that the prevalence of tapeworm carriers is higher among household members of NCC patients than in the rest of the population [27,51, 52]. For transmission of NCC the importance of a tapeworm carrier in the household and not of egg ingestion in strawberries or of contaminated flies changes the concept of control, since it is much easier and cheaper to treat tapeworm carriers than to modify sewage and irrigation in developing countries with huge territories.

A clear asociation exists between the presence of taeniosis and the severity of NCC, therefore the perception that *T. solium* tapeworms are silent guests causing no harm to humans is erroneous, and tapeworm carriers should be regarded as potential sources of contagion to both themselves and to those living in their close environment [53]. Just how important is the presence of a tapeworm carrier was demonstrated by the case of 4 orthodox Jewish families from New York, in which 4 neurological cases and 7 seropositive people were along two years after. Although these families did not ingest pork meat, the maid who cooked for these families was from Mexico and she had an intestinal *T solium* [54].

The information presented above clearly demonstrates a clustered distribution of persons with serological or clinical evidence of cysticercosis, infected pigs and tapeworm carriers, thus allowing to evaluate intervention measures: health education, self-detection of tapeworm carriers, mass treatment against human taeniosis and pigs vaccination. Regarding health education as a community-based intervention measure, a comprehensive study was undertaken in Chalcatzingo, Morelos with approximately 2000 inhabitants. An educational program was developed to identify the local knowledge of both diseases (taeniosis and cysticercosis) and of both parasites (the tapeworm and the cysticercus), in order to promote recognition of the parasites and knowledge of the transmission, and to improve hygienic behavior and sanitary conditions that foster transmission. This was performed by in-depth questionnaires developed by anthropologists. Based on the information obtained, an educational intervention was developed which included explanation of the life cycle, diseases, risk factors and control measures. For this purpose the anthropologists trained local leaders, selected among students, housewives, and teachers as well as the priest, to be in charge of promoting and providing health education, so that education remained in the community after the project ended. The effects of this educational intervention were evaluated by measuring changes in knowledge, attitudes and practices (Table 4) and prevalences of human taeniosis and swine cysticercosis before and after the campaign [56]. The prevalence in pigs at the start of the education intervention was 2.6% and 5.2% by tongue examination and western blot for antibody detection, respectively. Approximately one year after the intervention they were 0% and 1.2%, respectively, and remained so for almost 4 years. (Figure 6) [57].

Apparently an economic factor facilitated the success, since people learned that by having pigs restrained in certain areas without access to human feces or garbage they would not acquire the disease and thus could be sold at a higher price. In Coapeche, Veracruz, where swine cysticercosis was ascertained by western blot, none of the 53 pigs studied had antibodies or cysticerci. Latrines were present in 91% of houses and pigs were kept in restrained areas, demonstrating that adequate basic sanitary conditions and pig breeding practices are effective and practical to control *T. solium* in rural communities [58]. High standards of meat inspection and proper disposal of infected pig carcasses will also aid in preventing infected pigs from entering the food chain.

Effect detected by the anthropologic questionnaire	Before intervention	After intervention	At 6 months	At 42 months
Chalcatzingo (Health education)	%	%	%	%
Free roming pigs	29	9	6	4
Pigs that ingest feces	31	16	14	0
Outdoors fecalism	49	47	44	21
Atotonilco (Cestocidal treatment)	%	%	%	%
Free roming pigs	18	16	40	3
Pigs that ingest feces	20	22	15	3
Outdoors fecalism	50	45	45	39
Tetelilla (Both interventions)	%	%	%	%
Free roming pigs	48	32	17	14
Pigs that ingest feces	40	38	30	17
Outdoors fecalism	78	70	60	52

Table 4. Main effects of the intervention as per the anthropologic questionnaire

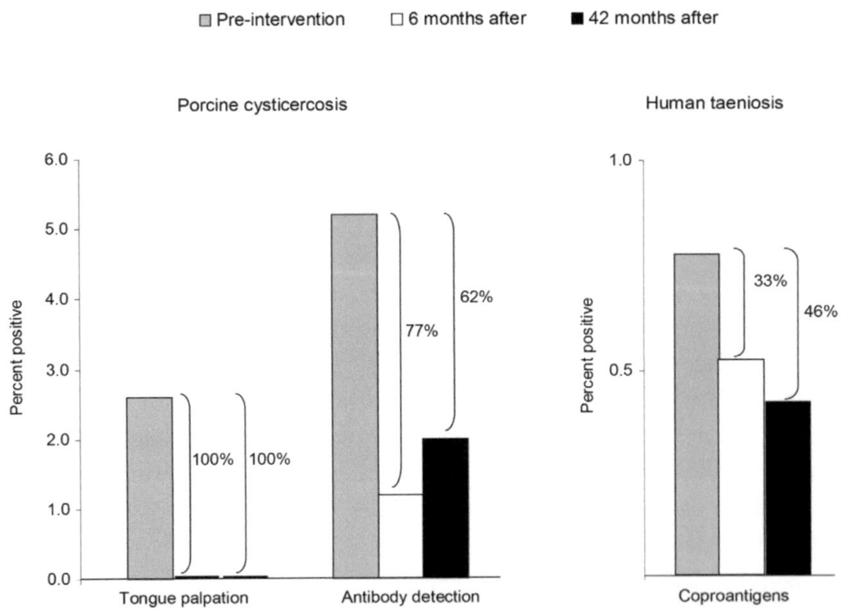

Figure 6. Effect of health education provided to the community of Chalcatzingo, Morelos, Mexico. Evaluation of porcine cysticercosis was measured by tongue palpation and serum antibodies detected by Western blot, while that of human taeniosis was measured by coproantigen detection. Assessment was performed before intervention (n = 1,404 for humans and 194 for pigs), 6 months later (n = 792 for humans and 165 for pigs), and 42 months later in 1996 (n = 605 for humans and 334 for pigs). Reproduced from [57].

Self-identification of tapeworm carriers as a community based intervention, alternative to health education, was evaluated in the municipality of Irapuato, Guanajuato. Clinical and animal health care practitioners and schoolteachers were trained in the life cycle, risk factors and control measures related to infection with *Taenia solium.* Over 120 small glass bottles, each containing a few tapeworm segments fixed in formaldehyde and an instructional guide were distributed among all clinical practitioners (physicians and nurses) working in health centers. The guide contained 10 key points on how to ask questions about tapeworm infections. The small bottles were shown during questionnaire administration to all people that attended the clinic for any medical reason in order to determine if they had seen such parasites in their feces or their family. Information on taeniosis and cysticercosis was also provided to the general population via different media. Seven tapeworm carriers were recorded in the official epidemiology surveillance system the year previous to the study, interestingly, the year after the study, 41 tapeworm carriers (37 *T. saginata*; 4 *T. solium*) were recorded. Thus six times more tapeworm carriers were notified after the study. All four persons with *T. solium* were treated, thereby eliminating the parasite and subsequently preventing new cases of human and swine cysticercosis that might have arisen [59]. This study demonstrates that self-detection is a feasible tool for control of *T. solium.*

The use of mass treatment with praziquantel to eliminate tapeworms from human carriers as a community-based intervention measure was evaluated in two studies. In a small community (559 inhabitants) in La Curva, Sinaloa, over 70% of the population over 5 years of age was treated with a 10 mg/kg dose. One year later, no infections with *Taenia* sp. eggs were found and no pigs with cysticercosis were detected. Seropositivity using ELISA was 11% before treatment and 7% afterwards, in the 30-39 year age group, antibody detection decreased from 30% to 7% suggesting that elimination of tapeworms reduces the possibility of contact with infective eggs. Interestingly, in the geographic section of the community where 3 of the 4 tapeworm carriers were found and treated, seropositivity was reduced from 19% to 2%, indicating that serum antibodies to *Taenia* antigens are short-lived and diminish, as contact with the parasite is lost [34]. In the second study performed in Atotonilco (3007 inhabitants), 87% of the community received a single dose of 5 mg/kg following a recommendation from WHO [60]. The prevalence of taeniosis was reduced by 53% after 6 months and by 56% after 42 months, as measured by CpAg ELISA or egg detection; late onset general seizures decreased by 70%. Anti-cysticercus antibodies in the human population were reduced by 75% after 42 months and antibodies in pigs also showed a significant reduction (55%) after 6 months [61]. In conclusion, the impact of mass chemotherapy against taeniosis to control cysticercosis in the short and long term was successfully demonstrated. Experience with praziquantel however suggested that it should not be given at doses lower than 10mg/kg. This population-based cestocidal treatment eliminated tapeworm carriers but generated symptomatology in a previously asymptomatic neurological case [62]. This observation highlights the importance of weighing targeted treatment, instead of mass drug administration, which can be used since potential tapeworm carriers are identified by direct questioning or by detection of parasite antigens or eggs, as well as by association with late onset epilepsy.

Another alternative for the control of cysticercosis is vaccination, especially because pigs are the only intermediate hosts that participate in the maintenance of the parasite in the environment. Based on the high protection obtained with recombinant antigens identified in *T. ovis* and *T. saginata* [63, 64], recombinant vaccines against *T. solium* were elaborated. For this cDNA from a genomic library from a *T. solium* tapeworm was prepared and with probes from *T. ovis* 18k and 45k antigens, the homologue recombinant DNAs were identified and cloned in *E. coli*. The oncosphere recombinant antigens were purified and used to vaccinate pigs in two independent trials performed in different institutions under controlled conditions. The first one was in 2000 and the second one in 2002. Each pig received 200ug of recombinant antigen TSOL18 or TSOL45 or the carrier, Glutathione S Transferase (GST) as a control group, with 1mg Quil A as adjuvant, intramuscularly each 15 days, in two occasions in the first experiment and thrice in the second one. For challenge, gravid proglottids were separated from a tapeworm recovered from a carrier. Proglottids were minced; eggs were obtained by sieving, washed, counted and used to challenge pigs 3 weeks after the 2nd or 3rd immunization, respectively. Each pig received orally 40,000 eggs in the first experiment, and 9,000 in the second one. Necropsies were performed 3-4 months after challenge infection, carcass musculature was sliced with hand-held knives or scalpels, and the number and viability of cysticerci were determined. Table 5 shows the results of both vaccination trials. Protection was calculated as the percent reduction in the mean number of cysticerci in each group in comparison with the mean number of cysticerci in the control group; as it can be seen, in both experiments TSOL18 give practically full protection. TSOL45 gave a high value of protection in the second experiment but no protection was detected in the first one [65].

Number of cysticerci in experiment 1 (infected with 40,000 eggs per pig)		X	Protection (%)
GST	167, 206, 234, 262, 415	257	
TSOL18	0, 0, 0, 0, 0	0	100
Number of cysticerci in experiment 2 (infected with 9,000 eggs per pig)		X	Protection (%)
GST or PBS	6, 10, 11, 13, 17, 26, 28, 40, 59, 64, 100,127	42	
TSOL18	0, 0, 0, 0, 1	0.2	99.5

Table 5. Number of cysticerci found in individual pigs

The humoral immune response of all pigs was evaluated against the cysticercal enriched glycoprotein antigen used for the diagnosis of human cysticercosis [42] specific diagnostic bands were obtained in all control pigs but not in immunized pigs that did not developed cysticerci. The immune response was also evaluated against the vaccinating antigen by ELISA; specific, complement-fixing antibodies against the recombinant antigens increased after challenge and thereafter decreased; Furthermore, these and oncosphere antigens from other taeniid cestodes, contain a protein sequence motif suggesting a tertiary structure similar to the fibronectin type III domain [66]. Vaccination results show that pigs became protected from acquiring cysticercosis in experimental conditions, therefore they were evaluated in field trials in Peru [67] and Cameroon [68]; similar high levels of protection were obtained.

4. Conclusion

Many epidemiological studies have shown a correlation between human cysticercosis, taeniosis and epilepsy and between seropositive people, infected pigs and disposal of feces and have identified community, behavioural and environmental practices that must be modified to prevent continued transmission of cysticercosis and taeniosis.

Table 6 summarizes those that the author considers the most relevant. Most importantly, these studies have shown that the main risk factor is the presence of a *Taenia* carrier in the immediate environment. A proposal to declare neurocysticercosis an international reportable disease has been published [69].

This proposal, if taken in account, could be helpful in the control of cysticercosis, since, if cases of cysticercosis and of taeniosis are reported in all countries, it will provide accurate quantification of the incidence and prevalence of neurocysticercosis at regional level, thus permitting the rational use of resources in eradication campaigns. Although NCC is endemic in several countries of Latin America, Sub-Saharan Africa and Asia [69], due to migration there are many patients with NCC that attend hospitals in several cities of the USA and, even more important is the fact that tapeworm carriers have been identified in USA and even in Muslim countries, therefore now cysticercosis is considered an emerging infectious disease in USA and in some of its states it is now a reportable disease. [19,70,71]. It should be noted that approximately 200 million people cross the Mexico-USA border each year, multiplying the opportunities of acquiring and transporting adult *T. solium* [72].

Personal measures
• After defecating check feces in search of a tapeworm
• If you have a tapeworm ask for treatment
• Wash hands after defecating
• Wash hands before eating and cooking
• Do not eat contaminated pork meat
Hygienic measures
• Avoid having outdoor fecalism
• If outdoor fecalism is necessary, cover, bury or burn the feces
• Cook sufficiently pork meat to kill possible parasites
• Freeze pork meat at least 5 days before cooking
• Wash properly fruit and vegetables
Pig breeding measures
• Avoid free roaming pigs
• Keep pigs in corrals
• Feed pigs with tortillas, bread and food leftovers
• Avoid access of pigs to letrines, feces and garbage
• Do not use pigpens as toilets
• Do not sell or buy pork meat with cysticerci

Table 6. Preventive measures against cysticercosis

The efforts and advancements described above, and others, drove Mexico onto a new stage regarding NCC: it is not anymore a public health problem. This parasitic disease was recognized as a public health problem when necropsy cases, published between 1947 and 1970, reported high frequencies of NCC. A recent publication [57] indicates that this disease has been controlled; the idea is supported by the dramatic decrease in the frequency of human NCC and human taeniosis obtained from the National Information System for Epidemiological Surveillance of the Ministry of Health in Mexico. The decrease was probably due to three reasons: 1) the abundant literature published by the Mexican scientific and medical communities working on cysticercosis; 2) the establishment of a National Program for the Control of *Taenia solium* since 1994; 3) the living conditions in Mexico have improved greatly in social, economy and health sectors.

Author details

Ana Flisser
Department of Microbiology and Parasitology, Faculty of Medicine,
National Autonomous University of Mexico (UNAM), Mexico DF

Acknowledgement

This chapter is dedicated to all the students and collaborators that I have had along 40 years in cysticercosis research. Gustavo Barradas, Unidad de Informatica y Telecomunicaciones, Facultad de Medicina, UNAM, provided technical support in the preparation of the manuscript.

5. References

[1] Flisser A. Neurocysticercosis in Mexico. Parasitology Today 1988;4:131-137.

[2] Bruschi F, Masetti M, Locci MT, Ciranni R, Fornaciari G. Cysticercosis in an Egyptian Mummy of the Late Ptolemaic Period. American Journal of Tropical Medicine and Hygiene 2006;74:598-599.

[3] Athenian Society. Aristophanes. The Knights. http://ebooks.adelaide.edu.au/a/aristophanes/knights/ The University of Adelaide Library, University of Adelaide, South Australia. The text appears to be derived from the edition published in 1912 by an anonymous translator (accessed 8 September 2012)

[4] Grove DL. A history oh human helminthology. CABI Intl Oxon UK1990. 355-383.

[5] Yoshino K. Studies on the post-embryonal development of *Taenia solium.* Part I. On the hatching of the eggs of *Taenia solium.* Journal of the Medical Association of Formosa 1933;32:139-141

[6] Yoshino K. Studies on the post-embryonal development of *Taenia solium.* Part II. On the migratory course of the oncosphere of *Taenia solium* within the intermediate host. Journal of the Medical Association of Formosa 1933;32:155-158

[7] Yoshino K. Studies on the post-embryonal development of *Taenia solium.* Part III. On the development of cysticercus cellulosae within the definitive intermediate host. Journal of the Medical Association of Formosa 1933;32:166-169.

[8] Yoshino K. On the evacuation of eggs from detached gravid proglottids of *Taenia solium* and on the structure of its eggs. Taiwan Igakkai Zasshi 1934:33:47-58.

[9] Rabiela MT, Ornelas Y, García-Allan C, Rodríguez del Rosal E, Flisser A. Evagination of *Taenia solium* cysticerci: a histologic and electron microscopy study. Archives of Medical Research 2000;31:605-607.

[10] Rabiela MT, Rivas A, Flisser A. Morphological types of *Taenia solium* cysticerci. Parasitology Today1989;5:357-359.

[11] Gómez-Izquierdo I. Locura por cisticercos del cerebro. Revista Médica 1901;13:205-207.

[12] Del Brutto OH, Rajshekhar V, White Jr, AC, Tsang VCW, Nash TE, Takayanagui OM, Schantz PM, Evans CAW, Flisser A, Correa D, Botero D, Allan JC, Sarti E, Gonzalez AE, Gilman RH, Garcia HH. Proposed diagnostic criteria for neurocysticercosis. Neurology 2001;57:177-183.

[13] Garcia HH, Evans CAW, Nash TE, Takayanagui OM, White AC, Botero D, Rajshekhar V, Tsang VCW, Schantz PM, Allan JC, Flisser A, Correa D, Sarti E, Friedland JS, Martinez SM, Gonzalez AE, Gilman RH, Del Brutto OH. Current consensus guidelines or treatment of neurocysticercosis. Clinical and Microbiological Reviews 2002;15:747-756.

[14] Del Brutto OH. Neurocysticercosis: A Review. Scientific World Journal 2012, doi:10.1100/2012/159821 http://www.ncbi.nlm.nih.gov/pmc/articles/PMC3261519/pdf/TSWJ2012-159821.pdf accessed 8 September 2012)

[15] WHO/FAO/OIE Guidelines for the surveillance, prevention and control of aeniosis/cysticercosis. Murrell KD (ed) 2005, 139pp

[16] Dixon HBF, Lipscomb FM. Cysticercosis: an analysis and follow up of 450 cases. Privy Council for Medical Research Special Report1961;229:1-58.

[17] MacArthur WP. Cysticercosis of the brain. British Medical Journal ii 1935;1229

[18] Flisser A, Rodríguez-Canul R, Willingham III AL. Control of the taeniosis/cysticercosis complex: future developments. Veterinary Parasitology 2006;139:283-292

[19] Schantz PM, Wilkins PP, Tsang VCW. Immigrants, imagings and immunoblots: the emergence of neurocysticercosis as a significant public health problem. In: Scheld MW, Craig WA, Hughes JM. (eds) Vol 2. ASM Press, Washington DC. 1998, p213-242

[20] Wandra T, Subahar R, Simanjuntak GM, Margono SS, Suroso T, Okamoto M, Nakao M, Sako Y, Nakaya K, Schantz PM, Ito A.Resurgence of cases of epileptic seizures and burns associated with cysticercosis in Assologaima, Jayawijaya, Irian Jaya, Indonesia, 1991-95. Transactions of the Royal Society for Tropical Medicine and Hygiene 2000;94:46-50.

[21] Schenone H, Villaroel F, Rojas A, Ramírez R. (1982). Epidemiology of human cysticercosis in Latin America. In: A. Flisser A. Willms K, Laclette JP, Larralde C, Ridaura C, Beltrán F (eds). Cysticercosis. Present State of Knowledge and Perspectives. SBN 0-12-260740-6. Academic Press, New York, pp. 25-38.

[22] Flisser A. Epidemiological studies of taeniosis and cysticercosis in Latin America. In: Cestode Zoonoses: Echinococcosis and cysticercosis, an emergent and global problem. Craig P, Pawlowski Z, (eds). IOS Press, NATO Science Series. Vol 341. Amsterdam. 2002 p.3-11.

[23] Velasco-Suarez M, Bravo-Becherelle MA, Quirasco F. Human cysticercosis: medical-social implications and economic impact. In: A. Flisser A. Willms K, Laclette JP, Larralde C, Ridaura C, Beltrán F (eds). Cysticercosis. Present State of Knowledge and Perspectives. ISBN 0-12-260740-6. Academic Press, New York, pp. 47-51.

[24] Flisser A, Gyorkos T. Contribution of immunodiagnostic tests to epidemiological /intervention studies of cysticercosis/taeniosis in Mexico. Parasite mmunology 2007;29:637-649.

[25] Flisser A, Bulnes I, Díaz ML, Luna R, Woodhouse E, Beltrán F, Ortega M, Larralde C. Estudio seroepidemiológico de la cisticercosis humana en poblaciones predominantemente indígenas y rurales del estado de Chiapas. Archivos de nvestigación Médica (México) 1976;7:107-113.

[26] Woodhouse, E., Flisser A. and Larralde, C. Seroepidemiology of human cysticercosis in México. In: A. Flisser A. Willms K, Laclette JP, Larralde C, Ridaura C, Beltrán F (eds). Cysticercosis. Present State of Knowledge and Perspectives. ISBN 0-12-260740-6. Academic Press, New York, pp. 11-24.

[27] Sarti E, Schantz PM, Lara-Aguilera R, Gómez H, Flisser A. *Taenia solium* Taeniasis and Cysticercosis in a Mexican Village. Tropical Medicine and Parasitology 1988;39:194-198.

[28] García-García ML, Torres M, Correa D, Flisser A, Sosa-Lechuga A, Velasco O, Mesa-Lucas A, Plancarte A, Avila G, Tapia R, Aguilar L, Mandujano A, Alcántara I, Morales Z, Salcedo A, Mañon ML, Valdespino-Gómez JL. Prevalence and risk of cysticercosis and taeniasis in a urban population of soldiers and their relatives. American Journal of Tropical Medicine and Hygiene 1999;61:386-389.

[29] Larralde C, Padilla A, Hernández M, Govezensky T, Sciutto E, Gutiérrez G, Tapia-Conyer R, Salvatierra B, Sepúlveda J. Seroepidemiology of cysticercosis in Mexico. Salud Pública (México) 1992;34:197-210.

[30] Sarti E, Schantz PM, Plancarte A, Wilson M, Gutiérrez IO, López AS, Roberts J, Flisser A. Prevalence and Risk Factors for *Taenia solium* Taeniasis and Cysticercosis in Humans and Pigs in a Village in Morelos, México. American Journal of Tropical Medicine and Hygiene 1992;46:677-683.

[31] Sarti E, Schantz PM, Plancarte A, Wilson M, Gutiérrez IO, Aguilera J, Roberts J, Flisser A. Epidemiological Investigation of *Taenia solium* Taeniasis and Cysticercosis in a Rural Village of Michoacan State, México. Transactions of the Royal Society of Tropical Medicine and Hygiene 1994;88:49-52.

[32] Keilbach NM, de Aluja AS, Sarti E. A Programme to Control Taeniasis-Cysticercosis (*T. solium*): Experiences in a Mexican Village. Acta Leidensia 1989;57:181-189.

[33] Díaz-Camacho S, Candil A, Uribe M, Willms K. Serology as an Indicator of *Taenia solium* Tapeworm Infection in a Rural Community in México. Transactions of the Royal Society of Tropical Medicine and Hygiene 1990;84:563-566.

[34] Díaz-Camacho S, Candil A, Suate V, Zazueta ML, Felix-Medina M, Lozano R, Willms K. Epidemiological Study and Control of *Taenia solium* Infections with Praziquantel in a Rural Village of México. American Journal of Tropical Medicine and Hygiene 1991;45:522-531.

[35] Cruz ME, Cruz I, Schantz PM, Dumas M. Headache and Cysticercosis in Ecuador, South America. Headache Journal 1995;35:93-97

[36] Garcia HH. Epidemiology of *Taenia solium* infection in Perú. In: IX International Congress of Parasitology, ICOPA IX, Monduzzi Editore SpA, Bologna, Italy, 1998, pp. 383-391.

[37] García-Noval J, Allan JC, Fletes C, Moreno E, De Mata F, Torres-Álvarez R, Soto de Alfaro H, Yurrita P, Higueras-Morales H, Mencos F, Craig PS. Epidemiology of *Taenia solium* Taeniasis and Cysticercosis in Two Rural Guatemalan Communities. American ournal of Tropical Medicine and Hygiene 1996;55:282-289.

[38] Garcia HH, Araoz R, Gilman RH, Valdez J, González AE, Gavidia C, Bravo ML, Tsang VCW, the Cysticercosis Working Group in Perú. Increased Prevalence of Cysticercosis and Taeniasis Among Professional Fried Pork Vendors and the General Population of a Village in the Perúvian Highlands. American Journal of Tropical Medicine and Hygiene 1998;59:902-905.

[39] Sánchez AL, Medina MT, Ljungstrom I. Prevalence of taeniasis and cysticercosis in a population of urban residence in Honduras. Acta Tropica 1998;69:141-149.

[40] Sánchez AL, Lindback J, Schantz PM, Sone M, Sakai H, Medina MT, Ljungstrom I. A population-based, case-control study of *Taenia solium* taeniosis and cysticercosis. Annals of Tropical Medicine and Parasitology 1999;93:247-258.

[41] Rodríguez-Canul R, Fraser A, Allan JC, Domínguez-Alpizar JL, Arfaez-Rodríguez F, Craig PS. Epidemiological Study of *Taenia solium* Taeniasis/Cysticercosis in a Rural Village in Yucatan State, México. Annals of Tropical Medicine and Parasitology 1999;93:57-67.

[42] Tsang VCW, Brand AJ, Boyer AE. An Enzyme-Linked Immunoelectrotransfer Blot Assay by Glycoprotein Antigens for Diagnosing Human Cysticercosis (*Taenia solium*). ournal of Infectious Diseases 1989;159:50-59.

[43] Schantz, P.M., Sarti, E., Plancarte, A., Wilson, M., Criales, J.L., Roberts, J. and Flisser, A. Community-based epidemiological investigations of cysticercosis due to *Taenia solium*: comparison of serological screening test and clinical findings in two populations in Mexico. Clinical Infectious Diseases 1994;18:879-885.

[44] Correa D, Sandoval M, Harrison LJS, Parkhouse ME, Plancarte A, Meza A, Flisser A. Human Neurocisticercosis: Comparison of Enzyme Immunoassay Capture Techniques Based on Monoclonal and Polyclonal Antibodies for the Detection of Parasite Products n Cerebrospinal Fluid. Transactions of the Royal Society of Tropical Medicine and Hygiene 1989;83:814-816.

[45] Garcia HH, Harrison LJS, Parkhouse RME, Montenegro T, Martínez SM, Tsang VCW, Gilman RH, The Cysticercosis Working Group in Peru. A Specific Antigen-Detection ELISA for the Diagnosis of Human Neurocisticercosis. Transactions of the Royal Society of Tropical Medicine and Hygiene 1998;92:411-414

[46] Aranda-Alvarez JG, Tapia-Romero R, Celis-Quintal G, Grijalva-Otero IE, Correa D. Human Cysticercosis: Risk Factors Associated with Circulating Serum Antigens in an Open Community of San Luis Potosi, México. Annals of Tropical Medicine and Parasitology 1995;89:689-692.

[47] Correa D, Sarti E, Tapia-Romero R, Rico R, Alcántara-Anguiano I, Salgado A, Valdez L, Flisser A. Antigens and Antibodies in Sera from Human Cases of Epilepsy or Taeniasis rom an Area of México where *Taenia solium* Cysticercosis is Endemic. Annals of Tropical Medicine and Parasitology 1999;93:69-74

[48] Fleury A, Hernández M, Fragoso G, Parkhouse RME, Harrison LJS, Sciutto E.. Detection of secreted cysticercal antigen: a useful tool in the diagnosis of inflammatory neurocysticercosis. Transactions of the Royal Society of Tropical Medicine and Hygiene 2003;97:542-546.

[49] Spindola-Felix N, Rojas-Wastavino G, Haro-Arteaga I, Cabrera-Bravo M, Salazar-Schettino PM. Parasite search in strawberries from Irapuato, Guanajuato and Zamora, Michoacan Mexico). Erchives of Medical Research 1996;27:229-231.

[50] Martinez-Maya JJ, de Aluja A, Gemmell M. Failure to incriminate domestic flies (Diptera: Muscidae) as mechanical vectors of *Taenia* eggs (Cyclophillidea: Taeniidae) in rural Mexico. ournal of Medical Entomology 2000;37:489–491.

[51] Flisser A. Risk factors and control measures for taeniosis/cysticercosis. In: Cestode Zoonoses: Echinococcosis and cysticercosis, an emergent and global problem. Craig P, Pawlowski Z, (eds). IOS Press, NATO Science Series. Vol 341. Amsterdam. 2002, p.335-342.

[52] Lescano AG, Garcia HH, Gilman RH, Guezala MC, Tsang VC, Gavidia CM, Rodriguez S, Moulton LH, Green JA, Gonzalez AE; Cysticercosis Working Group in Peru. Swine cysticercosis hotspots surrounding Taenia solium tapeworm carriers. American Journal of Tropical Medicine and Hygiene 2007;76:376-383

[53] Flisser A. Relación huésped-parásito en la cisticercosis humana y porcina (Trabajo de ngreso). Gaceta Médica de México 1987;123:157-164.

[54] Gilman RH, Del Brutto OH, García HH, Martínez M, the Cysticercosis Working Group n Perú. Prevalence of taeniosis among patients with neurocysticercosis is related to severity of infection. Neurology 2000;55:1062

[55] Schantz PM, Moore AC, Muñoz JL, Hartman BJ, Schaefer JA, Aron AM, Persaud D, Sarti E, Wilson M, Flisser A. Neurocysticercosis in an orthodox Jewish community in New York City, New England Journal of Medicine 1992;327:692-695.

[56] Sarti E, Flisser A, Schantz P, Gleizer M, Loya M, Plancarte A, Avila G, Allan J, Craig P, Bronfman M, Wijeyaratne P. Development and evaluation of a health education ntervention against *Taenia solium* in a rural community in Mexico. American Journal of Tropical Medicine and Hygiene 1997;56:127-132.

[57] Flisser A, Correa D. Neurocysticercosis may no longer be a public health problem in Mexico. PLoS Neglected Tropical Diseases 2010;4(12):e831.doi:10.1371

[58] Vázquez-Flores S, Ballesteros-Rodea G, Flisser A, Schantz P. Hygiene and restraint of pigs associated with absence of Taenia solium cysticercosis in a rural community of Mexico. Salud Pública de México 2001;43:574-576.

[59] Flisser A, Vázquez-Mendoza A, Martínez-Ocaña J, Gómez-Colín E, Sánchez Leyva R, Medina-Santillán R. Evaluation of a self-detection tool for tapeworm carriers for use in public health. American Journal of Tropical Medicine and Hygiene 2005;72:510-512.

[60] Pawlowski Z. Efficacy of low doses of praziquantel in taeniosis. Acta Tropica 1991;48:83-88.

[61] Sarti E, Schantz PM, Avila G, Ambrosio J, Medina-Santillán R, Flisser A. Mass Treatment Against Human Taeniasis for the Control of Cysticercosis: a Population-Based Intervention Study. Transactions of the Royal Society of Tropical Medicine and Hygiene 2000,94:85-89.

[62] Flisser, A., Madrazo, I., Puente, A., Schantz, P.M., Allan, J., Craig, P.S. and Sarti, E. 1993. Neurological symptoms in occult neurocysticercosis after single taeniacidal dose of praziquantel. Lancet. 342:748 (Letter).

[63] Gauci, C.G.P., Flisser, A. & Lightowlers, M.W. 1998. Taenia solium oncosphere protein homologous to host-protective *Taenia ovis* and *Taenia saginata* 18kDa antigens. International ournal for Parasitology 28: 757-760.

[64] Plancarte A, Flisser A, Gauci Ch, Lightowelers MW. Vaccination against *Taenia solium* cysticercosis in pigs using native and recombinant oncosphere antigens. International ournal of Parasitology 1999;29:643-647.

[65] Flisser A, Gauci CG, Martinez-Ocaña J, Zoli A, Garza-Rodriguez A, Dominguez-Alpizar JL, Maravilla P, Rodriguez-Canul R, Avila G, Aguilar-Vega L, Kyngdon C, Geerts S, Lightowlers MW. Protection against porcine cysticercosis induced by vaccination with recombinant oncosphere antigens. Infection and Immunity 2004;72:5292-5297

[66] Kyngdon CT, Gauci CG, Gonzalez AE, Flisser A, Zoli A, Read AJ, Martínez Ocaña J, Strugnell RA, Lightowlers MW. Antibody responses and epitope specificities to the Taenia solium cysticercosis vaccines TSOL18 and TSOL45-1A. Parasite Immunology 2006;28:191-199.

[67] Gonzalez AE, Gauci CG, Barber D, Gilman RH, Tsang VC, Garcia HH, Verastegui M, Lightowlers MW. Vaccination of pigs to control human neurocysticercosis. American ournal of Tropical Medicine and Hygiene 2005;72:837-839.

[68] Assana E, Kyngdon CT, Gauci CG, Geerts S, Dorny P, De Deken R, Anderson GA, Zoli AP, Lightowlers MW. Elimination of *Taenia solium* transmission to pigs in a field trial of the TSOL18 vaccine in Cameroon. International Journa of Parasitology 2010;40:515-519.

[69] Roman G, Sotelo J, del Bruto O, Flisser A, Dumas M, Wadia N, Botero D, Cruz M, Garcia H, de Bittencourt PRM, Trelles L, Arraigada C, Lorenzana P, Nash TE, Spina-Franca A. A Proposal to Declare Neurocysticercosis an International Reportable Disease. Bulletin World Health Organization. 2000;78:399-406.

[70] Aijaz F, Ahmed A. Cysticercosis in a Muslim woman. Journal of the Pakistan Medical Association 1993;43:23-24

[71] Townes JM, Hoffmann CJ, Kohn MA. Neurocysticercosis in Oregon, 1995-2000. Emerging Infectious Diseases 2004;10:508-510.

[72] Flisser A, Viniegra AE, Aguilar-Vega L, Garza-Rodriguez A, Maravilla P, Avila G. Portrait of human tapeworms. Journal of Parasitology 2004;90:914–916.

Chapter 10

Clinical Diagnoses of Neurocysticercosis

Arturo Carpio

Additional information is available at the end of the chapter

http://dx.doi.org/10.5772/52388

1. Introduction

Neurocysticercosis (NCC), the most common parasitic brain disease worldwide, is endemic in countries with poor sanitation, and is increasingly being reported in developed countries due to globalization and immigration. As of many decades ago innumerable papers have been published regarding the clinical diagnosis of NC. It has been typical to affirm that clinical manifestations are extremely heterogeneous because they depend on the number, location, size, viability, or evolutionary phase of the parasite, as well as on the immunological response of the patient [1,2]. One of the most intriguing aspects of NCC is that presumably a high percentage of the individuals harboring NCC remain asymptomatic [3]; however, among the symptomatic group, the only clinical manifestation in most patients with parenchymal NCC is seizures, and their neurological status is usually normal [2]. In some patients NCC develops clinical manifestations many years after the parasite lodges in the central nervous system [4], as either brain inflammation around the parasite or mass effect. It has also been stated that almost any neurological symptomatology may be found, ranging from mild headache or treatable acute seizures to very severe neurological manifestations, such as intracranial hypertension (ICH), dementia, or even death [5-8]. These assumptions are probably true, since empirical observation has shown that many of these factors are related to a specific clinical manifestation; however, to date there is no definitive study, using appropriate methodology, designed to address the precise role of each of these factors, or the interaction among them, on the development of symptoms or signs due to NC. This is why the clinical spectrum of symptomatic NCC is currently poorly understood [9].

2. Clinical manifestations of neurocysticercosis

A myriad of papers have reported a wide range of diverse symptoms and signs related to NC, such as manifestations of brainstem dysfunction, cerebellar ataxia, sensory deficits,

INTECH
open science | open minds

© 2013 Carpio, licensee InTech. This is a paper distributed under the terms of the Creative Commons Attribution License (http://creativecommons.org/licenses/by/3.0), which permits unrestricted use, distribution, and reproduction in any medium, provided the original work is properly cited.

involuntary movements, stroke-like symptoms, extrapyramidal signs, dementia, Bruns syndrome, Kluver-Bucy syndrome, cortical blindness, etc [2,10]; however, in some cases it is not possible to establish a clear cause-effect relationship between these pathologies and NC, and a fortuitous relationship among them may occur. Most of this information comes from retrospective data based on uncontrolled studies, historical case series, and anecdotal reports collected mainly from hospital neurological settings. A systematic review was conducted to estimate the clinical manifestation frequencies of symptomatic NCC [9]. The authors reviewed 1569 papers and only 21, based on minimal quality standards, were included in the final analysis. Most of the studies report clinical manifestations of NCC based on hospital medical charts, which don't present reliable information; the majority of them do not provided definitions of manifestations and, if they do, they vary from study to study. Among NCC patients seen in neurology clinics, about 79% had seizures/epilepsy, 38% severe headaches, 16% focal deficits, and 12% signs of increased intracranial pressure. Several other symptoms were also reported in less than 10% of the patients. The authors concluded that these estimates are only applicable to patients who are assisted in neurology clinics and likely over estimate the frequency of manifestations among all NCC cases [9]. Table 1 shows some representative studies which confirm the above mentioned clinical manifestations.

Clinical manifestations of NCC are determined mainly by the location of the parasite within the CNS, the evolutive phase of the parasite, and the immunological response of the patient, expressed as severity of disease activity. The clinical manifestations of parenchymal NCC are quite different from those of extraparenchymal NCC [11,12]. When the parasites are localized in the parenchyma, the main clinical manifestations are epileptic seizures or focal neurological deficits; if the parasites are localized inside the ventricles or the subarachnoid location there are signs and symptoms of cranial hypertension syndrome, cranial nerves abnormalities and hydrocephalus [12]. Regarding the parasite evolutive phase, the transitional or degenerative phase develops clinical manifestations due to the inflammatory reaction of the brain [13]. NCC predominantly affects adults in their third and fourth decade of life, and is relatively uncommon in children and the elderly [1,2] Reports of NCC are very rarely in children younger than 2 years of age because of the prolonged incubation period of *T solium.* Most often, the disease is recognized in children older than 7, due to this incubation period.

There is also clinical heterogeneity across geographical areas; most cases from the Indian subcontinent present single degenerative lesions, whereas those from Latin America present few viable cysts [14]. These differences are probably due to complex interactions between the host, parasite, and environmental factors [3]. Genetic differences in T. solium cysticerci have been reported from different countries [15,16] and may contribute towards the clinical variations among countries. A genetic susceptibility to NCC has been suggested by a reported positive association of HLA-DRBII 13 with single, contrast enhancing CT lesions [17]. However, familial aggregation of seizures in first degree relatives of NCC patients with seizures was not found [18].

Country (reference)	Clinical manifestations	No. Pts.	Age	NCC diagnostic criteria	design
Brazil, (Forlenza OV, 1997)	Seizures 60 5%. depression 52% intracranial hypertension 15%	38	18 to 59 years old	CT scans: small, multiple, calcifications or cystic, contrast enhanced or not, lesions within the parenchyma	historical cases from hospital records
Brazil (Loureiro MG et al, 1997)	Seizures 91%, headaches 23%, motor deficit 7%	44	All ages	Del Brutto et al diagnostic criteria *	historical cases from hospital records
Mexico (Ruiz M et al, 1997)	seizures, intracranial hypertension and learning disabilities	122	< 17 years old	CT scan (details not provided)	historical cases from hospital records
Mexico (Saenz B, et al, 2006)	Seizures 80% adults, 56% children headache 35% adults, 21%, children	206	All ages	CT scan or MRI (details not provided)	direct questionnaire or hospital records
USA (Rosenfeld EA et al, 1996)	Seizures 87%, headaches 32%, altered mental status 13%	47	1 to 15 years old	CT scan or MRI single or multiple parenchymal, intraventricular, spinal, or subarachnoid lesions that were contrast-enhancing, cystic, or calcified	historical cases from hospital records
Ecuador (Carpio A, et al. 2008)	Seizures 62%, headaches 70%, depression 17%	178	All ages	CT scan or MRI: One or more active or degenerative parenchymal cysts associated or not with an extraparenchymal location	prospective cohort study, definitions of clinical manifestations

* Reference 31

Table 1. Clinical manifestations of neurocysticercosis

3. Parenchymal neurocysticercosis

As previously stated, the most common clinical manifestation of parenchymal NCC is epileptic seizure, which occurs in 60-90% of cases. A clinical study including 336 patients [12], reported that seizures were the most common manifestation in the parenchymal location [88%), in comparison with the extraparenchymal location [20%); similarly, focal deficits or motor abnormalities were commonest in the parenchymal location [24% vs. 14%). Focal neurological deficits, when present, are usually transient, over a period of a few days, weeks, or months, with periods of remission and relapse, most likely due to different evolutionary stages of the parasite.

Clinical manifestations are clearly different when comparing by age [19]. Most cases of childhood NCC present mild to moderate symptomatology and single lesions [20-22]. A study [23] specifically carried out to compare the clinical manifestations between pediatric and adult NCC patients reported that seizures were more frequent in children [80.4% versus 56.1%), intracranial hypertension and headaches were more frequent in adults [27.2% versus 15.2% and 35.1% versus 21.7%, respectively), and focal deficits were 17% in adults and 12% in children. Although these age-related differences seem clear, a single effect of age is difficult to demonstrate, since various confounding factors are probably involved [19].

Most paediatric cases show a single transitional cyst, also named solitary cysticercus granuloma [2,24]. The single transitional cyst or single enhancing lesion on CT (SECTL) or hyperintense lesion on magnetic resonance imaging (MRI), is a common finding in patients with newly identified seizures in developing countries. These patients, mainly children and young adults, have some benign and transitory clinical manifestations, predominantly partial or partial secondary generalized seizures, and occasionally Todd's paresis or focal neurological deficits. SECTL tend to resolve spontaneously, without anticysticercal drugs or surgery, since the parasite is already in the degenerative phase and will eventually disappear or become calcified.

Symptomatology of altered mental state and psychiatric manifestations remains poorly described in the literature [9]. In two studies [25,26] which provided definitions of clinical manifestations, depression was reported about 53% and 15%, respectively. Differences on gender have also been identified. Inflammation surrounding parenchymal cysticerci is more intense in women [19]; and multiple degenerating parasites localized in the parenchyma are more frequently reported in young women. Regardless of the localization of the parasite, the inflammatory response, as expressed by cerebrospinal fluid (CSF) cellularity is also more intense in women [3]. A recent prospective study [19] confirms that there are significant gender and age differences in the local immune response, even after adjusting for differences in healthcare access.

4. Extraparenchymal neurocysticercosis

The extraparenchymal location (around 15–30% of cases) develops different clinical manifestations. Headache and signs of intracranial pressure are more frequent in the extraparenchymal location [88%), in comparison with the parenchymal location (10%). [12] When cysticerci are located inside the ventricular system, life-threatening acute intracranial hypertension as a result of hydrocephalus may occur; as a consequence, severe headache, dizziness and consciousness alteration are the predominant clinical manifestations [5,27].

Cysts in the subarachnoid space may lodge in the Sylvian fissure or basal cisterns and grow to a big size (racemose form), causing intracranial hypertension. This is associated with an intense inflammatory reaction, and fibrosis and progressive thickening of the leptomeninges at the base of the brain [13]. There is an obstruction of the CSF circulation, resulting in hydrocephalus and progressive intracranial hypertension. Inflammation of meninges, cranial nerve involvement, chiasmatic syndrome, and cerebral infarcts secondary to vasculitis may develop [5,6]. When hydrocephalus due to cysticercotic meningitis is present, the mortality rate is high (50%), and most patients die within 2 years after CSF shunting [6,8]. This is why ventricular and basal cisternal locations are considered to be malignant forms of NCC [28]. In cases with NCC meningitis, cerebrospinal fluid (CSF) may show mild elevation of protein, hypoglycorrhachia and lymphocytic pleocytosis, which is similar to other chronic basal meningitis, such as tuberculosis and mycosis.[2]

Spinal cord cysticercosis is rare. Patients experience nonspecific clinical manifestations, such us nerve root pain or spinal cord compression syndromes, according to the level of the lesion [29]. Severe forms of NCC may exceptionally occur, including cysticercotic encephalitis, which result in permanent neurologic sequel, such as amaurosis. Hydrocephalus and intraventricular NCC is extremely rare in children [23,30]

5. Immunological and imaging diagnosis

Two main techniques, the Enzyme-linked Immunosorbent Assay (Ab-ELISA) and Enzyme-Linked Immunoelectrotransfer Blot (EITB) Assay, are used for immunological diagnosis of NCC. ELISA test for antibodies or antigen detection have showed higher sensitivities and specificities in CSF than in sera [31]. EITB sensibility seems to be not significantly different in sera and CSF while specificity is higher in CSF [32]. Sensibility of either tests falls in cases of single cysts in parenchyma or when they are calcified [33]. In patients with reliable diagnosis of NCC by imaging studies, immunological test is not required, since a negative test will not discard a NCC. When imaging of extraparnechymal cysts is doubtful, determination of antigens by ELISA in CSF may be helpful [31].

Computed tomography and magnetic resonance imaging have been useful in the study of the parasite evolution within the brain parenchyma [2]. Once the oncosphere has passed into the parenchyma, it grows and evolves through vesicular, colloidal, granular-nodular, and calcified phases [13]. In the vesicular phase the larva lives inside a translucent liquid-filled cystic structure surrounded by a thin membrane. The CT scan depicts circumscribed, rounded, hypodense areas, varying in size and number, without enhancement by contrast media [34]. With the MRI, the vesicular larva appears with a CSF-like intensity signal on all sequences. Both MRI and CT may show a high intensity, 2-3 mm. mural nodule, depicting the scolex, in the interior of some vesicular cysts (Figure 1). It is better seen on fluid attenuated inversion recovery (FLAIR) sequence [35].

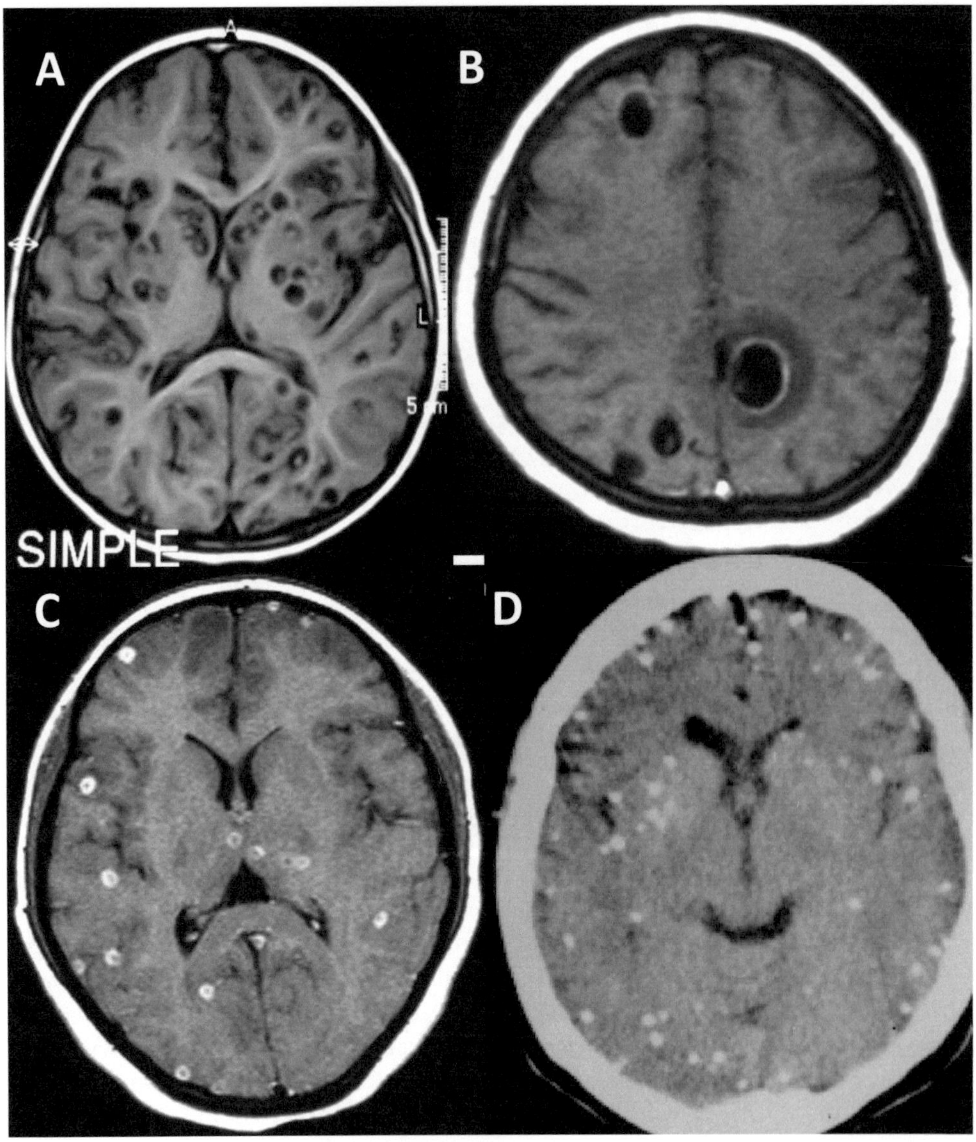

A: vesicular cysts B: colloidal cysts C: nodular cysts D: calcified cysts

Figure 1. Imaging of parenchymal neurocysticercosis

As the cyst degenerates, the CT scan shows an annular or nodular enhancement surrounded by perilesional edema. In this stage, the fluid content gives slightly higher signal than CSF and is sometimes isodense with the parenchyma on MRI-T1 and/or proton density-weighted, and high signal on T2 images. The capsule shows higher signal than the adjacent brain with thick ring enhancement on T1 images, while on T2 images there is a low ring signal surrounded by high signal lesion, due mostly to edema. Finally, when the cyst dies it may disappear or become an inactive calcified nodule of homogenous high density on CT, or low intensity on proton-weighted MRI [2] (Figure 1).

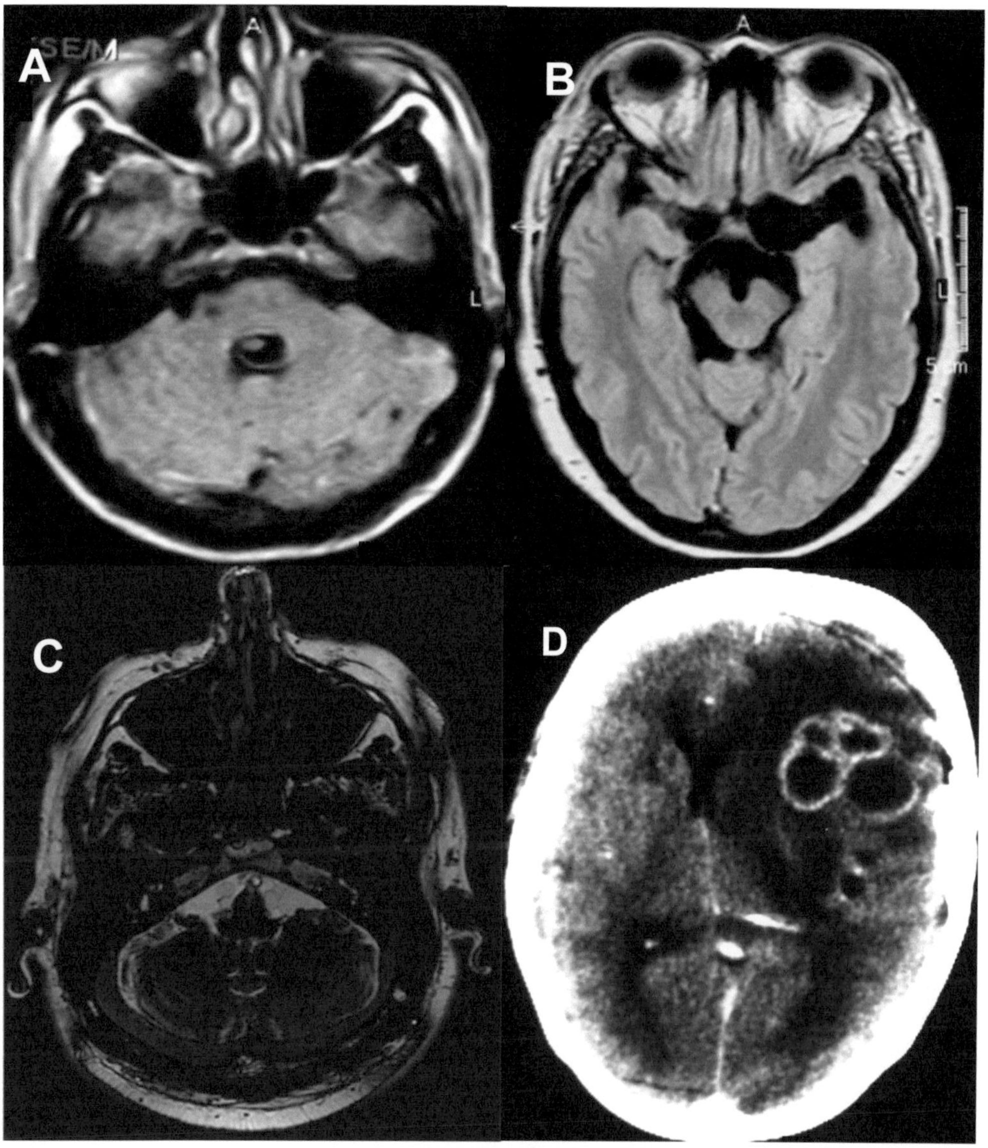

A: Cyst in the fourth ventricle B: Racemose cysts in the basal subarachanoid space C: cysts in the prepontine cisternal space (MRI FIESTA sequence) D: Racemose cysts in the degenerative stage

Figure 2. Imaging of extraparenchymal neurocysticercosis

Extraparenchymal NCC is more difficult to detect by imaging because the attenuation and signal intensity of the cyst's content is similar to that of CSF, the cystic wall is usually very thin and the cysts lack frequently of a scolex and generally not enhanced after contrast administration. In these cases, new MRI techniques such as fluid attenuated inversion recovery (FLAIR) and fast imaging employing steady-state acquisition (FIESTA) sequences, that seems to permit a better diagnosis (34-36) (Figure 2) . A common neuroimaging finding is hydrocephalus related to inflammatory occlusion of Luschka and Magendie foramina and basal fibrous arachnoiditis [36]. Cysts located within CSF cisterns usually have a multilobulated appearance (racemose form), displacing neighboring structures as a mass occupying lesion (Figure 2).

6. Difficulties with clinical diagnosis of neurocysticercosis

Del Brutto et al. proposed a diagnostic criterion for NCC in 2001 [37]. In spite of the fact that this proposal has not been validated so far, it has been an important contribution to current NCC knowledge. This proposal includes four categories of criteria—absolute, major, minor, and epidemiologic. A combination of these criteria results in degrees of diagnostic certainty: definitive and probable. Diagnosis of definitive NCC is made by the presence of one absolute criterion or of two major plus one minor or one epidemiologic criterion [37].

These diagnostic criteria may be useful to identify patients with mainly parenchymal forms of NC, but it is not for patients with extraparenchymal forms of NCC [31]. Among minor criteria are considered "manifestations suggestive of neurocysticercosis" which include seizures, focal neurologic deficits, increased intracranial pressure, and intellectual deterioration, which are predominantly related to parenchymal location of lesions, but not necessarily to extraparenchymal clinical manifestations such us those associated with intraventricular cysts or NCC meningeal inflammation. Among absolute criteria are considered "Cystic lesions showing the scolex on CT or MRI" or "spontaneous resolution of small single enhancing lesions" It is extremely rare to see scolex on CT or MRI inside the ventricles or the subarachnoid location, and it is also very difficult to demonstrate spontaneous resolution of small single enhancing lesions in the extraparenchymal location.

This diagnostic criteria proposal may be a source of bias even in the event of diagnosing parenchymal NC. For example, a patient who lives in any country where cysticercosis is endemic (epidemiologic criterion), with seizure or headache (1 minor criterion), a CT showing a calcification (one major criterion), and a positive serum enzyme-linked immunoelectrotransfer blot assay –EITB- (one major criterion), according to this proposal, should be categorized as "definitive NC". However, it could be erroneous to diagnose this patient as having NC, since headache is extremely unspecific, a positive EITB means just exposure to the parasite, and a calcification could correspond to many other pathologies, but not necessarily NC. The selection of these patients in some reports, especially those community-based, is probably over-diagnosing NC.

There are additional problems related to this proposal that could lead to a misleading diagnosis. According to these diagnosis criteria, two major criteria fulfill a definite NCC diagnosis criterion. In this context, a patient with a positive immunologic test for the detection of anticysticercal antibodies (major criterion) plus a plain X-ray films showing "cigarshaped" calcifications in thigh and calf muscles (major criterion) could be diagnosed as NC. It is very hard to accept that such a patient may unquestionably have cysticerci in the brain. Some authors have claimed that the generalized use of Del Brutto et al [38] criteria have created some distortion in the present perception of NCC [31] A broad consensus now exists that these criteria should be revised to incorporate current scientific knowledge, in order to achieve a new consensus on the diagnosis of NCC.

7. Conclusion

So far, diagnosis of NCC is mainly done by neuroimaging. New imaging techniques have improved detection of the scolex inside the cysts, which can be considered pathognomonic of neurocysticercosis There is no a typical clinical manifestation of NCC. Prospective cohort studies addressed to analyzing NCC clinical manifestations, including definitions and appropriate methodology, which make them comparable, are extremely scarce in the medical literature. Location of the parasite in the CNS, age, sex, and immunological response of the patient, all seem to play an important role in occurrence of symptoms and signs; however, the relative contribution of these factors, alone or in combination, is still unknown.

In the parenchymal location, seizures are the most frequent clinical manifestation, followed by headache, motor focal deficits, and psychiatric and cognitive symptomatology. These clinical manifestations may have periods of remission and exacerbation, according to the evolutionary phase of the parasite inside the parenchyma. Diagnosis of extraparenchymal NCC is even more difficult, considering that unspecific symptoms and signs of intracranial hypertension and meningitis may occur, with or without signs of CSF inflammation. The clinical manifestations due to parenchymal location are usually benign and are sometimes transitory in time; on the contrary, clinical presentation of the extraparenchymal location is life-threatening and may develop permanent sequels.

Properly-designed studies with similar methodology are needed to learn more about the natural history of the disease and the true distribution of clinical manifestations. There is also an urgent need to develop new consensus diagnosis criteria for NC.

Author details

Arturo Carpio
School of Medicine, University of Cuenca, Ecuador
G.H. Sergievsky Center, Columbia University, New York, USA

8. References

[1] Takayanagui OM, Jardim E. Clinical aspects of neurocysticercosis: analysis of 500 cases. Arq Neuropsiquiatr 1983;41:50–63.
[2] Carpio A. Neurocysticercosis: an update. Lancet Infectious Diseases. 2002;2:751-762.
[3] Fleury A, Escobar A, Fragoso G, Sciutto E, Larralde C. Clinical heterogeneity of human neurocysticercosis results from complex interactions among parasite, host and environmental factors. Trans R Soc Trop Med Hyg. 2010;104:243-250

[4] Dixon HBF, Lipscomb FM. Cysticercosis:an analysis and follow-up of 450 cases. Med Res Council spec.rep., no.299. London: Her Majesty's Stationery Office, 1961;1-58.

[5] Agapejev S, Pouza AF, Bazan R, Faleiros AT. Clinical and evolutive aspects of hydrocephalus in neurocysticercosis. Arq Neuropsiquiatr. 2007;65:674-80.

[6] Cárdenas G, Jung H, Ríos C, Fleury A, Soto-Hernández JL. Severe cysticercal meningitis: clinical and imaging characteristics. Am J Trop Med Hyg. 2010;82(1):121-5.

[7] Rodrigues CL, de Andrade DC, Livramento JA, Machado LR, Abraham R, et al. Spectrum of cognitive impairment in neurocysticercosis: differences according to disease phase. Neurology. 2012 Mar 20;78(12):861-866.

[8] Sotelo J, Marin C. Hydrocephalus secondary to cysticercotic arachnoiditis. A long-term follow-up review of 92 cases. J Neurosurg 1987;66:686–689.

[9] Carabin H, Ndimubanzi PC, Budke CM, Nguyen H, Qian Y, et al. Clinical manifestations associated with neurocysticercosis: a systematic review. PLoS Negl Trop Dis. 2011;5(5):e1152.

[10] Patel R, Jha S, Yadav RK. Pleomorphism of the clinical manifestations of neurocysticercosis. Trans R Soc Trop Med Hyg. 2006;100:134-141.

[11] Monteiro L, Almeida-Pinto J, Stocker A, Sampaio-Silva M. Active neurocysticercosis, parenchymal and extraparenchymal: a study of 38 patients. J Neurol 1993;241:15–21.

[12] Carpio A, Placencia M, Santillan F, Escobar A. A proposal for a classification of neurocysticercosis. Can J Neuro Sci 1994;21:43-47.

[13] Escobar A. The pathology of neurocysticercosis In, Palacios E, Rodriguez-Carbajal J, Taveras JM, eds. Cysticercosis of Central Nervous System. Springfield: Charles C Thomas, 1983. 27-54.

[14] Singh G. Neurocysticercosis in South-Central America and the Indian subcontinent. A comparative evaluation. Arq Neuropsiquiatr 1997;55:349–356.

[15] Maravilla, P., Gonzalez-Guzman, R., Zuniga, G., Peniche, A., Dominguez-Alpizar, J.L. et al. Genetic polymorphism in Taenia solium cysticerci recovered from experimental infections in pigs. Infect Genet Evol 2008;8:213-216.

[16] Vega, R., Pinero, D., Ramanankandrasana, B., Dumas, M., Bouteille, B., et al. Population genetic structure of Taenia solium from Madagascar and Mexico: implications for clinical profile diversity and immunological technology. Int J Parasitol 2003;33:1479-1485.

[17] Jain, S., Padma, M.V., Kanga, U., Mehra, N.K. and Maheshwari, N.C. Family studies and human leukocyte antigen class II typing in Indian probands with seizures in association with single small enhancing computed tomography lesions. Epilepsia 1999;40:232-238.

[18] Kelvin, E.A., Carpio, A., Hesdorffer, D.C., Bagiella, E., Leslie. et al. Investigation of familial aggregation of seizures in neurocysticercosis patients. Epilepsy Res 2009;84:67-71.

[19] Kelvin EA, Carpio A, Bagiella E, Leslie D, Leon P, Andrews H, et al. The association of host age and gender with inflammation around neurocysticercosis cysts. Ann Trop Med Parasitol. 2009;103:487-499.

[20] Rosenfeld EA, Byrd SE, Shulman ST. Neurocysticercosis among children in Chicago. Clin Infect Dis 1996;23:262–268.

[21] Ruiz-Garcia M, Gonzalez-Astiazara´n A, Rueda-Franco F. Neurocysticercosis in children. Clinical experience in 122 patients. Childs Nerv Syst 1997;13:608–612.
[22] Kelvin EA, Carpio A, Bagiella E, Leslie D, Leon P, et al. Seizure in people with newly diagnosed active or transitional neurocysticercosis. Seizure. 2011;20:119-125
[23] Sáenz B, Ruíz-Garcia M, Jiménez E, Hernández-Aguilar J, Suastegui R, et al. Neurocysticercosis: clinical, radiologic, and inflammatory differences between children and adults. Pediatr Infect Dis J. 2006;25:801-803.
[24] Singh G, Rajshekhar V, Murthy JM, Prabhakar S, Modi M, et al. A diagnostic and therapeutic scheme for a solitary cysticercus granuloma. Neurology. 2010;75(24):2236-2245.
[25] Forlenza OV, Vieira Filho AHG, Smith Nobrega JP, dos Ramis Machado L, Garcia de Varros N, et al. Psychiatric manifestations of neurocysticercosis: a study of 38 patients from a neurology clinic in Brazil. J Neurol Neurosurg Psychiatry 1997;62:612–616.
[26] Carpio A, Kelvin E, Bagiella E, Leslie D, Leon P, et al. The effects of albendazole treatment on neurocysticercosis: a randomized controlled trial. Journal of Neurology Neurosurgery and Psychiatry, 2008;79:1050-1055
[27] Citow JS, Johnson JP, McBride DQ, Ammirati M. Imaging feautures and surgery-related outcomes in intraventricular neurocysticercosis. Neurosurg Focus 2002;12:1-8
[28] Estañol B, Corona T, Abad P. A prognostic classification of cerebral cysticercosis: therapeutic implications. J Neurol Neurosurg Psychiatry 1986;49:1131-1134.
[29] Alsina GA, Johnson JP, McBride DQ, Rhoten PRL, Mehringer CM, et al. Spinal Neurocysticercosis. Neurosurg Focus 2002;12:1-7.
[30] Loureiro das Chagas MG, D'Oliveira A, Jr., Tavares-Neto J. Clinical aspects of neurocysticercosis at semi-desert region of the Brazialian northeast. Arq Neuropsiquiatr 2003;61: 398–402
[31] Fleury A, Hernández M, Avila M, Cárdenas G, Bobes RJ, et al. Detection of HP10 antigen in serum for diagnosis and follow-up of subarachnoidal and intraventricular human neurocysticercosis. J Neurol Neurosurg Psychiatry. 2007;78(9):970-974.
[32] Proaño-Narvaez JV, Meza-Lucas A, Mata-Ruiz O, García-Jerónimo RC, Correa D. Laboratory diagnosis of human neurocysticercosis: double-blind comparison of enzyme-linked immunosorbent assay and electroimmunotransfer blot assay. J Clin Microbiol. 2002;40(6):2115-2118.
[33] Singh G, Kaushal V, Ram S, Kaushal RK, Dhanuka AK, et al. Cysticercus immunoblot assay in patients with single, small enhancing lesions and multilesional neurocysticercosis. J Assoc Physicians India. 1999 May;47(5):476-9.
[34] Lucato LT, Guedes MS, Sato JR, et al. The role of conventional MR imaging sequences in the evaluation of neurocysticercosis: impact on characterization of the scolex and lesion burden. AJNR Am J Neuroradiol. 2007;28:1501-1504.
[35] Mont'Alverne Filho FE, Machado Ldos R, Lucato LT, Leite CC. The role of 3D volumetric MR sequences in diagnosing intraventricular neurocysticercosis: preliminar results. Arq Neuropsiquiatr. 2011;69:74-8.
[36] Fleury A, Carrillo-Mezo R, Flisser A, Sciutto E, Corona T. Subarachnoid basal neurocysticercosis: a focus on the most severe form of the disease. Expert Rev Anti Infect Ther. 2011;9(1):123-1 33.

[37] Del Brutto OH, Rajshekhar V, White Jr AC, Tsang VCW, Nash TE, Takayanagui OM, et al. Proposed diagnostic criteria for neurocysticercosis. Neurology 2001;57:177–183.
[38] Machado LR. The diagnosis of neurocysticercosis: a closed question? Arq Neuropsiquiatr. 2010;68(1):1-2.

Chapter 11

Neurocysticercosis and Epilepsy

Arturo Carpio

Additional information is available at the end of the chapter

http://dx.doi.org/10.5772/52389

1. Introduction

Neurocysticercosis (NCC) is a biological marker of poverty and underdevelopment [1]. The frequency of this brain parasitic disease is probably high worldwide, as well as epilepsy; however, little is known about the natural history of the infection in humans. Both, NCC and epilepsy, are an increasing burden on the welfare and economy of developing countries [2]. This is why knowledge of these diseases should be improved, in order to prevent them.

Acute symptomatic seizures are the most common clinical manifestation of NCC in those patients in whom a cysticercus is located in brain parenchyma [1-3]. Epilepsy attributable to NCC usually has a good prognosis in terms of seizure control and seizure remission [1,4]. Although some authors have suggested that anticysticercal treatment is associated with reduced seizure recurrence, there is no evidence that cysticidal treatment does more good than harm in addition to conventional antiepileptic treatment [2,5] According to new information, the traditional view of the relationship between NCC and epilepsy [2,3] can be questioned. Nowadays, NCC is considered a comorbid component of epilepsy [6]

2. Epidemiology of neurocysticercosis and epilepsy

In developed countries, the age-adjusted incidence of epilepsy ranges from 24 to 53/100,000 [7]. In developing countries (DC) the incidence of epilepsy on the basis of two studies carried out in South America in the last decade, ranged from 114 to 190/100,000 [8]; considerably higher than that reported in industrialized countries. New studies carried out in the last few years confirm high incidence: A hospital-based study of children in Tunisia reported the incidence of first unprovoked seizures to be 102/100,000 [9]. A population-based study carried out among children in Kenya, reported the incidence of epilepsy (two or more two unprovoked seizures) to be 187/100,000 [10]. In a population-based study among all ages in Honduras, Central America [11], the incidence of patients with non-febrile seizures was 92.7/100,000. Because of the broader case-inclusion criteria and uncertainty

INTECH
open science | open minds

© 2013 Carpio, licensee InTech. This is a paper distributed under the terms of the Creative Commons Attribution License (http://creativecommons.org/licenses/by/3.0), which permits unrestricted use, distribution, and reproduction in any medium, provided the original work is properly cited.

regarding age-specific distribution in these studies, there is no way to compare results from these incidence studies. Nonetheless, the incidence of epilepsy is probably higher in DC than in industrialized countries [7].

Reported prevalence of active epilepsy, based on methodology recommended by the International League Against Epilepsy (ILAE) Commission of Epidemiology and Prognosis [12] in DC, ranges from 3.9 to 15.7 per 1,000 person-years [13] These differences, however, are due to different approaches used by the studies and differences regarding the definitions of active epilepsy: Limiting assessment to those studies that provide information for age-adjusted rates, the average age adjusted prevalence of active epilepsy is 8.5/1,000, which is similar to the developed countries. This prevalence is low given the high incidence of epilepsy in DC and may be due to the fact that mortality of people with epilepsy is higher in comparison with that of developed countries. While studies from developed countries show a consistent pattern suggesting that the onset of epilepsy occurs at both extremes of life [7]; on the other hand, incidence in DC is highest among young and middle-aged adults [13], perhaps as a manifestation of diseases prevalent in these age-groups. This includes conditions such as brain injury and infectious and parasitic diseases endemic in these countries.

Taenia solium infection is widely endemic in poor countries, both in highlands or tropical areas, in Central and South America, and non-Muslim populations of Asia and Africa [1]. Cysticercosis is considered an emerging infectious disease in some developed countries; persons who have never left the United States as well as visitors to disease-endemic regions are at risk [2]. Data on the frequency of NCC from endemic countries have been compiled from clinic-based patients or autopsied cadavers. NCC was found, for example, in 2.8%-3.6% of all autopsies in some hospitals [14]. However, such statistics can be misleading because differences in availability of medical services and lack of comprehensive and consistent reporting in most countries still confound attempts to compare incidence and prevalence among countries [15]. Most reports fail to provide even minimal information regarding diagnostic criteria and definitions; consequently, these data are definitely biased and hardly representative of the general population.

Immunoserologic assays, such as enzyme-linked immunoelectrotransfer blot assay (EITB) or enzyme-linked immunosorbent assay (ELISA), detect antibodies against T. solium or cysticercus [1] Epidemiological surveys for human cysticercosis, using EITB as a marker of infection, report a seroprevalence from 8% to 12% in some regions of Latin American [16,17]. These assays are useful for identification of individuals who have had systemic contact with the parasite at some time. Seropositivity, however, does not necessarily mean an active systemic infection or central nervous system (CNS) involvement at any time [1,18]. Most seropositive individuals in these populations were asymptomatic. There are no prospective cohort studies providing information on the proportion of seropositive individuals that will develop seizures or other neurological symptoms. Some studies [17], but not all [19] have reported an association between seizures and seropositivity. Although a higher proportion of patients with epilepsy have been shown to be EITB positive when compared to those without epilepsy, the proportion of seropositivity in epileptic patients is similar to that reported in the general population in these same areas [17].

3. Definitions of epileptic seizures, epilepsy and neurocysticercosis

In order to understand the relationship between epilepsy and NCC, it is crucial to promote consistency in definitions to enhance research studies, facilitate comparison between populations, provide data useful for detection, treatment, and prevention, and to promote effective health care for people with epilepsy and NCC [2].

The natural history of the cysticerci in the CNS is not entirely understood. Computed tomography (CT) and magnetic resonance imaging (MRI) have been useful in the study of the evolution of the cysticercus within the brain parenchyma [20]. Once the oncosphere has passed into the parenchyma, it grows and evolves through vesicular, colloidal, granular-nodular, and calcified phases [21]. In the vesicular phase the host tends to show immune tolerance, and in most cases there is no surrounding parenchymal reaction; the larva lives inside a translucent liquid-filled cystic structure surrounded by a thin membrane, where it can remain viable from a few months to several years [22] The CT scan depicts circumscribed, rounded, hypodense areas, varying in size and number, without enhancement by contrast media [20].With the MRI, the vesicular larva appears with a CSF-like intensity signal on all sequences, with no surrounding high signal on T2-weighted images. Both MRI and CT may show a high intensity, 2-3 mm. mural nodule, depicting the scolex, in the interior of some parenchymal vesicular cysts.

As the cyst degenerates, it goes through a transitional stage: the contrast enhanced CT scan shows an annular (colloidal phase) or nodular [nodular phase) enhancement surrounded by irregular perilesional edema [1,20,22]. In this stage, the fluid content gives slightly higher signal than CSF and is sometimes isodense with the parenchyma on MRI-T1 and/or proton density-weighted, and high signal on T2 images. The capsule shows higher signal than the adjacent brain with thick ring enhancement on T1 images, while on T2 images there is a low ring signal surrounded by high signal lesion, due mostly to edema. Although these pathological changes are responsible for clinical manifestations, usually seizures and headache, they may not cause symptoms at all. Finally, when the cyst dies it may disappear or become an inactive calcified nodule of homogenous high density on CT, or low intensity on proton-weighted MRI [1].

Based on the abovementioned concepts a classification based on the viability and location of the parasite in the CNS of the host has been proposed: active, when the parasite is alive; transitional, if it is in the degenerative phase; inactive, if there is evidence of its death [20]. Each viability category was subdivided into parenchymal and extraparenchymal forms. The viability criterion is very important, as it allows us to analyze the natural history of the parasite, and, according to the parasite's evolutionary stage, the production of physiopathological changes in the host's CNS. On the basis of this classification, it is possible to relate clinical manifestations and therapeutic procedures to each category of the proposed classification. For example, seizures are the main symptom in the transitional parenchymal form due to the brain inflammatory reaction, whereas cranial nerve abnormalities and intracranial hypertension syndromes are more frequent in the subarachonoid and intraventricular forms.

According to the definitions suggested by the International League Against Epilepsy's Epidemiology Commissions [6,12] , epilepsy is defined as two or more unprovoked seizures occurring at least 24 hours apart. Unprovoked seizures may occur subsequent to a well-demonstrated antecedent condition, known to substantially increase the risk of epileptic seizures. New terminology and concepts proposed by the ILAE divide the causes of epilepsy into three broad categories: genetic, structural/metabolic, and unknown [23]. "The cause is considered structural/metabolic when a structural lesion (either static or progressive) or metabolic condition (e.g., inborn errors of metabolism) is present and is known to be associated with an increased risk of epilepsy." The cause is attributed to the condition that is most directly linked and proximate to the development of epilepsy, for example NCC, in the calcified phase.

An epileptic seizure is defined as "a transient occurrence of signs and/or symptoms due to abnormal excessive or synchronous neuronal activity in the brain" [24]. Epileptic seizures, even if recurrent, are not always synonymous with epilepsy per se [6]. Provoked or acute symptomatic seizures are seizures which occur "in close temporal association with an acute systemic, metabolic, or toxic insult or in association with an acute central nervous system (CNS) insult (infection, stroke, cranial trauma, intracerebral hemorrhage, or acute alcohol intoxication or withdrawal)," [12,25]. Such seizures are often isolated epileptic events associated with acute conditions, but may recur if the acute condition recurs, as happens in the transitional or degenerative form of NCC, due to the underlying inflammatory process

The interval between the insult and the seizure—which is used to separate acute symptomatic from unprovoked seizures—may vary according to the underlying clinical condition [23,25] . In the NCC case, this interval lasts while the inflammation signs due to the transitional or degenerative cysts persist (six months on average). Nonetheless, if seizures occur in the presence of parasites in viable or calcified phase, they are unprovoked and, if recurrent, should be considered epilepsy [1-3].

Seizures associated with NCC may be categorized as either acute symptomatic or as remote symptomatic seizures. Individuals with cysticerci in the transitional form or degenerative phase develop acute symptomatic seizures due to the acute inflammatory response of the brain; on the other hand, a patient with seizures who has active, viable cysts and/or inactive, non-inflammed calcified parasites may be categorized as having unprovoked seizures [3]. NCC has an unpredictable clinical course, which makes it difficult to categorize all cases into the proposed classification of the ILAE Commission. For instance, a patient with chronic recurrent seizures, whose imaging studies show several non-inflamed parenchymal calcifications, should be categorized as having remote symptomatic unprovoked seizures. The same patient, some years later, can experience a recurrence of parenchymal transitional cysts. This case should be considered to have multiple episodes of NCC now resulting in acute symptomatic seizures.

The recent ILAE report defines comorbidity as the co-occurrence of two or more separate medical conditions in the same individual and includes NCC as a comorbid condition associated with epilepsy [6]. Ultimately, in patients with NC, what matters most is to differentiate between provoked or acute symptomatic seizures and recurrent unprovoked seizures (epilepsy). This differentiation is very important, due to its implications concerning treatment and prognosis, as will be discussed below. Presumably, the inclusion of people with only acute symptomatic seizures as cases of epilepsy is one of the reasons for the high proportion of epilepsy reported in some studies [13].

4. Seizures as a main clinical manifestation of neurocysticercosis

In spite of the clinical heterogeneity and variability in the clinical forms of expression and evolution of NCC, all reports of medical literatures agree that seizures are the most common symptom of NC, occurring in 70-90% of patients [18,26]. However, seizure is more frequent when the parasite is located in the brain parenchyma of the patient, in comparison with the intraventricular or subarachnoid locations [20]. There is no uniformity in the reported distribution of seizure types in patients with NC. Some authors report a higher proportion of partial seizures, others conclude that generalized seizures are more frequent [1, 5, 27]. It seems that either generalized seizures or partial seizures with secondarily generalization are most commonly reported, while complex partial seizures are less frequent [1]

Seizures may occur at any evolutionary stage of the parasite. A recent prospective cohort study [28], whose aim was to describe seizure as a presenting symptom in individuals with recently diagnosed neurocysticercosis showed that most of the seizures in patients in the youngest age category (3–24 years old) appear to be provoked or acute symptomatic seizures due to transitional cysts in the brain parenchyma rather than new onset idiopathic ones. Thus, it appears that children are more likely to have NCC-related seizures than adults. The authors found transitional cysts to be associated with a significantly higher probability of seizure in the chi-square analysis; however, in the regression models that adjusted for patient age and gender as well as the number and location of the cysts, no specific cyst phase was found to be significantly associated with having seizures. Patients with cysts in the parietal lobe and with cysts in the frontal lobe were also more likely to present seizures.

It has been suggested that both age and gender influence the strength of the host's immune response. In a recent study [29] the odds of having transitional cysts were found to be 1.5-fold higher for the female patients than for the male; additionally, the number of transitional cysts was found to be 1.8-fold higher in the female patients than in the male, and this gender effect was not only statistically significant but also constant over time. It therefore appears that there are significant gender and age differences in the local immune response to NCC, even after adjusting for differences in healthcare access.

Some studies have also found familial aggregation of NCC infection [17, 30], as well as regional differences in the clinical manifestations of human NCC may indicate a role of host genetics [31]. However, in a recent study that investigated whether there is familial aggregation of seizures in first-degree relatives of NCC patients with seizure versus NCC patients without seizure as presenting symptom in a group of patients in Ecuador [32], there was no trend toward familial aggregation of seizures in NCC patients.

Neurologists from developing countries frequently see patients in whom the first seizure occurred many years before consultation; and when the second seizure occurs at the time of consultation, the imaging study shows one or more calcifications and one cyst in the transitional form with perilesional edema. We can assume that when the first seizures occurred, the patient had cysts in a transitional form, which eventually became calcified, and currently the patient has new acute seizures [1]. According to the ILAE Commission we should categorize these patients as having isolated epileptic events associated with a recurrent acute condition (transitional form) [3].

So far, the mechanism by which the calcified neurocysticercal lesions (CNL) cause seizures or epilepsy is not known [1,33,34] This has been attributed to residual perilesional gliosis that results in chronic epileptogenic foci [33]. CNL are frequently encountered on CT scans of asymptomatic individuals, and studies from Latin American countries report that the majority are incidental lesions [30,35] These observations would question the epileptogenicity of CNL. On the contrary, based on epidemiological studies, patients with epilepsy have a higher prevalence of calcified lesions than controls [19].

Another potential evidence for the epileptogenicity of CNL is the episodic appearance of edema surrounding the CNL after seizures. Some studies have suggested that perilesional oedema is associated with episodic seizure activity in patients with CNL [36] . The authors argue that episodic release of cysticercal antigens from the calcified lesions can lead to inflammation, perilesional edema, and seizures. These studies have not been replicated so far. Anyway, it is not clear whether this edema is causal or a consequence of the seizure [34]. Transient cortical edema after seizures, a rare neuroimaging finding, was described more than 20 years ago [37,38] but its mechanism has not been entirely clarified. The empirical observation of neurologists from NCC endemic countries is that perilesional oedema around calcification in patients with epilepsy are extremely rare and, when it happens, perilesional oedema disappears in a few days without any additional treatment, except for antiepileptic drugs.

Another study designed to analyze epileptogenesis in calcified neurocysticercosis using dynamic contrast-enhanced MRI [39], reported quantitative differences between symptomatic and asymptomatic groups in various perfusion indices. Median values of the rate transfer constant and leakage volume were higher in symptomatic patients than in asymptomatic patients, indicating a higher degree of blood brain barrier permeability in symptomatic individuals. This study also showed increased MMP-9 (R279Q) gene polymorphisms in subjects with seizures compared with those in asymptomatic and control subjects. Therefore, the epileptogenicity in patients with CNL could be related to degree of inflammation, which also may be partly determined by genetic factors. This study was carried out with a small sample of patients and should be confirmed in the future.

Single enhancing lesion and seizures. A single enhancing lesion on CT (SECTL) or hyperintense lesion on MRI is a common finding in patients with newly identified seizures in developing countries [40,41]. The patients, mainly children and young adults, have some benign and transitory clinical manifestations, predominantly partial or partial secondary generalized seizures, and occasionally Todd's paresis or focal neurological deficits. These lesions have been attributed mainly to cysticercosis or to tuberculosis; however, similar lesions have been reported in other inflammatory pathologies such as pyogenic abscess, histoplasmosis, blastomycosis and sarcoidiosis, post-infectious vasculitis, and to primary and metastatic brain tumors.

The natural history of these lesions usually takes one of two forms: it becomes isodense on CT, or isointense on MR, and then either resolves entirely, or a punctuate calcification may be left as a residue [41]. The time till resolution of the lesion is quite variable ranging from a few weeks to more than a year. SECTL are benign and tend to resolve spontaneously, without anticysticercal drugs or surgery, since the parasite is already in the degenerative phase and will eventually disappear or become calcified [1]. Treatment should be limited to medication required to control the acute symptoms, such as antiepileptic medication [2].

5. Neurocysticercosis as etiology of epilepsy

Analytical studies designed to establish associations and determinants of epilepsy have been scarce in DC. Comparing results of studies of etiology is difficult because of differences in definitions and lack of diagnostic criteria [3]. Most studies lack information on the latency between the first acute symptomatic seizure and the first unprovoked seizure, as well as age at onset of seizures and age at diagnosis. In studying etiology, it is preferable to use incident cases, not prevalent cases, because one cannot distinguish the potential etiological factors that preceded the onset of epilepsy from those which occurred after the disease developed. Cause and effect become confused. This is why It is extremely difficult to compare results of studies of epilepsy due to NC. These studies are few, and are frequently targeted at all seizures, instead of epilepsy alone. There are broad differences in the definition of NC, as well as failure to define criteria for diagnosis of either seizures or epilepsy.

Information available in developing countries shows that the proportion of idiopathic (60-70%) to symptomatic epilepsy (30-40%) is similar to that reported in studies from developed countries [8]. Among the symptomatic group, infection and parasitic diseases, particularly neurocysticercosis, perinatal brain damage, and head trauma are the most frequent disorders reported as a cause of epilepsy [5,42]. In a prospective cohort study of patients with newly-diagnosed epilepsy seen at the five main hospitals in the three major cities of Ecuador, perinatal brain damage (9%), neurocysticercosis (8.3%), central nervous system infections (4.2%), stroke (4.8%), and head trauma (4.2%) were the most frequent disorders reported as causes of epilepsy [42]. Although NCC is one of the most frequent antecedents among the symptomatic group, this disease is not necessarily the main cause of epilepsy, as has been previously suggested [11,17,43,44].

Hospital-based studies to analyze NCC as etiology of epilepsy are shown in Table 1. Studies of highly selected patients with seizures in neurologic services of hospital settings from some DC reported NCC as the main cause of epilepsy, accounting for 30% to 50% of patients [11,43]. In a study carried out in 212 patients with epilepsy, a rural sub-Saharan Africa area endemic for porcine cysticercosis [45], 2.4% were identified as definitive and 11% had lesions highly suggestive of NCC, using CT scan as part of the diagnoses. In another study from Africa, 37% of patients with epilepsy had NCC [46]. In studies from India, in which acute symptomatic seizures were excluded, only 11% (47) cases with epilepsy had NC; conversely, in a study of 572 patients with acute symptomatic seizures 67% had SECTL [48]. Another study was carried out in India [49] to determine the etiologic role of NCC in a hospital-based sample in 1026 patients with epilepsies divided according to the ILAE epidemiological criteria. NCC was diagnosed in imaging studies in 59% of those with acute symptomatic seizures, but only 2.0% with prevalent epilepsy, and none of the cases of incident epilepsy.

Author Country/year (reference)	# Pts.	Case Ascertainment	Type of study	NCC (%)
Medina et al México/1990 (11)	100	All seizures, CT scan	Prevalent cases	50%
Del Brutto et al Ecuador/1991 (43)	225	All seizures, CT scan	Prevalent cases	40%
Murthy et al India/1999 (48)	572	Acute seizures CT scan	Retrospect (SCTEL)	67 %
Sawhney et al India/1996 (47)	407	Single Sz. Excluded CT scan	Prevalent and incident cases	11 %
Singh G, et al India/2006 (49)	1026	Single, incident and prevalent seizures CT scan	Single Sz Prevalent cases Incident cases	59 % 2 % 0 %

Table 1. Neurocysticercosis as etiology of epilepsy: Hospital-based studies

The above mentioned studies confirm the necessity to differentiate between acute seizure and recurrent unprovoked seizures (epilepsy). It is likely that most of the patients with NCC have acute symptomatic seizures which do not necessarily evolve into epilepsy. Similarly, it is crucial to determine NCC as etiology of epilepsy in incident cases instead of prevalent ones. These are probably some of the reasons of over diagnosis of epilepsy in some hospital-based studies [3]

Community-based studies in which CT scan was used to diagnose NCC are shown in Table 2. In a study carried out in Ecuador [43], the authors concluded that NCC is associated with one in three cases of epilepsy and was possibly the cause of the excessive proportion of epilepsy in that population. However, only three (8%) of 24 people with epilepsy had "definitive" NCC. Another community survey [44] carried out in Peru showed that seroprevalence (using the enzyme-linked immunoelectrotransfer blot (EITB) assay] was positive in 24.2% (200/825); 15 of 39 individuals with seizures (38.5%) had lesions compatible with NCC on CT scan. The authors concluded that brain CT abnormalities compatible with

NCC were more frequent in individuals with seizures and in those with positive EITB for cysticercosis. Most of the patients who were diagnosed with NCC in this study had only calcifications (half of them had just one calcification); however, it is well known that brain calcifications do not necessarily mean NC. The small population samples of the above studies do not allow generalizations.

Author Country/year	Patients with epilepsy	Inclusion criteria	Diagnosis of NCC	NCC No. (%)
Montano, et al Perú/2005 (44)	39	All seizures Prevalent cases	CT scan, > 50% only 1 calcification	15 (38)
Del Brutto, et al Ecuador/2005 (43)	19	Recurrent seizures Prevalent cases	CT scan, All pts had only 1 calcification	5 (26)
Medina et al Honduras/2005 (11)	100	Recurrent seizures Prevalent cases	CT scan,	37(37)

Table 2. Neurocysticercosis as an etiology of epilepsy: Community-based studies

There are several studies in the medical literature that have reported an association between epilepsy and NCC based on positive serum antibodies to Taenia solium/cysticercosis [17,50,51]. Unfortunately, the presence of antibodies may indicate only previous exposure to or infection with the parasite, but not necessarily brain infection. This information has created some distortion in the current perception of NCC epidemiology. A systematic review of the literature on the frequency of NCC, diagnosed with neuroimaging, has been published [15]. Overall, 565 articles were retrieved and only 26 had reliable information to estimate the frequency of NCC in various populations worldwide. The authors concluded that the prevalence of NCC worldwide remains unknown; however, the proportion of NCC among persons with epilepsy was very consistent and estimated at 29.6% (95%CI: 23.5%–36.1%) from 12 studies conducted in Latin America, Sub-Saharan Africa, and Southeast Asia.

6. Inconsistencies in the relationship between neurocysticercosis and epilepsy

There are clinical inconsistencies in the link between epilepsy and NCC. Parasite location may be remote from the apparent epileptogenic region [3]. There is also no correlation between the NCC burden of lesions and the severity of the epilepsy. Patients with severe refractory seizures may have only one calcified lesion; on the other hand, there are patients with multiple cysts or calcifications but no seizures.

EEG has been found to be abnormal in 30-50% of patients with seizures due to NC. It is assumed that EEG findings have poor correlation with symptoms and CT lesions in patients with NCC [52.53]. A positive correlation between CT lesions and localizing or lateralizing

EEG abnormalities has been reported for only 15-30% of patients. Similarly, the correlation between seizure type and EEG abnormalities ranges from around 7% to 20% [53]. Discrepancies between clinical localization based on seizure semiology and location of the lesion on neuroimaging is a not uncommon feature in patients with NC. A non-causal relationship between epilepsy and cysticercosis in some cases might explain these apparent discrepancies [54,55]. Further prospective cohort studies, properly designed to study ictal and interictal EEG abnormalities in patients with seizures, correlated with the different evolutionary stages of the parasite, may clarify the relationship between NCC and epilepsy.

The coexistence of hippocampal atrophy and extrahippocampal pathological abnormalities, such as cortical dysgenesis and gliosis, referred to as "dual pathology", has been reported in 5 to 30% of patients with medically refractory partial seizures [56]. Dual pathology implies that both lesions somehow interact with each other and contribute to epileptogenesis through mechanisms still poorly understood. Some authors have also attributed hippocampal sclerosis to NCC [54.57,58]. Patients with calcifications due to NCC and mesial temporal lobe epilepsy (hippocampal sclerosis) became seizure free after anteromesial temporal lobectomy, without resection of the cysticercotic lesion [35], suggesting the two phenomena are independent. The presence of CNL does not influence the clinical and pathologic profile of patients with hippocampal atrophy. An irritative zone in the temporal lobe is more relevant in determining the severity, symptomatology and frequency of seizures than the number and location of calcifications [59]. The possibility of dual pathology related to NCC needs further clarification in prospective cohort studies.

NCC and epilepsy are common diseases in most developing countries. Because of their high prevalence, a causal as well as fortuitous relationship between the two conditions might exist [35,54,60] NCC is also an uncommon cause of intractable epilepsy, even in endemic regions and that it may only represent a coexistent pathology, according to a cross sectional study investigating the etiology of intractable epilepsy in 512 patients in Brazil [61].

7. Effect of antihelminthic drug treatment on recurrence of seizures

Treatment for NCC with antihelminthic drugs (AHD) such as praziquantel and albendazole has been available for at least 25 years, and since then its use has been controversial. Praziquantel was used for the first time in México [62]. Albendazole was used for the first time in China [63] .

To date, there are no controlled clinical trials to establish definitive doses and duration of treatment. A meta-analysis was published in 2005 [64], in which only 11 studies, among 764, were selected, only 6 with viable cysts and 5 with degenerative or coloidal cysts. The authors reported disappearance of viable cysts in 44% of patients who were treated with albendazole vs. 19% of the placebo group ($p < 0.025$). They also reported disappearance of degenerative cysts in 72% of patients of the albendazole group, and 63 % of the placebo group, but there was no statistical significance ($p < 0.38$). The Editors of the journal where this meta-analysis was published affirmed that selected studies were small and heterogeneous, and only 5 of 11 were good quality. They concluded that studies provided limited evidence of a modest effect of NCC treatment, since the effects of cysticidal treatment on neuroimaging end points were relatively small (OR <2.2) . A recent Cochrane review [65] of 21 randomized controlled clinical trials of cysticidal therapy concluded that with adults with viable cysts the use of albendazole is associated with a decrease in the number of cysts but not in the recurrence of seizures lesions.

One of the main reasons for which there is a lot of confusion in the medical literature and a supposed controversy regarding the effectiveness of AHD, is that most of the publications report "reduction of the number of lesions" as a valid endpoint to measure effectiveness of the treatment, which is misleading. We should wonder, for example, in the hypothetical event that a person with 10 viable cysts has been administered AHD, whether, as a consequence of the treatment, 8 parasite die (80% reduction of lesion/successful treatment?), but two cysts remain which may provoke seizures or headache: Is this a successful treatment? Maybe not.

The appropriate end point to evaluate the effectiveness of AHD could be the disappearance of cysts. Strictly speaking, even in the case that treatment with AHD may kill all parasites in a patient, it is not possible to talk about "cure" because, as we know, most cysts once they die became calcifications, a permanent sequel, which could aggravate seizures long life If we compare those studies in which one of the end points to evaluate effectiveness of AHD is disappearance of cysts (table 3), including the results of the abovementioned meta-analysis, where about 30% to 40% of patients had disappearance of cysts [66-68]. Therefore, there is no controversy; we can affirm that, according to available evidence based medicine, AHD are effective in one third of patients, approximately.

8. Risk of seizure recurrence in patients with neurocysticercosis

Some authors report that NCC patients with acute symptomatic seizures have a good prognosis in terms of remission of seizures [69-73]; others report that most patients have a high risk of seizure recurrence, and suggest that prognosis improves after antihelminthic treatment. [66]. Prospective cohort studies have determined the risk of seizure recurrence after a first seizure due to NCC is between 17% to 56%, depending on the viability of the parasite. The risk is greater in the transitional forms and it diminishes in the viable or calcified forms [73-76]. Overall, the risk of seizure recurrence involves around one third of patients.

It has also been suggested that seizure control in patients with NCC is improved and that the chance of remaining seizure-free after the withdrawal of antiepileptic drugs is greater after a course of AHD, when compared with seizure control in those in whom the disease is left untreated [66]. However, current reliable information has shown that AHD treatment in patients with seizures due to NCC is not associated with the recurrence of seizures at all [67,68] (Table 3).

Regarding the duration for which antiseizure medication should be continued following an acute NCC episode, some clinicians routinely continue antiseizure medication for 1 year, but shorter and longer intervals have been recommended [1]. One assumes that the risk of seizures is substantial as long as there is an active ongoing process as characterized by persistence of edema around the degenerating lesion. Because of this, CT scan is a useful tool for these treatment decisions. It is appropriate to monitor cyst activity with CT scanning and to continue antiseizure medication until resolution of the acute lesion. After this time antiseizure medication may be discontinued [1]. Seizures occurring in individuals after resolution of edema and resorption or calcification of the degenerating cyst should be considered unprovoked and, in this situation, long-term antiseizure medication is warranted.

Author/year, reference	Treatment groups (No. patients)	Cysts disappearance* No./%	Seizures recurrence** No./%
Garcia H, et al. 2004 (66)	Albendazole (55) Placebo (54)	21 (38%) 8 (15%)	32 (56%) 32 (54%)
Carpio A, et al. 2008, (73)	Albendazole (51) Placebo (50)	18 (35%) 6 (12%)	19 38%) 27 (48%)
Das K, et al. 2007 (68)	Albendazole (148) Placebo (150)	10 (7%) 12 (8%)	40 (27%) 24 (16%)

* CT scan at 6 months after finishing treatment

** Seizures recurrence at one year follow-up

Table 3. Effects of cysticidal drugs on resolution of parenchymal viable cysts and seizures recurrence in patients with neurocysticercosis (randomized, placebo-controlled studies)

It seems that interpretation of risk of seizures after neurocysticercosis is difficult. These difficulties are increased in those patients who have mixed forms, including active, transitional, and calcified lesions. Further studies should be performed in order to estimate recurrence risk in those patients with seizures due to calcifications alone, in comparison with patients with acute seizures due to transitional cysts.

9. Conclusions

Epilepsy and NCC are common diseases in poor countries, and NCC is increasingly diagnosed in developed countries due to migration from endemic regions. However, reliable data concerning prevalence and incidence of NCC is lacking worldwide.

Seizures are the most common symptom in patients with the parenchymal location of the parasite. Seizures may occur at any evolutionary stage of the parasite, but acute symptomatic seizures are more frequent in the transitional form, due to the inflammatory response of the brain. Most people with NCC have acute symptomatic seizures that do not necessarily evolve into epilepsy. This is one of the reasons that epilepsy is over diagnosed in some studies. The ILAE's Commission on Epidemiology includes NCC as a comorbid condition associated with epilepsy.

There are inconsistencies in the link between epilepsy and NC. Because of the high prevalence of each condition, a causal as well as fortuitous relationship between the two pathologies might exist. NCC is not necessarily the main cause of epilepsy in endemic countries, although it is one of the most frequent antecedents among adult patients with symptomatic epilepsy.

Several studies have reported an association between epilepsy and NCC based on positive serum antibodies to Taenia solium/cysticercosis. This information has created distortion in the perception of NCC epidemiology

Seizures in the context of edema and a degenerative lesion should be considered acute symptomatic even if they occur many months after presentation. After resolution of the acute lesion antiseizure medication may be discontinued. Seizures occurring after resolution of edema or calcification of the degenerating cyst should be considered unprovoked and, in this situation, long term antiepileptic medication is warranted. There is no correlation between treatment with antihelminthic agents and seizure recurrence

The prognosis of seizure in patients with NCC is good. In about two thirds of the patients with acute symptomatic seizures due to NCC the seizures do not recur [67] People with acute seizures NCC should be treated with antiseizure medication until cyst resolution on CT scan. The risk of seizure recurrence (epilepsy) occurs in the inactive or calcified form of NC.

Recommendations: Further research should be undertaken in order to clarify: -the natural history of T.Solium/cysticercosis disease, -the variability of antihelminthic treatment efficacy, -the factors that contribute to clinical heterogeneity of NC, -immunological response of the host. It is also recommended to standardize a common methodology, including definitions, in order to propose new diagnoses criteria for NCC.

Health authorities should focus on prevention and eradication of taeniasis/cysticercosis in order to decrease the number of individuals with seizures/epilepsy and other consequences.

Author details

Arturo Carpio
School of Medicine, University of Cuenca, Ecuador
G.H. Sergievsky Center, Columbia University, New York, USA

10. References

[1] Carpio A. Neurocysticercosis: an update. Lancet Infectious Diseases. 2002;2:751-762.

[2] Pal DK, Carpio A, Sander JWAS. Neurocysticercosis and Epilepsy. J Neurol Neurosurg Psychiatry 2000;68:137-143

[3] Carpio A, Escobar A, Hauser WA: Epilepsy and cysticercosis: a critical review. Epilepsia 1998;39:1025-1040.

[4] Ferreira LS, Li LM, Zanardi VA, Guerreiro MM. Number and viability of parasite influence seizure frequency in children with neurocysticercosis. Arq Neuropsiquiatr. 2002;60(4):909-911

[5] Martinez, H.R., Rangel-Guerra, R., Arredondo-Estrada, J.H., et al. Medical and surgical treatment in neurocysticercosis. A magnetic resonance study of 161 cases. Journal of Neurological Science 1995;130:25-34

[6] Thurman DJ, Beghi E, Begley CE, Berg AT, Buchhalter JR, et al. ILAE Commission on Epidemiology. Standards for epidemiologic studies and surveillance of epilepsy. Epilepsia. 2011;52 Suppl 7:2-26.

[7] Hauser WA, Hesdorffer DH. Epilepsy: frequency, causes and consequences. New York: Demos Press; 1990.

[8] Bharucha NE, Carpio A, Gallo Diop A. Epidemiology of Epilepsy in Developing Countries . In: Engel P. Pedley T, editors. Epilepsy. A comprehensive textbook, 2nd ed. Phladelphia: Lippincot Williams & Wilkins. 2008:89-101

[9] Banerjee PN, Hauser WA. Incidence and prevalence. In: Engel P. Pedley T, editors. Epilepsy. A comprehensive textbook, 2nd ed. Philadelphia: Lippincot Williams & Wilkins; 2008:45-56.

[10] Mungala-Odera V, White S, Meehan R, et al. Prevalence, incidence and risk factors of epilepsy in older children in rural Kenya. Seizure. 2008;17:396-404..

[11] Medina MT, Duron RM, Martinez L, et al. Prevalence, incidence, and etiology of epilepsies in rural Honduras: the Salama study. Epilepsia 2005;46:124–131.

[12] Commission on Epidemiology and Prognosis of the International League Against Epilepsy. Guidelines for epidemiologic studies on epilepsy. Epilepsia 1993;34:592–596.

[13] Carpio A, Hauser WA. Epilepsy in the developing world. Current neurology and neuroscience reports. 2009;9(4):319-26

[14] Lino RS, Jr., Faleiros AC, Vinaud MC, Oliveira FA, Guimaraes JV, et al. Anatomopathological aspects of neurocysticercosis in autopsied patients]. Arq Neuropsiquiatr 2007;65:87–91.

[15] Ndimubanzi PC, Carabin H, Budke CM, Nguyen H, Qian YJ, et al. A systematic review of the frequency of neurocyticercosis with a focus on people with epilepsy. PLoS Negl Trop Dis. 2010 Nov 2;4(11):e870

[16] Fleury, A., Morales, J., Bobes, R.J., Dumas, M., Yanez, O., et al. An epidemiological study of familial neurocysticercosis in an endemic Mexican community. Trans. R. Soc. Trop. Med. Hyg. 2006;100:551-558.

[17] Goodman K, Ballagh SA, Carpio A. Case control study of seropositivity for cysticercosis in Cuenca, Ecuador. Am J Trop Med Hyg 1999;60:70-4.

[18] Garcia HH, Gilman R, Martìnez M, Twang VCW. Cysticercosis as a major cause of epilepsy in Peru. Lancet 1993;341:197-200.

[19] Garcia-Noval J, Moreno E, de Mata F, et al. An epidemiological study of epilepsy and epileptic seizures in two rural Guatemalan communities. Ann Trop Med Parasitol 2001;95:167–175.

[20] Carpio A, Placencia M, Santillán F, Escobar A. A Proposal for a classification of neurocysticercosis. Can J Neuro Sci. 19942;1:43-47.

[21] Escobar A. The pathology of neurocysticercosis In, Palacios E, Rodriguez-Carbajal J, Taveras JM, eds. Cysticercosis of Central Nervous System. Springfield: Charles C Thomas, 1983. 27-54.

[22] Zee CS, Go JL, Kim PE, DiGiorgio CM. Imaging of neurocysticercosis. Neuroimaging Clin N Am 2000;10:391-407.

[23] Berg AT, Scheffer IE. New concepts in classification of the epilepsies: entering the 21st century. Epilepsia. 2011;52(6):1058-62.

[24] Fisher RS, van Emde Boas W, Blume W, Elger C, Genton P, et al. Epileptic seizures and epilepsy: definitions proposed by the International League Against Epilepsy (ILAE) and the International Bureau for Epilepsy (IBE). Epilepsia 2005;46:470–472.

[25] Beghi E, Carpio A, Forsgren L, Hesdorffer DC, Malmgren K, et al. Recommendation for a definition of acute symptomatic seizure. Epilepsia. 2010;51(4):671-5.

[26] Carabin H, Ndimubanzi PC, Budke CM, Nguyen H, Qian Y, et al. Clinical Manifestations Associated with Neurocysticercosis: A Systematic Review. PLoS Negl Trop Dis 2011;5(5): e1152. doi:10.1371/journal.pntd.0001152.

[27] Murthy, J.M., Reddy, V.S. Clinical characteristics, seizure spread patterns and prognosis of seizures associated with a single small cerebral calcified CT lesion. Seizure. 1998;7:153-157.

[28] Kelvin EA, Carpio A, Bagiella E, Leslie D, Leon P, et al. Seizure in people with newly diagnosed active or transitional neurocysticercosis. Seizure. 2011;20:119-25

[29] Kelvin EA, Carpio A, Bagiella E, Leslie D, Leon P, Andrews H, et al. The association of host age and gender with inflammation around neurocysticercosis cysts. Ann Trop Med Parasitol. 2009;103:487-99.

[30] Fleury A, Escobar A, Fragoso G, Sciutto E, Larralde C. Clinical heterogeneity of human neurocysticercosis results from complex interactions among parasite,host and environmental factors. Trans R Soc Trop Med Hyg. 2010;104:243-50

[31] Singh G. Neurocysticercosis in South-Central America and the Indian subcontinent. A comparative evaluation. Arq Neuropsiquiatr 1997;55:349–56.

[32] Kelvin, E.A., Carpio, A., Hesdorffer, D.C., Bagiella, E., Leslie, D. et al. Investigation of familial aggregation of seizures in neurocysticercosis patients. Epilepsy Res 2009;84:67-71

[33] Rathore C, Radhakrishnan K. What causes seizures in patients with calcified neurocysticercal lesions? Neurology. 2012;78(9):612-3.

[34] Antoniuk SA, Bruck I, Dos Santos LH, Pintarelli VL, Navolar FB, et al. Seizures associated with calcifications and edema in neurocysticercosis. Pediatr Neurol. 2001;25(4):309-311.

[35] Leite JP, Terra-Bustamante VC, Fernandes RM, Santos AC, Chimelli L, et al. Calcified neurocysticercotic lesions and postsurgery seizure control in temporal lobe epilepsy. Neurology. 2000;55(10):1485-1491.

[36] Nash TE, Pretell EJ, Lescano AG, et al. Cysticercosis Working Group in Peru. Perilesional brain oedema and seizure activity in patients with calcified neurocysticercosis: a prospective cohort and nested case-control study. Lancet Neurol. 2008;7:1099-1105.

[37] Jayakumar PN, Taly AB, Mohan PK. Transient computerised tomographic (CT) abnormalities following partial seizures. Acta Neurol Scand. 1985;72(1):26-9.

[38] Bansal BC, Dua A, Gupta R, Gupta MS. Appearing and disappearing CT scan abnormalities in epilepsy in India--an enigma. J Neurol Neurosurg Psychiatry. 1989;52(10):1185-1187.

[39] Gupta RK, Awasthi R, Rathore RK, Verma A, Sahoo P, et al. Understanding epileptogenesis in calcified neurocysticercosis with perfusion MRI. Neurology. 2012;78(9):618-625.

[40] Rajshekhar V, Jeyaseelan L. Seizure outcome in patients with a solitary cerebral cysticercus granuloma. Neurology. 2004;62(12):2236-40.

[41] Singh G, Rajshekhar V, Murthy JM, Prabhakar S, Modi M, et al. A diagnostic and therapeutic scheme for a solitary cysticercus granuloma. Neurology. 2010 Dec 14;75(24):2236-45.

[42] Carpio A, Hauser WA. Remote symptomatic epilepsies and epileptic syndromes: Etiological spectrum. In: Murthy JMK, Senanayke N (Eds). Epilepsy in the Tropics. Landes Bioscience, Georgetown, USA, 2006:72-84.

[43] Del Brutto OH, Santibanez R, Idrovo L, et al. Epilepsy and neurocysticercosis in Atahualpa: a door-to-door survey in rural coastal Ecuador. Epilepsia. 2005;46:583-587

[44] Montano SM, Villaran MV, Ylquimiche L, et al. Neurocysticercosis. Association between seizures, serology, and brain CT in rural Peru. Neurology 2005;65:229–233.

[45] Winkler AS, Blocher J, Auer H, et al. Anticysticercal and antitoxocaral antibodies in people with epilepsy in rural Tanzania.Trans R Soc Trop Med Hyg. 2008;102:1032-1038.

[46] Foyaca-Sibat H, Cowan LD, Carabin H, Targonska I, Anwary MA, et al. Accuracy of Serological Testing for the Diagnosis of Prevalent Neurocysticercosis in Outpatients with Epilepsy, Eastern Cape Province, South Africa. PLoS Negl Trop Dis 2009;3(12): e562. doi:10.1371/journal.pntd.0000562,

[47] Sawhney MI, Lekhra OP, Shashi JS, Prabhakar S, Chopra JS. Evaluation of epilepsy management in a developing country: a prospective study of 407 patients. Acta Neurol Scand 1996;94:19-23

[48] Murthy JM, Yangala R. Acute symptomatic seizures - incidence and etiological spectrum: a hospital-based study from South India. Seizure. 1999;8(3):162-165.

[49] Singh G, Singh P, Singh I, et al. Epidemiologic classification of seizures associated with neurocysticercosis: observations from a sample of seizure disorders in neurologic care in India. Acta Neurol Scand. 2006;113:233-240.

[50] Prasad KN, Prasad A, Gupta RK, et al. Neurocysticercosis in patients with active epilepsy from the pig farming community of Lucknow district, north India. Trans R Soc Trop Med Hyg. 2009;103:144-150.

[51] Blocher J, Schmutzhard E, Wilkins PP, Gupton PN, Schaffert M, et al. A cross-sectional study of people with epilepsy and neurocysticercosis in Tanzania: clinical characteristics and diagnostic approaches. PLoS Negl Trop Dis. 2011;5(6):e1185.

[52] Chayasirisobhon, S., Menoni, R., Chayasirisobhon, W., et al. Correlation of electroencephalography and the active and inactive forms of neurocysticercosis. Clinical Electroencephalography. 1999;30:9-11.

[53] Cukiert, A., Puglia, P., Scapola, H.B., et al. Congruence of the topography of intracraneal calcifications and epileptic foci. Arq Neuropsiquiatr 1993;52:289-294.

[54] Sakamoto AC et al. Cysticercosis and Epilepsy. In, Kotagal P, Luders HO, eds. The Epilepsies: Etiologies and Prevention. San Diego: Academic Press, 1999. 275-282.

[55] Singh, G., Sachdev, M.S., Tirath, A., Gupta, A.K., Avasthi, G. Focal cortical-subcortical calcifications (FCSCs) and epilepsy in the Indian subcontinent. Epilepsia. 2000;41:718-726.

[56] Cendes, F., Cook, M.J., Watson, C., et al. Frequency and characteristics of dual pathology in patients with lesional epilepsy. Neurology 1995;45:2058-2064.

[57] Singla M, Singh P, Kaushal S, Bansal R, Singh G. Hippocampal sclerosis in association with neurocysticercosis. Epileptic Disord. 2007;9(3):292-9

[58] Rathore C, Thomas B, Kesavadas C, Radhakrishnan K. Calcified neurocysticercosis lesions and hippocampal sclerosis: potential dual pathology? Epilepsia. 2012;53(4):e60-2.

[59] Kowacs PA, Rogacheski E, Muzzio J, Werneck LC: The role of the irritative zone and of the number and distribution of calcifications in the severity of epilepsy associated with intracranial calcifications. Arq Neuropsiquiatr 2006;64:905–911.

[60] Terra-Bustamante VC, Coimbra ER, Rezek KO, et al.: Cognitive performance of patients with mesial temporal lobe epilepsy and incidental calcified neurocysticercosis. J Neurol Neurosurg Psychiatry 2005:76:1080–1083.

[61] Velasco TR, Zanello PA, Dalmagro CL, Araújo D Jr, Santos AC, et al. Calcified cysticercotic lesions and intractable epilepsy: a cross sectional study of 512 patients. J Neurol Neurosurg Psychiatry. 2006;77(4):485-488.

[62] Robles C, Chavarrıa M. Presentacion de un caso clınico de cisticercosis cerebral tratado medicamente con un nuevo farmaco: Praziquantel. Salud Publica de Mexico 1979;epoca V;XXI(5).pp. 603-618.

[63] Xiao ZX, Zhao CY, Liu LP. Albendazole treatment in cerebral cysticercosis. Chin J Int Med. 1986;25:100-102

[64] Del Brutto, O. H. Roos, K. L. Coffey C. S. Garcıa, H. H.. Meta-analysis: cysticidal drugs for neurocysticercosis: albendazole and praziquantel. Annals of Internal Medicine. 2006;45:43–51,.

[65] Abba K, Ramaratnam S, Ranganathan LN. Anthelmintics for people with neurocysticercosis. Cochrane Database Syst Rev. 2010 Mar 17;(3):CD000215.

[66] Garcia H, Pretell E, Gilman R, et al. A trial of antiparasitic treatment to reduce the rate of seizures due to cerebral cysticercosis. N Engl J Med 2004; 350:249-258..

[67] Carpio A, Kelvin E, Bagiella E, et al. The effects of albendazole treatment on neurocysticercosis: a randomized controlled trial. J Neurol Neurosurg Psychiatry, 2008;79:1050-1055

[68] Das K, Mondal GP, Banerjee M, Mukherjee BB, Singh OP. Role of antiparasitic therapy for seizures and resolution of lesions in neurocysticercosis patients: an 8 year randomised study. J Clin Neurosci. 2007;14(12):1172-1177.

[69] Singhi P, Ray M, Singhi S, et al. Clinical spectrum of 500 children with neurocysticercosis and response to albendazole therapy. J Child Neurol 2000;15:207-213.

[70] Manreza ML. Epilepsia e neurocisticerose. In, Guerreiro CAM, Guerreiro MM, Cendes F, Lopes-Cendes I, eds. Epilepsia. Sao Paulo: Lemos Editorial. 2000. 255-264

[71] Ferreira LS, Zanardi VA, Scotoni AE, Li LM, Guerreiro MM. Childhood epilepsy due to neurocysticercosis: a comparative study. Epilepsia. 2001;42:1438-1444.

[72] Goel D, Mittal M, Bansal KK, Singhal A. Natural history of solitary cerebral cysticercosis cases after albendazole therapy: a longitudinal follow-up study from India. Acta Neurol Scand. 2010;121(3):204-208.

[73] Carpio A, Hauser W: Prognosis for seizure recurrence in patients with newly diagnosed neurocysticercosis. Neurology 2002;59:1730–1734.

[74] De Souza A, Thennarasu K, Yeshraj G, et al.: Randomized controlled trial of albendazole in new onset epilepsy and MRI confirmed solitary cerebral cysticercal lesion: effect on long-term seizure outcome. J Neurol Sci 2009;276:108–114.

[75] Sharma P, Garg RK, Verma R, Singh MK, Shukla R. Risk of seizure recurrence in patients of new-onset partial seizure having a solitary cysticercus granuloma of brain or normal neuroimaging. J Neurol Sci. 2011;15;301:21-26.

[76] Thussu A, Chattopadhyay A, Sawhney IM, Khandelwal N: Albendazole therapy for single small enhancing CT lesions (SSECTL) in the brain in epilepsy. J Neurol Neurosurg Psychiatry 2008;79:272–275.

Chapter 12

Epilepsy and Neurocysticercosis in Sub-Saharan Africa

Andrea Sylvia Winkler

Additional information is available at the end of the chapter

http://dx.doi.org/10.5772/53289

1. Introduction

In sub-Saharan Africa neurocysticercosis (NCC), which represents the infection of a human brain with the larva (=cysticercus) of the pork tapeworm (=*Taenia solium*), and epilepsy due to various causes are among the most frequent neurological disorders/syndromes. To date, NCC in the context of sub-Saharan Africa has not attracted much attention despite the fact that the prevalence rates of human and porcine cysticercosis seem to increase and both diseases are treatable. Epilepsy represents the most common neurological disorder in many parts of sub-Saharan Africa and NCC seems to be a major cause of it in *Taenia solium* cysticercosis endemic areas. Diagnosing NCC among people with epilepsy is vital as this not only prevents further morbidity and mortality through potential aggravation of the disease, but also leads to a different treatment approach: from a mere symptomatic treatment with administration of antiepileptic medication only to a curative approach, assuming that once the parasite has been cleared epileptic seizures will cease. However, in the diagnosis and treatment of NCC neuroimaging plays a crucial role and this has to be considered when dealing with affected individuals form resource-poor settings, where neuroimaging is not available. Therefore special diagnostic and therapeutic guidelines for sub-Saharan Africa have to be developed, but so far national and international stakeholders have not taken this into consideration. This chapter aims at raising awareness of both NCC and epilepsy in sub-Saharan African, appealing to the international community to consider NCC in resource-poor settings as a separate entity regarding its diagnostic and therapeutic approach with the need for clearly defined guidelines in the described context.

1.1. Definition of epilepsy and acute symptomatic epileptic seizures

A condition characterized by recurrent (two or more) afebrile epileptic seizures that is unprovoked by any immediate identified cause and thus is not due to an acute intracranial or extracranial condition is termed epilepsy [1]. A person who has had a seizure within the

INTECH
open science | open minds

© 2013 Winkler, licensee InTech. This is a paper distributed under the terms of the Creative Commons Attribution License (http://creativecommons.org/licenses/by/3.0), which permits unrestricted use, distribution, and reproduction in any medium, provided the original work is properly cited.

last five years and those on anticonvulsant medication are considered to have "active epilepsy" [1,2]. The definition of active epilepsy does not have implications on starting antiepileptic treatment. Some African researchers suggest starting treatment if the last seizure was within the previous year [3]. We advocate for a more flexible initiation of antiepileptic treatment. Treatment of epilepsy always has to be considered on a multifactorial basis and includes the risk of recurrence based on seizure pathology (e.g., generalized versus focal epilepsy), seizure frequency, associated disease and available antiepileptic treatment, among others.

Epileptic seizures that are based on intracranial pathologies, such as parasitic disease, cerebrovascular accidents or trauma, and stop after the underlying cause, e.g. the associated oedema, has resolved, are called acute symptomatic epileptic seizures and have to be differentiated from epileptic seizures in the context of "chronic" epilepsy. In "chronic epilepsy" brain lesions may still be present, but they belong to the entity of neurological sequelae such as calcifications after parasitic diseases or chronic lesions in the context of cerebrovascular accidents or trauma, among others. These lesions most likely will not undergo further changes and therefore the "chronic" epilepsy type is treated symptomatically with antiepileptic drugs. In acute symptomatic epileptic seizures treatment of the primary cause is mandatory, if possible, but antiepileptic drugs are often added. After the acute phase withdrawal of antiepileptic treatment is desirable, but has to be decided on a case-to-case basis.

1.2. Prevalence of epilepsy in sub-Saharan Africa

In sub-Saharan Africa, epilepsy is among the most common neurological disorders. Its devastating impact on individuals suffering from it as well as on affected African communities was described as early as 1960 in Mahenge, southern Tanzania [4]. These early anecdotal reports were corroborated by a large-scale hospital-based study in Nigeria in the 1970s [5]. Since then, prevalence data on epilepsy have been collected in community-based studies throughout Africa with varying results depending on the study population and the methodologies used (mainly on active epilepsy), ranging from 5.2-74.4/1000 with a median of 15/1000 inhabitants [6,7]. This is compared to high-income countries where the prevalence of active epilepsy is estimated to be about 4-8/1000 inhabitants [8]. Interestingly, hotspots of highly prevalent epilepsy have been reported in various African countries such as Benin, the Ivory Coast, Cameroon, Nigeria, Senegal and Tanzania [6,9]. Causes for these high prevalence rates have so far not been identified, but they are deemed to be partly genetic in nature, most likely with a consistent environmental factor that affects genetically predisposed individuals [6].

Our own data from a hospital-based study on neurological disorders in northern Tanzania show epileptic seizures to be the most prevalent neurological disorder [10,11]. Of the 740 patients with neurological symptoms/signs, 272 (36.8%) had at least one epileptic seizure during their stay at the hospital or immediately before admission to the hospital. Febrile seizures (82/272; 30.2%) accounted for the majority of epileptic seizures. This was followed by symptomatic epileptic seizures (72/272; 26.5%), which were mainly due to cerebral infections, then epilepsy (65/272; 23.9%) as defined by the International League Against Epilepsy [1]. Assumed symptomatic seizures without an obvious cause that did not meet the criteria of epilepsy occurred in 15.4% (42/272) and pseudoseizures were witnessed in 4.0% (11/272). The mortality rate of the patients with epileptic seizures was high with 18.8% (51/272). Peak mortality rates were found in people with symptomatic disease and those with assumed symptomatic epileptic seizures, at 38.9% (28/72) and 31.0% (13/42), respectively. These results clearly show where the burden of neurological disorders in sub-Saharan Africa, in our case northern Tanzania, lies and have implications for the objective of delivering appropriate care for patients suffering from epileptic seizures [10].

The high prevalence rates of epileptic seizures/epilepsy found in the above hospital-based study were also confirmed in a community-based setting. Of the 7399 people who were visited in a community-based study in the same area the above hospital-based study was conducted 83 people were diagnosed with epilepsy and of those 64 had active epilepsy (last seizure within the last 5 years; [12]). The point prevalence of epilepsy within the study population of 7399 people was 11.2/1000 (95% CI 8.9-13.9/1000) with an age-adjusted prevalence of 13.2/1000. The prevalence of active epilepsy was 8.7/1000 (95% CI 6.7-11.0/1000) with an age-adjusted rate of 9.1/1000. The majority of patients suffered from generalized epilepsies. Not surprisingly, three quarters of the people with epilepsy had never accessed any health facilities [12].

Our findings confirm high prevalence rates of epileptic seizures/epilepsy in the hospital and the community, which agrees with the results of previous epidemiological studies of epilepsy in sub-Saharan Africa [5,6,9,13-19]. Most studies conducted in parts of Africa and Latin America indicate higher prevalence rates of epilepsy than have been found in high-income countries, but these prevalence rates can vary within a single country, as shown in Benin, the Ivory Coast, Senegal and Tanzania [6,9,19]. In a recent large-scale study from Kenya, it was shown that the active prevalence was only 4.5/1000, and therefore in the range of prevalence rates of high-income countries, with a high heterogeneity of prevalence rates across different areas ranging from below 1.0/1000 to 12.9/1000 [3]. Active epilepsy was defined as at least one seizure during the last year (the usual definition is one seizure during the last five years; see 1.1.) which may account for the lower prevalence rate found.

1.3. Classification of epileptic seizures/epilepsy in resource-poor settings

Classifying epileptic seizures/epilepsy in resource-poor countries can be challenging, bearing in mind that the availability of diagnostic tools such as appropriate serological investigations, electroencephalography and neuroimaging can be scare or, especially in rural Africa, absent altogether. Whether the seizures reported in rural Africa are primarily generalized or focal in nature is still a matter of debate and depends upon the setting and methodology used (e.g. hospital-based versus community-based), the country of investigation, the questionnaires used (different sensitivities and specificities) and the diagnostic tools available [6]. While members of the International League Against Epilepsy have developed consensus papers on the best classification of epileptic seizures [20] and epilepsies [21,22] that are considered international standards, they mainly refer to high-income countries, which only include 20% of all people with epilepsy worldwide [23,24]. In contrast, appropriate classification systems for epileptic seizures/epilepsy in low-income countries seem to be virtually absent. Seizure semiology, the description of which can be incomplete due to language and sociocultural barriers, and important seizure related issues such as possible aetiologies and concomitant diseases (e.g. perinatal neurological sequelae) are relevant for the classification of epileptic seizures/epilepsy in these countries and should form parts of an adapted classification system. The growing relevance of global neurology together with the already substantial burden of epileptic seizures/epilepsy in sub-Saharan Africa calls for an expert-led committee to decide on an appropriate classification system for epileptic seizures/epilepsy for clinical use in low-resource countries.

We suggest a classification system that is based on clinical grounds alone, and mainly refers to the description of seizures provided by the patients and their relatives along with relevant information from past medical histories, birth and family histories and a thorough neurological examination. Electroencephalography and neuroimaging are not usually at hand in resource-poor settings and therefore are not included in the classification system. The classification system suggested is based on the classification of epileptic seizures and epilepsy as stipulated by the International League Against Epilepsy [1,20-22]. Based on our experience while working in northern Tanzania we identified four main categories of epileptic seizures/epilepsy that have different needs for further investigation, treatment and follow-up, showing variable prognoses ([25,26]; Figure 1).

Generalized types of seizure:

1. *Generalized seizures within a specific age range:* primary generalized seizures that start within a specific age group (mainly between 6 and 25 years). Seizures in this group can also be termed idiopathic generalized epilepsy.
   Cause: none obvious
   Prognosis: good
   Investigations: keep to a minimum
2. *Generalized seizures outside a specific age range:* primary generalized seizures that start outside the specific age range of most of the idiopathic generalized epilepsies where no symptoms/signs on clinical examination suggest a secondary cause.
   Cause: none obvious, seizures may be "cryptogenic".
   Prognosis: variable
   Investigations: further investigations necessary (electroencephalography, neuroimaging)

Partial types of seizure that clinically appear as generalized seizures:

3. *Generalized seizures with diffuse brain damage:* secondary generalized seizures that start in a generalized way, but diffuse brain damage with mental retardation is obvious. The large majority of patients are children.
   Cause: mostly known (e.g. birth defect)
   Prognosis: variable
   Investigations: keep to a minimum

4. *Generalized seizures with focal signs:* secondary generalized seizures with a focal start, clear unilateral seizures or focal neurological signs upon examination but without signs of diffuse brain damage.
Cause: may become obvious upon further investigation
Prognosis: depends on the underlying cause
Investigations: further investigations necessary (electroencephalography, neuroimaging)

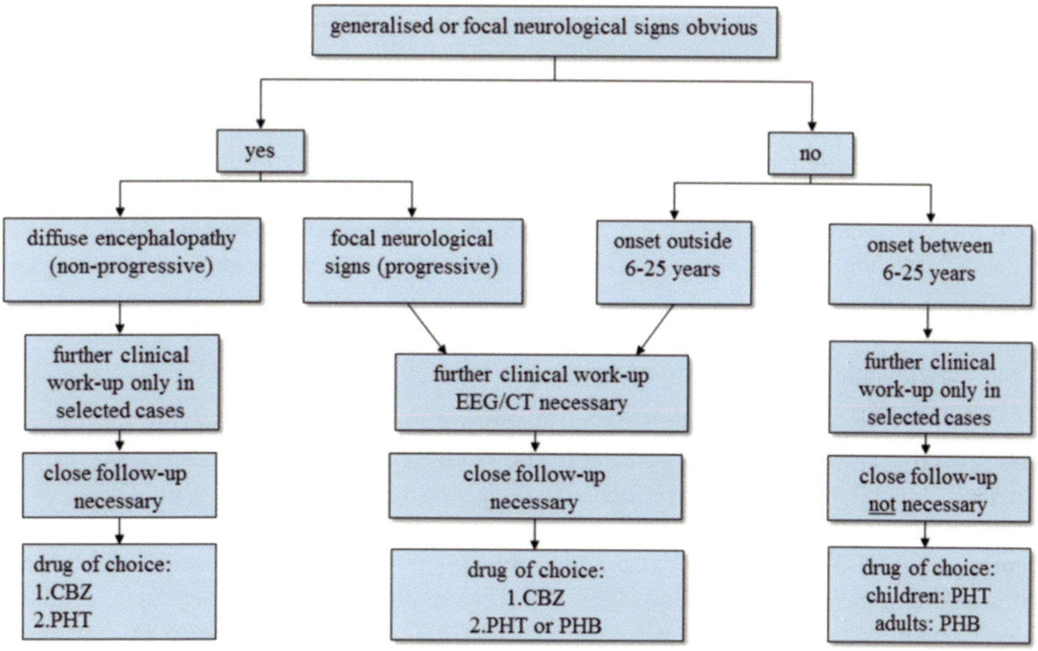

Figure 1. Algorithm on how to classify people with epilepsy in resource-poor countries regarding diagnostic and therapeutic implications. Primary generalised seizures are split according to the age of onset (see text); these two groups have a different diagnostic and therapeutic approach. Patients with primary generalised seizures that start outside 6-25 years are more likely to have cerebral lesions than patients whose epilepsies start within 6-25 years where idiopathic epilepsy prevails, and therefore need further investigation. In people with epilepsy and diffuse brain damage, diagnostic tests are rarely needed as the extent of the cerebral sequelae is known and the condition is not progressive. In contrast, in people with epilepsy who show focal signs without diffuse brain damage, further diagnostic steps are essential in order to identify the underlying, potentially treatable cause. In all four groups, treatment depends mainly on the age of the patient, seizure activity, seizure frequency, the presence of mental handicap and the presence of focal neurological signs, bearing in mind that the choice of antiepileptic medication is limited. CBZ = carbamazepine, PHT = phenytoin, PHB = phenobarbitone.

We opted for a simply structured, easy-to-understand classification system that mainly consists of the four groups of epileptic seizures/epilepsy described above based on seizure description, clinical information and a physical examination (Figure 1). Our classification shares many similarities with the International League Against Epilepsy classifications [1, 20-22], especially the International Classification of Epileptic Seizures [20], but it has been tailored to fit local circumstances. This was deemed important in order to gain information on possible causes, necessary investigations within a resource-poor setting, best antiepileptic treatments and prognoses of seizure disorders (Figure 1).

The "generalized types of seizure" (groups 1 and 2; Figure 1) were divided according to age at onset. They presented as classic primary generalized seizures without any suggestion of focal neurological signs or focal seizure onset. The subdivision of primary generalized seizures into those that start within a specific age range (6-25 years;[27]) and those that start outside of this age range was deemed important as the approach used for each is different (Figure 1). Idiopathic epilepsy types include distinct seizure syndromes with distinct ages of onset, although mainly within the postulated age group of 6-25 years [27-29]. Primary generalized seizures outside of this age range, either below about 6 years or above about 25 years, can still be idiopathic in nature, although seizures caused by brain lesions, especially in a resource-poor setting, may prevail. Our hospital-based study showed that symptomatic seizures are frequent. When looking at the exact age distribution, 70.8 % (51/72) of the patients with symptomatic seizures were aged either below 6 years or above 25 years when presenting with symptomatic seizures [10]. Therefore, for people with epilepsy presenting with primary generalized seizures that fall into these age groups, further investigations with electroencephalography and neuroimaging seem to be important (Figure 1).

The "partial types of seizure with the clinical appearance of generalized seizures" (groups 3 and 4; Figure 1) were divided according to the extent of brain damage associated with the seizures. Mental retardation and intellectual decline due to serious brain disorders in children of resource-poor countries are much more frequent compared to resource-rich countries [30,31]. These are often associated with epileptic seizures that are difficult to treat and have an unfavourable prognosis [32]. Thus, this group of people with epilepsy deserves special attention, and therefore has been summarized as a separate group (group 3). In children with more widespread brain damage, antiepileptic drugs with sedative effects such as phenobarbitone could further hamper intellectual development. Often, additional diagnostic tests do not add to the management of these young patients as the cause of cerebral sequelae is known and the condition is not progressive (Figure 1). "Over-diagnosing" patients in this context can cause unnecessary financial burden to the families.

Epilepsy in resource-poor countries is often associated with brain lesions of various origins, with infection and trauma being the most important causes in this setting [2, 33]. These patients can show focal neurological signs and/or present with clinically obvious secondary generalized seizures, but, in contrast to group 3, they do not show signs of more widespread brain damage. Often, a patient is previously healthy before a special event precedes the onset of seizures, although this is not mandatory. Further diagnostic procedures in these patients are important in order to identify the underlying, potentially treatable cause of the epilepsy (Figure 1).

In summary, we have identified four major groups of epileptic seizures on clinical grounds that are relevant to the diagnosis of epilepsy in sub-Saharan Africa. The suggested investigations within a resource-poor setting, treatment and prognosis differ between the groups, and a classification of affected patients within the most appropriate group could help guide the clinician towards the appropriate management of people with epilepsy within a rural African setting.

1.4. Treatment gap of epilepsy in sub-Saharan Africa

In many African countries, epileptic seizures/epilepsy represent a tremendous socio-economic burden, partly due to the chronicity of the disease, and therefore not only have repercussions on individuals but also on their families and the community they live in. The figures released by the WHO are convincing: 50 million people worldwide suffer from epilepsy; 80% of them live in resource-poor countries [23] and of these up to 90% are untreated or treated insufficiently [34]. Newer figures indicate that 63 million people live with epilepsy in low- and middle-income countries [35]. This 90% treatment gap was corroborated by studies from northern and southern Tanzania showing that 76% and 95% of people with epilepsy, respectively, had not been treated [12,19]. Dramatic global disparities in this treatment gap were identified by a systematic review which showed that 75% and fewer than 10% of PWE from low-income and high-income countries, respectively, were untreated or insufficiently treated for their epilepsy [36]. A recent study from Kenya demonstrated an epilepsy treatment gap of 62% using serum antiepileptic drug levels as a measure of compliance and found that self-reporting of compliance to antiepileptic medication was very unreliable when compared to the serum antiepileptic drug levels [37,38].

Although access to modern medicine is limited for people with epilepsy who live in sub-Saharan Africa, traditional medicines are widely used as they represent the only treatments that are accessible to most of the affected population. The lack of awareness of local and international policy makers, poor infrastructure, long travel distances, the insufficient or only intermittent availability of antiepileptic medications, the lack of education among people with epilepsy, their families and the communities, the predominance of traditional belief systems and the scarcity of trained medical personnel may be responsible for this large treatment gap [39,40]. Another important but often neglected cause of this treatment gap is social stigma. In many countries of sub-Saharan Africa, epilepsy has mystical connotations, which is another reason why the majority of people with epilepsy resort to traditional medicines before even considering modern medicine. In many societies, epilepsy is viewed as punishment for sins or breaking taboos, a curse, bewitchment or demoniac possession, as well as a contagious disease, resulting in the rejection and discrimination of affected individuals [41]. A recent study from Zambia showed that people with epilepsy are disadvantaged regarding social and economic matters compared to people with other chronic diseases without an attached stigma, such as asthma, diabetes mellitus, hypertension and rheumatic heart disease [42]. The aforementioned aspects all contribute to the fact that the majority of people with epilepsy go untreated. This treatment gap is the main cause of individual suffering and the socio-economic burden of the disease, necessitating improvements in therapeutic strategies [6,43,44]. A pre-requisite for successful treatment also includes a good knowledge of the possible aetiologies of seizure disorders as treatment can largely depend on underlying pathologies.

1.5. Causes of epileptic seizures/epilepsy in sub-Saharan Africa

Causes of epileptic seizures/epilepsy are highly variable across different regions of sub-Saharan Africa and depend on geographical, climatic, political, social and hygienic conditions. However, the main and most important causes of epilepsy seem to be very similar throughout sub-Saharan Africa and have been studied in great detail, both in hospital and community settings, showing that a positive family history (genetic predisposition), a past history of febrile convulsions, perinatal neurological disorders, head injuries, cerebrovascular accidents and infections of the central nervous system account for most cases of epilepsy [6]. Also included are a variety of protozoon (the most important being cerebral malaria) and helminthic infections, of which *Taenia solium* (its larval stage causing cysticercosis) has attracted considerable attention in sub-Saharan Africa over the past few years. Therefore, epileptic seizures/epilepsy in the context of NCC will be described in more detail in the following paragraphs in order to provide adequate information on clinical characteristics, diagnosis and treatment in the context of sub-Saharan Africa.

2. Prevalence of neurocysticercosis in sub-Saharan Africa

NCC represents the most common helminthic infection of the central nervous system [45] and is endemic in most countries of Latin America, Asia and sub-Saharan Africa. NCC is not only one of the major causes of acquired epileptic seizures/epilepsy in low-resource countries, but it is also of increasing concern in so far non-endemic countries, such as Europe and the United States, due to globalization and the migration of infected people [46-50].

Community-based estimation of the prevalence of NCC is difficult as neuroimaging would have to be applied to a large population putting seemingly healthy people at risk of radiation and therefore has been performed rarely so far [51]. In contrast, the prevalence of human *Taenia solium* cysticercosis in communities has been assessed as this requires blood analysis only. In cysticercosis endemic areas of the Democratic Republic of Congo, Burkina Faso and Zambia the prevalence of *Taenia solium* cysticercosis as measured with an antigen-ELISA was 22%, 10% and 5.8%, respectively [52-54]. Indirect approaches are used to get an impression about the prevalence of people with NCC in a certain population and often people suffering from epileptic seizures or epilepsy are included into these studies. The prevalence of epilepsy has shown to be high in a *Taenia solium* cysticercosis endemic area from Burkina Faso which found an epilepsy lifetime prevalence of 4.5% [55]. A recent meta-analysis on the prevalence of NCC in people with epilepsy, including 12 studies mainly from Latin America, India and sub-Saharan Africa, found that NCC was the cause of epilepsy in almost 30% of people with epilepsy [56].

If extrapolating the above results to the entire population of sub-Saharan Africa (850 million people; [57]) and assuming a prevalence of epilepsy of 4-13/1000 [3,12], approximately 3.4 to 11.05 million people would suffer from epilepsy. Thirty per cent of it is due to NCC yielding 1.02-3.32 million people with epilepsy due to NCC in sub-Saharan Africa. Epilepsy makes up for approximately 80% of the symptoms in NCC [58] and therefore 1.28-4.15 million people would suffer from symptomatic NCC including all neurological signs/symptoms (see

2.4.). We also know that symptomatic NCC is only the tip of the iceberg and that the majority of people with NCC are asymptomatic. We assume conservatively 50% of all NCC cases to be asymptomatic [59]. Therefore the total of all people suffering from NCC in sub-Saharan Africa would be somewhere between 2.56-8.30 million. These figures would however come down if only areas confirmed with endemic *Taenia solium* cysticercosis would be considered. Currently a number of 631 776 908 people has been assumed to live in the *Taenia solium* cysticercosis endemic areas of sub-Saharan Africa (endemic countries: [60]; populations in these endemic countries: [61]) yielding an NCC-based epilepsy population of 0.76-2.46 million and a population suffering from symptomatic NCC of 0.95-3.08 million. The same amount of people would suffer from asymptomatic NCC, if assuming that 50% of all cases are asymptomatic.

Latent NCC cases when harbouring *Taenia solium* cysticerci can become symptomatic at any time due to the natural course of disease or in the context of treatment received for intestinal parasites [62]. These people are also at risk of developing symptomatic disease through mass drug administration for soil-transmitted helminths and schistosomiasis, among others [63-66]. Praziquantel and albendazole, two antihelminthic drugs (see 2.6.1.), are at the heart of mass drug administration and may be able to convert latent NCC to symptomatic NCC by destroying the parasite and potentially provoking brain oedema [65,66]. Anecdotal reports of sudden onset of serious neurological signs and/or death after mass drug administration have been noted, but to date no large-scale studies on the topic of the side effects after mass drug administration in carriers of latent cysticerci have been performed. Such studies are desperately needed to evaluate the risk of symptomatic NCC with potentially ensuing death in many hundreds of thousands of people in sub-Saharan Africa. For more details on the calculation of how many people in sub-Saharan Africa would potentially be at risk of developing neurological side effects after mass drug administration of praziquantel and albendazole refer to Winkler [67].

NCC not only imposes a huge socioeconomic burden onto the health systems of affected African nations (see 2.3.), but also indicates that people who potentially could be cured from their epilepsy by antihelminthic medication are practically left untreated. Data on sub-Saharan prevalence rates of NCC in people with epileptic seizures/epilepsy are mainly based on serological results and only exist from a few countries with results of over 40% (Cameroon) depending on the serological tests used [68-70]. A recent meta-analysis that only included African studies showed a significant association between epilepsy and cysticercosis with an odds ratio of 3.4 [71]. More details on the prevalence of NCC (serology and imaging) are available from South African studies [68], where one study found 50.6% of newly diagnosed people with epilepsy showing lesions of NCC on neuroimaging [72]. The only neuroimaging-based study in sub-Saharan Africa outside South Africa was performed from our own group. Definite NCC lesions on computed tomography (CT) were demonstrated in 2.4% (5/212) of people with epilepsy, lesions highly suggestive of NCC were present in 11.3% (24/212) and lesions compatible with NCC were found in 4.2% (9/212). The NCC lesions were significantly more frequent in people with epilepsy compared to the controls [73].

Although it was clearly demonstrated that NCC in people with epilepsy from sub-Saharan Africa is prevalent, there is still some controversy regarding the manifestation of NCC in different age groups. In a recently conducted study, there was a trend of people with epilepsy and NCC being older and having their first seizure later compared to people with epilepsy without NCC [74]. Other studies also report that NCC is the cause of late-onset epilepsy [75-78]. A possible reason might be that older people with epilepsy are more susceptible to the infection. However, especially the calcified stage of NCC was found to be more common in younger people with epilepsy, whereas cysts were found to be more common in older people with epilepsy [73,74]. This may be explained by a different immunoresponse to the infection with age. The age of first manifestation of NCC seems however difficult to obtain, especially in sub-Saharan Africa, as children are often excluded from neuroimaging studies for obvious ethical reasons, although several reports have demonstrated the presence of NCC among children [79-83].

2.1. Neurocysticercosis in people with HIV/AIDS

Most NCC endemic areas are also endemic for HIV/AIDS and interaction of the two diseases, as known for HIV/AIDS and malaria and HIV/AIDS and tuberculosis, would seem plausible. Indeed, acceleration of the clinical course of HIV/AIDS in patients co-infected with *Taenia solium* cysticerci has been suggested based on the manipulation of the immune system by the parasite [84,85]. In South Africa, NCC has been described as one of the most important focal brain lesion in people with HIV/AIDS with neurological signs depending on the location of the lesion. Interestingly intraventricular NCC seems to be especially common in patients with HIV/AIDS from South Africa presenting with epileptic seizures and signs of increased intracranial pressure, among others. Treatment with ventriculo-peritoneal shunts carries a bleak prognosis, whereas antihelminthic medication together with steroids shows a better outcome in these patients. These reports from South Africa are fairly worrying and repeated regular treatment with short courses of praziquantel together with steroids have been advocated for HIV/AIDS patients from highly endemic areas to reduce the rate of re-infection which may accelerate the course of disease, if left untreated [84]. However, to date no systematic studies on co-infection with *Taenia solium* cysticerci and HIV have been conducted in sub-Saharan Africa. Observations from South Africa indicate that co-infection is high [84,85]. Conversely, studies from India and Mexico have shown that seroprevalence of *Taenia solium* cysticercosis in patients with HIV/AIDS is lower than in the non-HIV/AIDS population, which may point to an impaired immunoreaction with unreliable detection of *Taenia solium* cysticercosis antibodies [86,87]. The fact of unreliable *Taenia solium* cysticercosis serodiagnosis could present a substantial problem in the HIV/AIDS population with focal neurological signs in whom tuberculous meningitis/tuberculoma and toxoplasmosis, two diseases with different therapeutic approaches, represent the most important differential diagnoses.

2.2. Monetary burden of neurocysticercosis in sub-Saharan Africa

A comprehensive estimate of the monetary burden of cysticercosis in the *Taenia solium* cysticercosis hyperendemic Eastern Cape Province of South Africa indicated the monetary burden per capita to be between US$ 2.6 and US$ 4.8, which is substantial when compared to annual health expenditures of US$ 41.3 per capita for people living in poor dwellings in that province. The overall monetary burden was calculated to vary from US$ 18.6 million to US$ 34.2 million depending on the method used to estimate productivity losses. The epilepsy prevalence of the Eastern Cape Province, the proportion of people with epilepsy seeking medical care and the proportion of epilepsy cases attributable to NCC as well as the proportion of work time lost due to NCC were found to have the most influence on the estimated monetary burden [88]. The total societal costs due to *Taenia solium* cysticercosis in the main pig breeding region of West Cameroon (West, Southwest and Northwest Provinces) was also recently estimated [89]. Based on an epilepsy prevalence of 3.6%, the number of people with NCC-associated epilepsy was estimated at 50 326, representing 1.0% of the local population, whereas the number of pigs diagnosed with cysticercosis was estimated at 15 961 (based on lingual examination results), which corresponds to 5.6% of the local pig population. The total annual costs due to *Taenia solium* cysticercosis in West Cameroon were estimated at € 10.3 million, of which 4.7% were due to losses in pig production and 95.3% to direct and indirect losses caused by human *Taenia solium* cysticercosis. The monetary burden per case of human NCC amounted to € 194 and the average number of Disability-Adjusted Life Years (DALYs) lost was 9.0 per thousand persons per year which was higher than estimates for some other neglected tropical diseases [89].

2.3. Staging, pathology and clinical characteristics of neurocysticercosis

In humans, after the ingestion of *Taenia solium* eggs, oncospheres hatch and penetrate the gut wall. They are transported via the bloodstream and cysticerci form within a few weeks/months, mainly in subcutaneous tissue (painless, palpable, cystic lesions), skeletal muscle (lesion may not be palpable), the eye and the central nervous system, particularly in the brain but also in the spinal cord ([90]; Figure 2). Differences in phenotype of cysticercosis between various regions of the world have been described, indicating that the subcutaneous form of cysticercosis is most frequent in Asia, least prevalent in Latin America and that reports of its occurrence are conflicting in sub-Saharan Africa [67]. Especially cysticercosis of the eye and central nervous system are of clinical importance, where cysticerci can cause inflammation and/or space-occupying lesions with a mass effect and/or obstruction with resulting hydrocephalus.

In the brain, immature cysticerci appear within 1-4 weeks after the ingestion of eggs (stage 1). After approximately 1 month, this phase is followed by the maturation of cysticerci, which happens with surprisingly little or no inflammation (stage 2). This stage can last for more than 10 years and cysticerci survive by disarming host defences. Neurological symptoms and/or signs are not usually reported. Stage 3 (2-10 years or more after cysticerci maturation) is characterized by an intense host immunoresponse leading to the degeneration of cysticerci (granuloma), which may now cause neurological symptoms and/or signs [91]. The reasons for cysticerci to eventually be recognized by the host and thereby to go from stage 2 to stage 3 have not been understood so far. Antihelminthic treatment seems to accelerate this transition, as often the administration of antihelminthic medication causes perifocal oedema surrounding the parasite [62]. In stage 4, the inflammatory response has resolved, either without scarring or leaving behind residual calcifications ([91]; Figure 2).

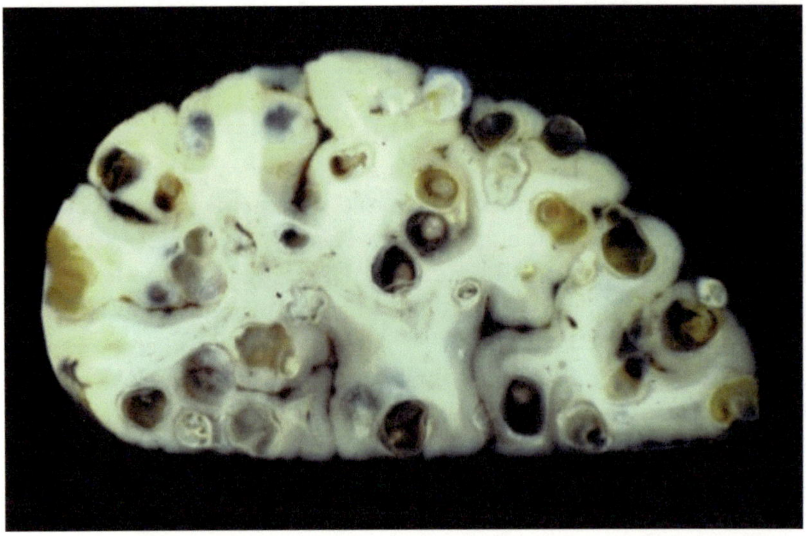

Courtesy of Prof. Theodore Nash who has also given permission for reproduction, Laboratory of Parasitic Diseases, National Institutes of Allergy and Infectious Diseases, National Institutes of Health, Bethesda, Maryland, USA.

Figure 2. Cross-section of a human brain showing various stages of neurocysticercosis, including cysts showing the scolex (stage 2), granulomas with surrounding inflammation (stage 3) and calcifications (stage 4). For more details refer to section 2.4. in the main body of the text.

NCC can cause a variety of symptoms and signs depending on the number, size, stage and location of the pathological changes as well as the host's immunoresponse and the parasite's genotype, or it can also be clinically asymptomatic. Post-mortem studies have shown that in up to 50% of people with NCC the cerebral lesions were asymptomatic [59]. There may be single or multiple cysticerci in the brain (intraparenchymal NCC, approximately 80%; Figure 2) and, in extreme cases, encephalitis (Figure 2) may ensue. Single enhancing (intraparenchymal) lesions (SEL) represent a separate entity that has been described mainly in patients from the Indian subcontinent. Differential diagnosis is difficult and may encompass tuberculoma, toxoplasmosis, brain abscess and tumours, among others. A lesion < 2 cm in diameter without gross perifocal oedema and subsequent growth is likely to represent a degenerating *Taenia solium* cysticercus. Patients mainly present with partial onset seizure with or without generalisation and have a high risk of seizure recurrence. Contrary to India, multiple lesions mainly of the intraparenchymal type seem to prevail in people with NCC from Latin America, sub-Saharan Africa and other Asian countries although scientific publications on NCC-related neuroimaging from sub-Saharan Africa and Asian countries other than India are rare [67,92,93].

Cysticerci can also occur in the ventricular system and/or the subarachnoid space (extraparenchymal NCC, approximately 20%), which is often associated with intraparenchymal NCC. Ventricular disease may cause ependymitis and/or increased intracranial pressure. Arachnoiditis, especially in the basal cisterns, which can lead to communicating hydrocephalus, vasculitis and/or compression of cerebral vessels, can result from subarachnoid disease. Intramedullary cysticerci can be found in the spinal cord, causing focal neurological symptoms/signs, and extramedullary cysticerci can cause radicular symptoms and/or signs [94].

If cerebral cysticerci or calcifications are intraparenchymal, epileptic seizures and/or epilepsy may ensue [95,96]. During stage 3 of cyst degeneration new-onset acute symptomatic epileptic seizures can occur that usually resolve after the inflammation has died down, which is very characteristic of this phase. In the case of remaining calcifications, recurrent epileptic seizures, i.e. epilepsy, can develop, although fortunately most patients remain asymptomatic ([91,97]; see 1.1.). The majority of cysticerci calcify, but cysticerci may also become invisible on CT and magnetic resonance imaging (MRI). Although the parasite is assumed dead, intermittent flares of oedema around calcifications have been described and they seem to be associated with increased seizure activity. The mechanisms of oedema occurrence however is not fully understood, but increased antigen accessibility with subsequent enhanced immunoresponse have been suggested. Another cause for the development of epilepsy after cyst resolution is the development of perilesional gliosis around calcifications secondary to prior inflammation [97].

A systematic review on the clinical manifestations in people with NCC showed that the majority of symptomatic adult cases (78.9%) had epileptic seizures [58]. This may be the only presentation, especially in people with single enhancing granulomatous lesions that bears a good prognosis compared to infection with multiple cysticerci [92]. Epileptic seizures were followed by headaches in 27.7% of people [58]. Headache in people with NCC can be acute or chronic, and presents as tension-type or migraine-like episodes [98,99]. Headache can also indicate raised intracranial pressure [90]. Furthermore, adults with NCC also present with focal neurological signs (11.8%), signs of intracranial hypertension (16.3%), meningitic symptoms (5.6%), gait abnormalities (5.6%) and altered mental state/psychiatric symptoms (28.1%), among others [58]. Forlenza et al. [100] examined 38 cases with NCC and found cognitive decline in 87.5% and psychiatric illness in 65.8% of them, with depression and psychosis being the most frequent psychiatric disorders. These findings were corroborated by a study from Brazil which showed that cognitive impairment was ubiquitous in 40 patients with NCC and that dementia was obvious in 12.5% [101]. A recent interesting and well conducted study, although small in sample size, showed that people with new-onset epileptic seizures and NCC performed worse on cognitive tests including scores for attention, processing speed, learning and memory compared to controls with and without epilepsy (people with epilepsy unrelated to NCC and healthy neighbourhood controls). However, the difference was only significant for the attention score (people with epilepsy and NCC compared to epilepsy controls). Over time (6 month-follow up) people with NCC-based epilepsy, who were all treated with albendazole, had significant improvement in psychomotor speed and working memory, but there were no significant changes in any of the cognitive test scores above, although a general trend for better performance after treatment was visible. Both epilepsy groups were controlled for seizure frequency and antiepileptic medication was kept constant during the study period [102].

In children with NCC from a series of studies conducted in Latin America, mainly single colloidal parenchymal cysts were seen, but heavy infection was also described. Calcifications were seen less often and the development of hydrocephalus, and basal subarachnoid disease seemed to be rare [83,103,104]. The most frequent clinical presentation in children is epileptic seizures followed by headaches and signs of elevated intracranial pressures. The only major difference compared to adults was that children portrayed relatively little psychiatric symptoms [58].

2.4. Diagnosis of neurocysticercosis including information on sub-Saharan Africa

A suspected diagnosis of NCC (e.g. epileptic seizures in a patient from an area endemic for *Taenia solium* cysticercosis) should be confirmed with a combination of neuroimaging and serology, if possible. On neuroimaging cysts, granulomas and/or calcifications will support the clinically based suspicion of NCC. However, these lesions may also be caused by other pathogens and pathological processes and therefore combination with *Taenia solium* cysticercosis serology is highly desirable. Both, neuroimaging and *Taenia solium* cysticercosis serology are often not available in resource-poor settings, but routine cerebrospinal fluid analysis may point the direction and can be obtained from patients without major impairment of consciousness. Cerebrospinal fluid analysis in NCC very often is unremarkable, but it may also show signs of parasitic disease, especially in multicystic disease and intraventricular/subarachnoid forms of NCC, including slightly elevated cell count (usually not exceeding 100 cells/μl, demonstrating mononuclear pleocytosis and eosinophilia) and increased protein levels in the range of 50 to 300 mg/dl. Glucose levels are usually normal [105].

Today a wide array of serological tests for *Taenia solium* cysticercosis exist such as the antigen/antibody enzyme-linked immunosorbent assay (ELISA) and immunoblots which can be performed in serum and/or cerebrospinal fluid of suspected cases [90,106-111]. However, a positive test only indicates cysticercosis but not necessarily NCC, and the sensitivity and specificity for current infection with *Taenia solium* cysticercus and prior exposure to the parasite can vary considerably according to the test used [106, 108, 112]. In addition, polymerase chain reaction (PCR) methods for the diagnosis of *Taenia solium* cysticercosis are under development, but so far are not part of routine diagnosis due to varying levels of sensitivities and specificities [113,114]. Also, these techniques, with high-cost equipment and need for regular maintenance may not be suitable for countries of sub-Saharan Africa.

When it comes to the availability of *Taenia solium* cysticercosis serological tests in sub-Saharan Africa the information is scarce and relies on personal communication. I therefore suggest that one of the tasks of the next Cysticercosis Working Group in Eastern and Southern Africa (CWGESA) meeting should be the establishment of an accurate list of *Taenia solium* cysticercosis immunodiagnostic tests available in countries of sub-Saharan Africa. The information I have got so far, even after communicating with various stakeholders, is not much different form the information published in Winkler et al. [110] and therefore would need updating by talking to reference people of the individual countries. In summary, in Mozambique and South Africa *Taenia solium* cysticercosis antibody-ELISA has been available for some years (personal communication with Dr Lee Willingham, WHO, Geneva, Switzerland). My own cysticercosis project in collaboration with the Department of Infectious Disease and Tropical Medicine of the University of Munich and funded by the German Research Foundation is currently transferring capacity for *Taenia solium* cysticercosis antibody-ELISA to the CWGESA Regional Reference Centre for Immunodiagnosis of *Taenia solium* Infections at the University of Zambia, to Gulu University of Uganda and to Muhimbili University of Health and Allied Sciences of Tanzania. There are also plans to transfer the new T24 recombinant-based antibody-ELISA test developed by the U.S. Centers for Disease Control and Prevention to Zambia, Mozambique and Madagascar (personal communication with Dr Lee Willingham, WHO, Geneva, Switzerland) and according to the latest information training of personnel has started (personal communication with Dr Patricia Wilkins, U.S. Centers for Disease Control and Prevention, Atlanta, USA). Diagnostic possibilities for *Taenia solium* cysticercosis in terms of immunoblot currently do not exist in countries of sub-Saharan Africa. A *Taenia solium* cysticercosis antigen-ELISA has been performed over the last years in Zambia at the CWGESA Regional Reference Centre for Immunodiagnosis of *Taenia solium* Infections at the University of Zambia. Member countries of the CWGESA send samples for antigen-ELISA testing to this reference laboratory. Recently, antigen-ELISA facilities have also been established in Mozambique, Madagascar, South Africa, Burkina Faso and Cameroon (personal communication with Dr Lee Willingham, WHO, Geneva, Switzerland). Confirmation whether these tests are still functional has not been obtained from the individual countries, but could be included into the working schedule of the next CWGESA meeting.

Although positive serological and/or DNA-based tests may give the first indication, the gold standard of NCC diagnosis is neuroimaging, including CT and/or MRI, both of which are generally not available in sub-Saharan Africa. In neuroimaging, only a lesion showing the scolex (= head of the parasite) is classified as a definite NCC lesion and considered pathognomonic [90,106,107,109]. Active NCC is defined as the presence of any cystic lesions (with or without scolex) or lesions with ring enhancement. In contrast, parenchymal calcifications are classified as inactive [95,97].

Cysts are best visualized on MRI, whereas CT is the imaging of choice for calcifications. Cyst fluid shows the same signal than cerebrospinal fluid and is hypointense (dark signal) on T1-weighted images as well as fluid attenuated inversion recovery (FLAIR) sequences and hyperintense (bright) on T2-weighted images. In the vesicular stage of NCC, there is no surrounding oedema. Cysts are usually 1-2 cm in diameter and the scoleces inside the cysts 1-2 mm. The latter is isointense relative to brain parenchyma (Figure 3a). During the degenerative process with thickening of the cyst wall, increased protein content of the cyst fluid and surrounding inflammatory signs, the signal intensity of the cyst fluid is higher than that of cerebrospinal fluid on T1-weighted images, but still hypointense compared to parenchyma, and hyperintense on T2-weighted images (colloid vesicular stage), whereas the cyst wall is hyperintense on T1- and hypointense on T2-weighted sequences. As the degeneration goes on with proliferation and retraction of the cyst wall and reabsorption of the fluid (granular nodular stage) the granuloma becomes isointense and eventually hyperintense on T1- and hypointense on T2-weighted images. Ring-enhancement or total enhancement of the degenerative cysticerci after application of contrast indicates inflammation and subsequent disruption of the blood-brain barrier with leakage of plasma into cerebral tissue and is best visualized on T1-weighted images (Figure 3b). Perifocal oedema is best seen on FLAIR sequences (bright signal) and T2-weighted images (less bright signal). Calcifications (nodular calcified stage) often go unnoticed on MRI or may appear as small iso- or hypointense lesions on T1- and T2-weighted images [115]. Subarachnoid NCC shows multiple cystic masses in the basal cisterns or Sylvian fissure, among other locations. The masses may be lobulated and compress adjacent structures. Signal intensity usually compares with that of cerebrospinal fluid on all magnetic resonance sequences and is best seen as dark signal in T1-weighted and FLAIR images (Figure 3c). Ventricular NCC shows best on T1-weighted sequences, because on T2-weighted images the high signal intensity of the cyst fluid is indistinguishable from that of the cerebrospinal fluid (refer to chapter on extraparenchymal NCC) [115]. On CT scan cysts are hypodense (Figure 4a) and granuloma may be isodense to the parenchyma and only be seen after administration of contrast (Figure 4b). Calcifications are hyperdense (Figure 4c). Extraparenchymal NCC can easily be missed on CT, especially the ventricular form.

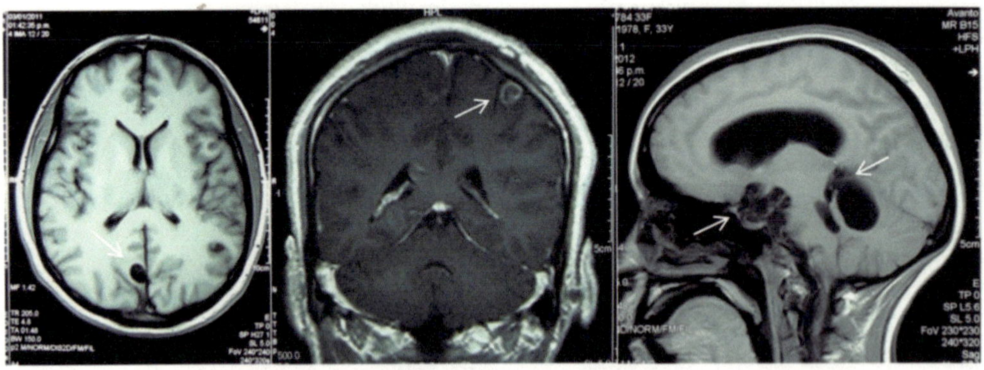

a) b) c)

All pictures are courtesy of Prof. Hector H. Garcia, Department of Microbiology, School of Sciences, and Director Center for Global Health - Tumbes, Universidad Peruana Cayetano Heredia, Lima, Peru.

Figure 3. a-c): magnetic resonance images of neurocysticercosis lesions; 3a) axial T1-weighted image showing a pathognomonic cyst with scolex (approximate diameter of 1 cm) in the right occipital lobe; 3b) coronal T1-weighted contrast enhanced image, showing a cystic lesion with an enhancing rim in the left parietal lobe; 3c) sagittal T1-weighted image showing extraparenchymal subarachnoid cysticercosis with multiple, lobulated cystic lesions predominantly in the subarachnoid space (prepontine, suprasellar cistern and cisterna ambiens) as well as probable intraventricular lesions with potential dilation of the 4th ventricle.

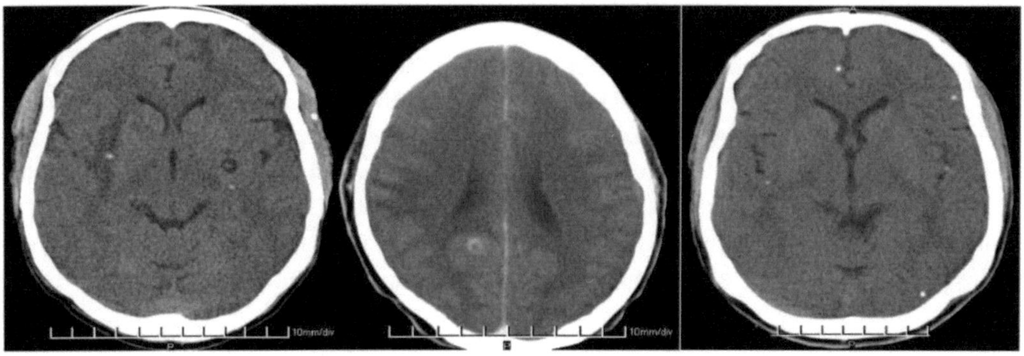

a) b) c)

Permission for reproduction has been obtained from SpringerWienNewYork. The pictures were originally published in Winkler AS, Willingham L 3rd, Sikasunge CS, Schmutzhard E. Epilepsy and neurocysticercosis in sub-Saharan Africa. Middle European Journal of Medicine 2009; 121 (suppl 3): 3-12.

Figure 4. a-c) axial computed tomography images of various stages of neurocysticercosis lesions; 4a) pathognomonic subcortical cyst left showing the scolex with a close-by calcification; calcified subcortical cyst right with perifocal/perilesional oedema; calcification in the left temporal muscle; 4b) "ring enhancing lesion" due to a degenerating subcortical cyst in the right occipital lobe; 4c) several scattered intraparenchymal calcifications most likely in the context of neurocysticercosis.

In a resource-rich setting the combination of MRI and CT makes a lot of sense to neither miss cystic lesions or granulomas nor calcifications. Combination of neuroimaging and immunodiagnostic test is strongly advised and their results together with clinical, pathological and epidemiological criteria as well as response to treatment with antihelminthic drugs are summarized in the diagnostic criteria for NCC suggested by Del Brutto et al. [107,109,116]. If neither immunodiagnostic tools nor neuroimaging are available, extirpation of subcutaneous nodules and a thorough ophthalmological examination may support the suspected diagnosis [107,109,116]. Due to an emphasis on neuroimaging and serological tests, the Del Brutto criteria seem to be rather impractical for its use in resource-poor settings and may need adjustment to suit local circumstances.

2.5. Treatment of neurocysticercosis with a focus on sub-Saharan Africa

In the treatment of NCC, symptomatic (steroids, antiepileptic medication, analgesics) and potentially curative treatment (antihelminthic medications) has to be differentiated. Indication and contraindication for antihelminthic treatment as outlined below must be observed. Neuroimaging is mandatory to start treatment with antihelminthic drugs and therefore antihelminthic treatment is not indicated in most patients from sub-Saharan Africa (except South Africa), where neuroimaging is absent. If there is any doubt as to the appropriateness of antihelminthic treatment, symptomatic treatment should be favoured. In addition, the treatment approach in acutely symptomatic and life-threatening disease is different form the more chronically symptomatic condition (see 2.5.1.).

2.5.1. Antihelminthic and/or anti-oedematous treatment

Currently, there are no standard treatment guidelines for NCC; therefore treatment has to be tailored to the individual case. Only active disease needs treatment with antihelminthic drugs and/or steroids. Dosages and the duration of treatment can be highly variable and mainly depend on the number, size, location and developmental stage of the cysts, their surrounding inflammatory oedema, clinical symptoms/signs (their acuteness and severity) as well as potential risk factors of treatment. On the one hand, care needs to be taken not to "over-treat" as the administration of antihelminthic drugs can cause cerebral oedema and worsen symptoms and, on the other hand, one has to be prepared to extend treatment for some months as the penetration of drugs into cysts can be poor. The follow-up of patients has to be ensured, ideally with neuroimaging, but this may not be available in resource-poor settings [90,95,117]. Although treatment has to be flexible, there are some rules of thumb that should be followed. The administration of antihelminthic drugs may elicit or increase pre-existing cerebral oedema and therefore is contraindicated in cases with increased intracranial pressure, subarachnoidal NCC in close proximity to blood vessels and NCC encephalitis (Figure 2). In these conditions, steroids should be administered alone and may later be combined with antihelminthic drugs. In intraparenchymal active NCC without signs of increased intracranial pressure, steroids should be administered simultaneously with antihelminthic treatment, at least for the first week. The antihelminthic drug of choice is albendazole, which unfortunately is not often available in sub-Saharan Africa. The suggested dose is 15 mg/kg per day for 8-15 days. Praziquantel can also be used to treat NCC, although it is not as effective as albendazole [118], but it can be found in most sub-Saharan countries. Its recommended dose is 50 mg/kg per day for 15-30 days [90,94,117]. Metabolism of praziquantel and albendazole is increased with simultaneous usage of antiepileptic drugs, in particular phenytoin and carbamazepine, and the levels of praziquantel are reduced when the drug is administered together with steroids. Co-administration with cimetidine may increase the bioavailability of praziquantel [90,94]. Alternatively the dose of praziquantel may be increased or its course shortened and repeated. Also, in resource-poor settings, patients may not be particularly compliant with treatment. The best solution would be to keep the patient in hospital for the time of treatment, but due to financial expenses the patient may not agree. To minimise costs an elegant solution may be a high-dose short-term treatment with 100 mg/kg praziquantel in three divided doses every two hours followed by corticosteroids. This treatment regimen has been demonstrated to be successful in single cyst disease, but unfortunately efficacy could not be demonstrated in patients with multiple cysts, which is the phenotype that prevails in sub-Saharan Africa [67,119,120]. Even with normal dosage and course of treatment cure rates with antihelminthic drugs in general seem to be low. In untreated patients, 40% of cysts are cleared and in treated patients 60% of cysts disappear after one course of treatment. Furthermore, rebound inflammation may occur after abrupt withdrawal of antihelminthic medication and/or steroids and may be due to overcompensation of the immune system after removal of treatment with anti-inflammatory medication [117].

Steroids should be initiated together with antihelminthic drugs in intraparenchymal disease and ideally should be administered for as long as the patient is symptomatic (e.g. chronic progressive headache, acute symptomatic epileptic seizures) but at least for the first days antihelminthic treatment is given. So far steroid doses in the treatment of NCC have not been standardized [121]. Prednisone is recommended at a dosage of 1 mg/kg per day either p.o. or i.v.. Alternatively, dexamethasone can be used at 12-24 mg/d, maximum of 30 mg/day, p.o. or i.v.. Metabolism of both drugs may be increased by antiepileptic medication [90,94]. Steroids are used in all condition where cerebral oedema is present or may develop. To date there are only four controlled trials of the use of steroids in NCC and all of them were conducted in single enhancing granulomatous lesions (see 2.4.). Treatment regimens consisted of prednisolone 1 mg/kg for 10 days with a 4-day taper with and without antiepileptic treatment, prednisolone 1 mg/kg for 7 days with a 3-day taper without antiepileptic treatment and methylprednisolone 1 g/1.72 m^2 for 5 days without antiepileptic treatment. All studies showed a decrease in epileptic seizures and three showed a significant clearance of cysts on CT [122-125].

In summary, only confirmed active intraparenchymal and symptomatic (e.g. epileptic seizures) disease requires treatment with triple therapy, i.e. antihelminthic medication, steroids and antiepileptic medication. For antiepileptic treatment see 2.6.2. Once the parasite has gone into the transitional stage, antihelminthic drugs may no longer be needed as the parasite is already attacked and destroyed by the host. Current advice is that the symptomatic patient of the transitional stage should be maintained on symptomatic treatment only, i.e. steroids and antiepileptic medication [126]. There is however some controversy over the topic of treatment of the transitional stage and new results are expected shortly (personal communication with Prof. Hector H. Garcia, Universidad Peruana Cayetano Heredia, Lima, Peru). In inactive symptomatic disease the patient should receive antiepileptic mediation only if seizures are present. If perilesional oedema is obvious, steroids may be beneficial, although there are only anecdotal reports [121]. Treatment of extraparenchymal disease is much more tedious than that of intraparenchymal disease, and in most cases requires lengthy treatment regimens with antihelminthic medication and steroids or operative procedure if cysts are located in the ventricles [117]. For more details refer to the chapter of extraparenchymal NCC…

Furthermore, treatment of affected individuals only represents one facet in the multifaceted approach towards the eradication of NCC. Another important step is the prevention (reducing the number of free-roaming pigs, the vaccination of pigs) and treatment of porcine cysticercosis as well as the treatment of *Taenia solium* taeniosis (human tapeworm infection; [47,67,127,128]). In addition, increasing hygienic standards in affected communities, meat inspections, educating farmers and health education within communities should be top priorities in the fight against NCC. For more details refer to the chapter of ...

2.5.2. *Antiepileptic treatment*

Antiepileptic treatment should be initiated if seizure activity is recurrent, irrespective of whether epileptic seizures occur within the setting of stage-3 symptomatic cysts or stage-4 calcifications after clearance of the parasite (see 2.2.). According to the latest guidelines of the International League Against Epilepsy [129], treatment should be initiated after the first epileptic seizure if seizures are caused by an underlying lesion. In resource-poor settings without access to neuroimaging, an underlying lesion in the context of NCC can only be assumed if certain factors such as neurological signs on examination or a contact history with a tapeworm carrier or pigs are present. In some hospitals, electroencephalography may be available and focal activities on electroencephalograms may help decide when to start treatment.

Antiepileptic medication is limited in sub-Saharan Africa. The mainstay of antiepileptic treatment is phenobarbitone, although phenytoin and carbamazepine can also be found in rural African hospitals, but their supply is often erratic. Valproate is stocked only occasionally, and most times is not delivered through the national pharmacies, but relies on private donations. Dosing and potential side effects of antiepileptic medication available in sub-Saharan Africa are given in Table 1.

Antiepileptic medication (indication)	**Starting dose**	**Titration (~usual adult maintenance dose)**	**Side effects (list non-exhaustive)**	**Route of administration**
Phenobarbitone (all forms of epilepsy; may be tried in atypical absences, atonic and tonic seizures)	1. 30 mg p.o. 2. (rapid) 50 mg i.v., s.c. or i.m. every 6 h diluted 1:10 with inj. water 3. (status) 20 mg/kg i.v. diluted 1:10 with inj. water (start with 200-400 mg) (maximum rate: 100 mg/min)	30 mg p.o. every 3 days (long half-life) (~60-180 mg/day)	neurological/psychiatric: fatigue, drowsiness, lethargy, pronounced cognitive decline, learning disabilities, headaches, ataxia, nystagmus, dysarthria, depression, agitation, aggression, hyperkinesia (children), confusion (elderly); other: megaloblastic anaemia (may be treated with folic acid**), constipation, rickets and osteomalacia (vitamin D deficiency**), impotence; vitamin K deficiency** and withdrawal seizures in new-borns; teratogenicity rapid titration in status: respiratory depression	oral, i.v., s.c., i.m.
Carbamazepine (partial (simple and complex) and secondary generalised tonic-clonic seizures; some primary generalised seizures; not in absences and myoclonic seizures)	200 mg p.o.	200 mg p.o. every 3-5 days (~800-2000 mg/day)	skin: from transient erythematous rash*** (frequent) to Stevens-Johnson syndrome, photosensitivity lupus erythematosus; blood: leucopenia, thrombocytopenia, agranulocytosis, aplastic anaemia; cardiovascular: conduction disturbances, thromboembolism; gastro-intestinal: nausea, vomiting, cholestatic jaundice, hepatitis, constipation, diarrhoea,	oral

Antiepileptic medication (indication)	Starting dose	Titration (~usual adult maintenance dose)	Side effects (list non-exhaustive)	Route of administration
			anorexia; genito-urinary: renal failure, proteinuria, impotence; neurological/psychiatric: dizziness, drowsiness, headache, ataxia, confusion, agitation, visual disturbances (double vision often associated with peak plasma levels), dyskinesia, paraesthesia, depression, activation of psychosis; other: alopecia, arthralgia, fever, lymph node enlargement, gynaecomastia, galactorrhoea, pulmonary hypersensitivity, hyponatraemia, oedema, osteomalacia; teratogenicity;	
Phenytoin (all forms of epilepsy except absence seizures and myoclonic seizures)	1. 300 mg p.o. 2. (rapid) 600 mg p.o. for 3 days 3. (status) 1.5 g i.v. diluted 1:10 with inj. water (first 250 mg as bolus over 10 minutes, next 500 mg in 0.5 to 6 hours, next 750 mg in 1-24 hours according to clinic) (maximum rate: 20 mg/min)	25-50 mg p.o. per day (~200-500 mg/day*)	skin and gum: gingival hypertrophy and tenderness, coarse facies, hirsutism, acne, rash***, lupus erythematosus, Stevens-Johnson syndrome, toxic epidermal necrolysis; blood: megaloblastic anaemia (may be treated with folic acid**) leucopenia, thrombocytopenia, agranulocytosis, aplastic anaemia; gastro-intestinal: nausea, vomiting, hepatitis, liver failure; neurological/psychiatric: vertigo, double vision, nystagmus, tremor, confusion, dizziness, headache, insomnia dyskinesia; ataxia, slurred speech, nystagmus and blurred vision (are signs of overdosage); peripheral neuropathy, irreversible cerebellar atrophy; other: fever, polyarthritis, lymphadenopathy, rickets and osteomalacia (lowered plasma calcium concentration); teratogenicity; rapid titration in status: cardiac dysrhythmias, hypotonia	oral, i.v. (beware of phlebitis)

Antiepileptic medication (indication)	Starting dose	Titration (~usual adult maintenance dose)	Side effects (list non-exhaustive)	Route of administration
Valproate (all forms of epilepsy; drug of choice in primary generalised epilepsy, generalised absences and myoclonic seizures; may be tried in atypical absences, atonic and tonic seizures, Salaam attacks; has got similar efficacy to that of phenytoin and carbamazepine in partial epilepsy)	1. 600 mg p.o. 2. (status) 3.6 g i.v. diluted approx. 1:10 with inj. water (first 1.2 g as bolus over 10 minutes, second 1.2 g as bolus over 10 minutes, next 1.2 g in 12-24 hours according to clinic) (maximum rate: 100-200 mg/min)	150-300 mg p.o. every 3 days (~ 900-3000 mg/d)	skin: rash, toxic epidermal necrolysis, Stevens-Johnson syndrome, vasculitis, hirsutism, acne; blood: thrombocytopenia, inhibition of platelet aggregation, leucopenia, pancytopenia, red cell hypoplasia, fibrinogen reduction; gastro-intestinal: nausea, vomiting, increased appetite and weight gain, impaired hepatic function leading rarely to fatal hepatic failure****, rarely pancreatitis*****, hyperammonaemia; neurological/psychiatric: ataxia, tremor, dizziness, sedation (rarely lethargy and confusion associated with too high an initial dose), increased alertness, occasionally aggression, hyperactivity and behavioural disturbances, extrapyramidal symptoms, dementia, acute valproate-induced encephalopathy******; other: irregular periods, amenorrhoea, gynaecomastia, hearing loss, Fanconi's syndrome, fatigue, hair loss, oedema	oral, i.v.

*has a narrow therapeutic index and the relationship between dose and plasma concentration is non-linear; small dosage increases in some patients may produce large rise in plasma concentration with acute toxic side-effects; a few missed doses or a small change in drug absorption may result in a marked change in plasma concentration.
**consider vitamin administration together with antiepileptic medication
***discontinue; if mild re-introduce cautiously, but discontinue immediately if recurrence
****withdraw treatment immediately if vomiting, anorexia, jaundice or/and loss of seizure control occurs
*****measure plasma amylase in acute abdominal pain
******withdraw treatment immediately if within the first week of starting medication impairment of consciousness, increased seizure frequency, dysarthria and/or, asterixis occurs

Table 1. Antiepileptic medication available in sub-Saharan Africa: indication, drug loading, titration and maintenance doses as well as side effects (in the order of their availability; adjusted from [67])

Epileptic seizures in the context of NCC are of the secondary generalized type, but very often clinical examination does not reveal neurological signs. Therefore, in practice, it is difficult to differentiate epileptic seizure due to NCC from other types of seizures. Given the limited supply of medication, the most appropriate antiepileptic medication for seizures caused by NCC would be carbamazepine which is effective for partial seizures and secondary generalised seizures. It has generally fewer side-effects than phenytoin or the barbiturates, but reversible blurring of vision, dizziness and unsteadiness are dose-related and may be dose-limiting (Table 1). If carbamazepine is absent or if it is not tolerated, phenobarbitone and phenytoin can also be administered. However side effects may limit their use (Table 1). Therefore, if in a patient with normal neurological examination additional tests such as a positive result on *Taenia solium* cysticercosis antigen serology and/or neuroimaging indicate a focal start of the seizure, the patient should be started on carbamazepine first. As most people with epilepsy in sub-Saharan Africa do not have access to these investigations, treatment has to be started according to the suspected origin of the seizures and based on the experience of the involved physician. Also, phenobarbitone, despite its unpleasant side effect profile, has been shown to be a highly effective drug when it comes to seizure control. Surprisingly, many adults tolerate it fairly well, but its use has to be very restrictive in children and women of child bearing age because of possible cognitive decline and withdrawal seizures in the new-born, respectively (Table 1). A recent study from a *Taenia solium* cysticercosis endemic area of northern Tanzania showed that compliant people with epilepsy and NCC were well controlled on antiepileptic monotherapy with a trend towards better seizure control under carbamazepine compared to phenobarbitone. However, sample size in the groups was small and a final conclusion as to which of the two drugs leads to better seizure control in people with epilepsy and NCC cannot be drawn with certainty [74].

In addition to choosing the right antiepileptic medication, communication with the patients and their families is vital. The treatment gap for people with epilepsy in sub-Saharan Africa is substantial and it is most important to take its causative factors into consideration when counselling people with epilepsy (see 1.4.). It is also mandatory that patients who are started on antiepileptic medication and their families are informed about potentially ensuing side effects as well as the temporary nature of some of them in order to enhance compliance with medication. Follow-up appointments in short interval are advisable in the early phase of antiepileptic treatment. When informing patients about their treatment it has to be emphasized that withdrawal seizures can occur when stopping antiepileptic medication abruptly and that once their seizures abate the medication still has to be continued until the physician decides to withdraw the medication. There are no guidelines as to withdrawal of antiepileptic mediation in the context of NCC and therefore this has to be decided on a case-to-case basis. Usually withdrawal is considered when the epilepsy is in remission, i.e. the patient has to be seizure free for two years, although one year may be considered enough in resource-poor settings. Predictors for remaining seizure-free after withdrawal of antiepileptic medication seem to be normal neurological examination and use of carbamazepine prior to withdrawal [130], indicating outcome after drug withdrawal may be favourable in people with epilepsy and NCC. However, longitudinal studies on withdrawal of antiepileptic medication in people with epilepsy and NCC in sub-Saharan Africa have not been performed so far, but would definitely be needed to be able to develop guidelines on withdrawal of antiepileptic medication in this population.

2.5.3. Treatment in the absence of neuroimaging

The majority of patients in resource-poor settings have neither got access to neuroimaging nor to *Taenia solium* cysticercosis immunodiagnostic tests. Although positive results on *Taenia solium* cysticercosis antigen-ELISA may indicate active disease [131], treatment with antihelminthic medication must not be initiated on the basis of serology alone as cyst stage and presence of oedema cannot be estimated. Oedema can potentially be aggravated by antihelminthic medication resulting in deterioration of the patient's condition and, in the worst case, death may ensue caused by cerebral herniation leading to compression of the brainstem with severe compromise of vital functions. Therefore, I strongly suggest that in the absence of neuroimaging patients should be treated symptomatically only, i.e. anti-pain medication and antiepileptic drugs (see 2.5.2.).

The administration of steroids as symptomatic treatment in patients with signs and symptoms of increased intracranial pressure, such as chronic progressive headache in the context of suspected but not imaging-confirmed NCC, is debatable and has to be decided on an individual basis. A classical scenario where steroid administration may be advisable is in patients with acute symptomatic seizures who come from a *Taenia solium* cysticercosis endemic area. High doses of steroids may be started in these patients and tapered once symptoms abate. At the same time antiepileptic medication should be started on which the patient will be maintained until fit for withdrawal (see 2.5.2.). In this context, it is however crucial to exclude the most important differential diagnoses such as cerebral malaria, bacterial and tuberculous meningitis as well as encephalitis, among others, for which a spinal tap is necessary. The result of cerebrospinal fluid analysis is usually unequivocal for bacterial meningitis and in that case steroids are not to be started without antibacterial treatment. The result of cerebrospinal fluid analysis in tuberculous meningitis and viral encephalitis may be similar to that in NCC (although most patients with intraparenchymal NCC show normal results on cerebrospinal fluid; see 2.4.) with an unspecific medium increase in cell count and no major other obvious abnormalities, especially in a resource-poor setting where protein and glucose often are not measured. The eosinophils may be elevated in NCC, but this is not mandatory. Therefore differential diagnosis may prove difficult, but a trial of steroids will not harm patients with tuberculous meningitis or viral encephalitis as brain oedema may be present and administration of steroids to these patients may actually improve their symptoms [132,133].

Even after satisfactory symptomatic treatment the question remains whether withholding antihelminthic treatment in patients with NCC will have disadvantages in terms of cyst clearance or seizure control. Results are controversial. Garcia et al. showed that treatment with albendazole in addition to antiepileptic medication significantly cleared the parasite and reduced seizure frequency, especially those with generalisation, when compared to the control group that received antiepileptic medication only [134]. In contrast, in another study the same combination of albendazole and antiepileptic treatment in people with NCC was not superior to therapy with antiepileptic drugs alone. The combination treatment led to increased hospital admission, increased seizure frequency, more cases of encephalopathy and deaths. A greater proportion of lesions calcified compared to the group that was treated with antiepileptic drugs alone, in which more lesions resolved completely [135].

In summary, treatment of NCC in the absence of neuroimaging has to be decided on an individual basis and depends on clinical symptoms and/or signs, whether acute or chronic, and on the physician's experience as well as local practice. Most patients with NCC can be maintained on antiepileptic medication alone, but steroid application may be considered in the severely ill patient bearing in mind the implication of potential differential diagnoses.

3. Conclusions and outlook

This chapter demonstrates clearly the importance of epileptic seizures/epilepsy and NCC for sub-Saharan Africa in terms of prevalence and burden of each of the two disorders, but it also emphasizes NCC as an important cause of acute symptomatic seizures and secondary epilepsy in many African countries. *Taenia solium* cysticercosis is a potentially eradicable disease and successful implementation of treatment of human taeniosis and porcine cysticercosis (please refer to other chapters in the book) as well as enforcement of hygienic measure, such as building of latrines and hand washing after toilet use, among others, may prevent many cases of epileptic seizures/epilepsy and therefore reduce individual suffering as well as socioeconomic losses to African societies. Although eradication of the disease has to be the ultimate aim, treatment of affected individuals for now should be in the forefront of activities of African physicians who attend to people with epileptic seizures/epilepsy. I have suggested how people with epileptic seizures/epilepsy and/or NCC in resource-poor settings should be approached, but want to emphasize that this is my personal opinion/experience based on many years of work as a trained neurologist in sub-Saharan Africa. Conveying my own opinion in this chapter my aim was to stimulate discussion across disciplines and nations. Hopefully national and international stakeholders, such as the ministries of health of African countries and The World Health Organization, have by now become aware that NCC and the ensuing epilepsy in sub-Saharan African represent a "silent epidemic". Affected people deserve standardized treatment maximizing its benefits but at the same time minimizing its drawbacks. In that sense I am hopeful that in the near future guidelines on how to treat people with epilepsy and/or NCC will be decided by an expert-led commission and enforced as standard of care in sub-Saharan countries by the respective national and internal stakeholders.

List of abbreviations

CT; computed tomography
CWGESA; Cysticercosis Working Group in Eastern and Southern Africa
FLAIR; fluid attenuated inversion recovery
HIV/AIDS; human immunodeficiency virus/acquired immunodeficiency syndrome
MRI; magnetic resonance imaging

NCC; neurocysticercosis

Author details

Andrea Sylvia Winkler*
Department of Neurology, Klinikum rechts der Isar, Technical University Munich, Munich, Germany

Acknowledgement

I am extremely grateful to the patients of the Epilepsy Clinics of Haydom Lutheran Hospital (northern Tanzania) and Mahenge Hospital (southern Tanzania) for helping me gain all my experience which a good part of this book chapter is based on. I am further indebted to all my African, European and Canadian colleagues and friends who have always encouraged me to take up "neurology of sub-Saharan Africa" as my special field of research. I am also extremely thankful to the German Research Foundation (DFG) and the Bill and Melinda Gates foundation for supporting further work into the subject of epilepsy and NCC.

4. References

[1] International League Against Epilepsy (ILAE). Commission on Epidemiology and Prognosis of the International League Against Epilepsy. Guidelines for epidemiologic studies on epilepsy. Epilepsia 1993; 34: 592–596.
[2] Senanayake N, Román GC. Epidemiology of epilepsy in developing countries. Bulletin of the World Health Organization 1993; 71: 247–258.
[3] Edwards T, Scott AG, Munyoki G, Odera V, Chengo E, Bauni E, Kwasa T, Sander LW, Neville BG, Newton CR. Active convulsive epilepsy in a rural district of Kenya: a study of prevalence and possible risk factors. The Lancet Neurology 2008; 7: 50–56.
[4] Aall-Jilek LM. Epilepsy in the Wapogoro tribe in Tanganyika. Acta Psychiatrica Scandinavica 1965; 41: 57–86.
[5] Osuntokun BO. The pattern of neurological illness in tropical Africa. Experience at Ibadan, Nigeria. Journal of the Neurological Sciences 1971; 12: 417–442.
[6] Preux PM, Druet-Cabanac M. Epidemiology and aetiology of epilepsy in sub-Saharan Africa. The Lancet Neurology 2005; 4: 21–31.
[7] Forsgren L. Estimations of the prevalence of epilepsy in sub-Saharan Africa. The Lancet Neurology 2008; 7: 21–22.
[8] Forsgren L, Beghi E, Oun A, Sillanpää M. The epidemiology of epilepsy in Europe - a systematic review. European Journal of Neurology 2005; 12: 245–253.
[9] Rwiza HT, Kilonzo GP, Haule J, Matuja WBP, Mteza I, Mbena P, Kilima PM, Mwaluko G, Mwang'ombola R, Mwanijande F, Rweyemamu G, Matowo A, Jilek-Aall LM. Prevalence and incidence of epilepsy in Ulanga, a rural Tanzanian district: a community-based study. Epilepsia 1992; 33: 1051–1056.

---

* Corresponding Author

[29] Wolf P. Historical aspects of idiopathic generalized epilepsies. Epilepsia 2005; 46: 7–9.

[30] Couper J. Prevalence of childhood disability in rural KwaZulu-Natal. South African Medical Journal 2002; 92: 549–552.

[31] Ashwal S, Russman BS, Blasco PA, Miller G, Sandler A, Shevell M, Stevenson R; Quality Standards Subcommittee of the American Academy of Neurology; Practice Committee of the Child Neurology Society. Practice parameter: diagnostic assessment of the child with cerebral palsy: report of the Quality Standards Subcommittee of the American Academy of Neurology and the Practice Committee of the Child Neurology Society. Neurology 2004; 62: 851–863.

[32] Aneja S, Ahuja B, Taluja V, Bhatia VK. Epilepsy in children with cerebral palsy. Indian Journal of Pediatrics 2001; 68: 111–115.

[33] Everitt AD, Sander JWAS. Classification of the epilepsies. Time for a change? European Journal of Neurology 1999; 42: 1–10.

[34] Scott RA, Lhatoo SD, Sander JWAS. The treatment of epilepsy in developing countries: where do we go from here? Bulletin of the World Health Organization 2001; 79: 344–351.

[35] Ngugi AK, Bottomley C, Kleinschmidt I, Sander JW, Newton CR. Estimation of the burden of active and life-time epilepsy: a meta-analytic approach. Epilepsia 2010; 51: 883–890.

[36] Meyer AC, Dua T, Ma J, Saxena S, Birbeck G. Global disparities in the epilepsy treatment gap: a systematic review. Bulletin of the World Health Organization 2010; 88: 260–266.

[37] Mbuba CK, Ngugi AK, Fegan G, Ibinda F, Muchohi SN, Nyundo C, Odhiambo R, Edwards T, Odermatt P, Carter JA, Newton CR. Risk factors associated with the epilepsy treatment gap in Kilifi, Kenya: a cross-sectional study. The Lancet Neurology 2012; 11: 688–696.

[38] Winkler AS. Measuring the epilepsy treatment gap in sub-Saharan Africa. The Lancet Neurology 2012; 11. 655–657.

[39] Winkler AS, Mayer M, Schnaitmann S, Ombay M, Mathias B, Schmutzhard E, Jilek-Aall L. Belief systems of epilepsy and attitudes towards people living with epilepsy in a rural community of northern Tanzania. Epilepsy & Behavior 2010a; 19: 596–601.

[40] Winkler AS, Mayer M, Ombay M, Mathias B, Schmutzhard E, Jilek-Aall L. Attitudes towards African traditional medicine and Christian spiritual healing regarding treatment of epilepsy in a rural community of northern Tanzania. African Journal of Traditional, Complementary and Alternative Medicines 2010b; 7: 162–170.

[41] Jilek-Aall L. Morbus sacer in Africa: some religious aspects of epilepsy in traditional cultures. Epilepsia 1999; 40: 382–386.

[42] Birbeck G, Chomba E, Atadzhanov M, Mbewe W, Haworth A. The social and economic impact of epilepsy in Zambia: a cross-sectional study. The Lancet Neurology 2007; 6: 39–44.

[43] Sander JWAS, Shovron SD. Epidemiology of the epilepsies. Neuroepidemiology 1996; 61: 433–443.

[44] Jallon P. Epilepsy in developing countries. Epilepsia 1997; 38: 1143–1151.

[45] Del Brutto OH. Helminthic infections of the central nervous system. In: Noseworthy JH (ed). Neurological therapeutic principles and practice. Abingdon, Oxon (UK): Informa Health Care; 2006. pp 1133-1152.

[46] Wallin M, Kurtzke J. Neurocysticercosis in the United States: review of an important emerging infection. Neurology 2004; 63: 1559–1564.

[47] Willingham AL III, Harrison LJ, Fèvre EM, Parkhouse ME. Inaugural meeting of the Cysticercosis Working Group in Europe. Emerging Infectious Diseases 2008; 14: e2.

[48] Del Brutto OH. A review of cases of human cysticercosis in Canada. Canadian Journal of Neuroscience 2012a: 39: 319–22.

[49] Del Brutto OH. Neurocysticercosis among international travelers. Journal of Travel Medicine 2012b; 19: 112–17.

[50] Del Brutto OH. Neurocysticercosis in Western Europe: a re-emerging disease? Acta Neurologica Belgica 2012c; April 18 [Epub ahead of print]

[51] Fleury A, Gomez T, Alvarez I, Meza D, Huerta M, Chavarria A, Carrillo Mezo RA, Lloyd C, Dessein A, Preux PM, Dumas M, Larralde C, Sciutto E, Fragoso G. High prevalence of calcified silent neurocysticercosis in a rural village of Mexico. Neuroepidemiology 2003; 22: 139–145.

[52] Carabin H, Millogo A, Praet N, Hounton S, Tarnagda Z, Ganaba R, Dorny P, Nitiéma P, Cowan LD; Evaluation du Fardeau Economique de la Cysticercose Au Burkina Faso (EFECAB). Seroprevalence to the antigens of *Taenia solium* cysticercosis among residents in three villages in Burkina Faso: a cross-sectional study. PLoS Neglected Tropical Diseases 2009; 3: e555.

[53] Kanobana K, Praet N, Kabwe C, Dorny P, Lukanu P, Madinga J, Mitashi P, Verwijs M, Lutumba P, Polman K. High prevalence of Taenia solium cysticercosis in a village community of Bas-Congo, Democratic Republic of Congo. International Journal of Parasitology 2011; 41: 1015–1018.

[54] Mwape KE, Phiri IK, Praet N, Muma JB, Zulu G, Van den Bossche P, de Deken R, Speybroeck N, Dorny P, Gabriël S. *Taenia solium* infections in a rural area of Eastern Zambia-a community based study. PLoS Neglected Tropical Diseases 2012; 6: e1594

[55] Nitiéma P, Carabin H, Hounton S, Praet N, Cowan LD, Ganaba R, Kompaoré C, Tarnagda Z, Dorny P, Millogo A, Efécab. Prevalence case-control study of epilepsy in three Burkina Faso villages. Acta Neurologica Scandinavica 2012; 126: 270–278.

[56] Ndimubanzi PC, Carabin H, Budke CM, Nguyen H, Qian YJ, Rainwater E, Dickey M, Reynolds S, Stoner JA. A systematic review of the frequency of neurocyticercosis with a focus on people with epilepsy. PLoS Neglected Tropical Diseases 2010; 4: e870.

[57] World Bank 2011. http://data.worldbank.org/sites/default/files/adi_2011-web.pdf Last accessed July 2012

[58] Carabin H, Ndimubanzi PC, Budke CM, Nguyen H, Qian Y, Cowan LD, Stoner JA, Rainwater E, Dickey M. Clinical manifestations associated with neurocysticercosis: a systematic review. PLoS Neglected Tropical Diseases 2011; 5: e1152.

[59] De Almeida SM, Torres LFB. Neurocysticercosis—retrospective study of autopsy reports, a 17-year experience. Journal of Community Health 2011; 36: 698–702.

[60] WHO 2010. Working to overcome the global impact of neglected tropical diseases. First WHO report on neglected tropical diseases.

http://whqlibdoc.who.int/publications/2010/9789241564090_eng.pdf
[61] World Atlas 2010.
http://www.worldatlas.com/aatlas/populations/ctypopls.htm "Last accessed July 2012
[62] Ramos-Zúñiga R, Pérez-Gómez HR, Jáuregui-Huerta F, López-Hernández MD, Valera-Lizárraga JE, Paz-Vélez G, Becerra-Valdivia A. Incidental Consequences of Antihelmintic Treatment in the Central Nervous System. World Neurosurgery 2012 Feb 10 [Epub ahead of print]
[63] Johnson RB. Potential hazard of mass praziquantel use. American Journal of Medicine 1986; 80: A88.
[64] Torres JR, Noya O, de Noya BA, Mondolfi A. Seizures and praziquantel. A case report. Revista do Instituto de Medicina Tropical São Paulo. 1988; 30: 433–436.
[65] Flisser A, Madrazo I, Plancarte A, Schantz P, Allan J, Craig P, Sarti E. Neurological symptoms in occult neurocysticercosis after single taeniacidal dose of praziquantel. The Lancet. 1993; 342: 748.
[66] Garcia HH, Gonzalez I, Mija L. Neurocysticercosis uncovered by single-dose albendazole. New England Journal of Medicine 2007; 356: 1277-1278.
[67] Winkler AS. Neurocysticercosis in sub-Saharan Africa: A review of prevalence, clinical characteristics, diagnosis and management. Pathogens & Global Health 2012 (in print).
[68] Mafojane NA, Appleton CC, Krecek RC, Michael LM, Willingham AL 3rd. The current status of neurocysticercosis in eastern and southern Africa. Acta Tropica 2003; 87: 25–33.
[69] Zoli A, Shey-Njila O, Assana E, Nguekam JP, Dorny P, Brandt J, Geerts F. Regional status, epidemiology and impact of *Taenia solium* cysticercosis in western and central Africa. Acta Tropica 2003a 87: 35–42.
[70] Zoli AP, Nguekam JP, Shey-Njila O, Nsame Nforninwe D, Speybroeck N, Ito A, Sato MO, Dorny P, Brandt J, Geerts S. Neurocysticercosis and epilepsy in Cameroon. Transactions of the Royal Society of Tropical Medicine and Hygiene 2003b; 97: 683–686.
[71] Quet F, Guerchet M, Pion SDS, Ngoungou EB, Nicoletti A, Preux PM. Meta-analysis of the association between cysticercosis and epilepsy in Africa. Epilepsia 2010; 51: 830–837.
[72] Campbell CD, Farrell VJR. Brain scans, epilepsy and cerebral cysticercosis. South African Medical Journal 1987; 72: 885–886.
[73] Winkler AS, Blocher J, Auer H, Gotwald T, Matuja W, Schmutzhard E. Epilepsy and neurocysticercosis in rural Tanzania – an imaging study. Epilepsia 2009d; 50: 987–993.
[74] Blocher J, Schmutzhard E, Wilkins PP, Gupton P, Schaffert M, Auer H, Gotwald T, Matuja W, Winkler AS. A cross-sectional study of people with epilepsy and neurocysticercosis: clinical characteristics and diagnostic approaches. PLoS Neglected Tropical Diseases 2011; 5: e1185.
[75] Rigatti M, Trevisol-Bittencourt PC. Causes of late-onset epilepsy in an epilepsy clinic of Santa Catarina—Southern Brazil. Arquivos de Neuro-Psiquiatria 1999; 57: 787–792.
[76] Medina MT, Rosas E, Rubio-Donnadieu F, Sotelo J. Neurocysticercosis as the main cause of late-onset epilepsy in Mexico. Archives of Internal Medicine 1990; 150: 325–327.
[77] Del Brutto OH, Santibáñez R, Idrovo L, Rodrìguez S, Díaz-Calderón E, Navas C, Gilman RH, Cuesta F, Mosquera A, Gonzalez AE, Tsang VC, García HH. Epilepsy and neurocysticercosis in Atahualpa: a door-to-door survey in rural coastal Ecuador. Epilepsia 2005; 46: 583–587.

[78] Nicoletti A, Bartoloni A, Sofia V, Bartalesi F, Chavez JR, Osinaga R, Paradisi F, Dumas JL, Tsang VC, Reggio A, Hall AJ. Epilepsy and neurocysticercosis in rural Bolivia: a population-based survey. Epilepsia 2005; 46: 1127–1132.
[79] Mitchell WG, Crawford TO. Intraparenchymal cerebral cysticercosis in children: diagnosis and treatment. Pediatrics 1988; 82: 76–82.
[80] Thomson AJ. Neurocysticercosis—experience at the teaching hospitals of the University of Cape Town. South African Medical Journal 1993; 83: 332-334.
[81] Ferreira LS, Zanardi VA, Scotoni AE, Li LM, Guerreiro MM. Childhood epilepsy due to neurocysticercosis: a comparative study. Epilepsia 2001; 42: 1438–1444.
[82] Singhi P, Singhi S. Neurocysticercosis in children. Journal of Child Neurology 2004; 19: 482–492.
[83] Sáenz B, Ruíz-Garcia M, Jiménez E, Hernández-Aguilar J, Suastegui R, Larralde C, Sciutto E, Fleury A. Neurocysticercosis: clinical, radiologic, and inflammatory differences between children and adults. The Pediatric Infectious Disease Journal 2006; 25: 801–803.
[84] Foyaca-Sibat H, Ibanez-Valdes L de F. Intraventricular neurocysticercosis in HIV positive patients. International Journal of Neurology, 2003a; 2(1). http://www.ispub.com/journal/the_internet_journal_of_neurology/volume_2_number_1_37/article/intraventricular_neurocysticercosis_in_hiv_positive_patients.html Last accessed July 2012
[85] Foyaca-Sibat H, Ibanez-Valdes L de F. Neurocysticercosis in HIV-positive patients. International Journal of Infectious Diseases 2003b; 2(2). http://www.ispub.com/journal/the-internet-journal-of-infectious-diseases/volume-2-number-2/neurocysticercosis-in-hiv-positive-patients.html Last accessed July 2012
[86] Jessurun J, Barron-Rodriguez LP, Fernandez-Tinoco G, Hernandez-Avila M. The prevalence of invasive amebiasis is not increased in patients with AIDS. AIDS 1992; 6: 307–309.
[87] Parija SC, Gareesh AR. A serological study of cysticercosis in people with HIV. Revista do Instituto de Medicina Tropical de São Paulo 2009; 51: 185–189.
[88] Carabin H, Krecek RC, Cowan LD, Michael L, Foyaca-Sibat H, Nash T, Willingham AL. Estimation of the cost of *Taenia solium* cysticercosis in Eastern Cape Province, South Africa. Tropical Medicine and International Health 2006; 11: 906–916.
[89] Praet N, Speybroeck N, Manzanedo R, Berkvens D, Nsame Nforninwe D, Zoli A, Quet F, Preux PM, Carabin H, Geerts S. The disease burden of *Taenia solium* cysticercosis in Cameroon. PLoS Neglected Tropical Diseases 2009; 3: e406.
[90] Serpa JA, Yancey LS, White AC Jr. Advances in the diagnosis and management of neurocysticercosis. Expert Review of Anti-Infective Therapy 2006; 4: 1051–1061.
[91] Davis LE. Neurocysticercosis. In: Power C, Johnson RT (eds). Emerging neurological infections. Boca Raton: Taylor & Francis; 2005. pp 261-287.
[92] Singh MK, Garg RK, Nath G, Verma DN, Misra S. Single small enhancing computed tomographic (CT) lesions in Indian patients with new-onset seizures: a prospective follow-up in 75 patients. Seizure. 2001; 10: 573–578.

[93] Singh G, Rajshekhar V, Murthy JMK, S. Prabhakar S, Modi M, Khandelwal N, Garcia HH. A diagnostic and therapeutic scheme for a solitary cysticercus granuloma. Neurology 2010; 75: 2236–2245.

[94] Mansur MM 2010. Cysticercosis. http://emedicine.medscape.com/article/215589-overview Last accessed July 2012

[95] Nash TE, Singh G, White AC, Rajshekhar V, Loeb JA, Proaño JV, Takayanagui OM, Gonzalez AE, Butman JA, DeGiorgio C, Del Brutto OH, Delgado-Escueta A, Evans CA, Gilman RH, Martinez SM, Medina MT, Pretell EJ, Teale J, Garcia HH. Treatment of neurocysticercosis: current status and future research needs. Neurology 2006; 67: 1120–1127.

[96] White AC. Why are there seizures in neurocysticercosis: Is it in the genes? The Journal of Infectious Diseases 2010; 202: 1152–1153.

[97] Nash TE, Del Brutto OH, Butman JA, Corona T, Delgado-Escueta A, Duron RM, Evans CA, Gilman RH, Gonzalez AE, Loeb JA, Medina MT, Pietsch-Escueta S, Pretell EJ, Takayanagui OM, Theodore W, Tsang VC, Garcia HH. Calcific neurocysticercosis and epileptogenesis. Neurology 2004; 62: 1934–1938.

[98] Cruz ME, Schantz PM, Cruz I, Espinosa P, Preux PM, Cruz A, Benitez W, Tsang VCW, Fermoso J, Dumas M. Epilepsy and neurocysticercosis in an Andean community. International Journal of Epidemiology 1999; 28: 799–803.

[99] Mishra D. Cysticercosis headache: an important differential of childhood headache disorder in endemic countries. Headache 2007; 47: 301–302.

[100] Forlenza OV, Filho AH, Nobrega JP, dos Ramos Machado L, de Barros NG, de Camargo CH, da Silva MF. Psychiatric manifestations of neurocysticercosis: a study of 38 patients from a neurology clinic in Brazil. Journal of Neurology, Neurosurgery and Psychiatry 1997; 62: 612–616.

[101] Ciampi de Andrade D, Rodriques CL, Abraham R, Castro LH, Livramento JA, Machado LR, Leite CC, Caramelli P. Cognitive impairment and dementia in neurocysticercosis: a cross-sectional controlled study. Neurology 2010; 74: 1288–1295.

[102] Wallin MT, Pretell EJ, Bustos JA, Caballero M, Alfaro M, Kane R, Wilkin J, Sullivan C, Fratto T, Garcia HH. Cognitive changes and quality of life in neurocysticercosis: a longitudinal study. PLoS Neglected Infectious Diseases 2012; 6: e1493.

[103] Morales NM, Agapejev S, Morales RR, Padula NA, Lima MM. Clinical aspects of neurocysticercosis in children. Pediatric Neurology 2000; 22: 287–291.

[104] Antoniuk S, Bruck I, Santos LH, Souza LP, Fugimura S. Neurocysticercosis in children: clinical study and follow-up of 112 patients. Revista de Neurologia 2006; 42(suppl 3): S97–101.

[105] Sotelo J, Del Brutto OH. Review of neurocysticercosis. Neurosurgical Focus 2002; 12: e1.

[106] Pal DK, Carpio A, Sander JWAS. Neurocysticercosis and epilepsy in developing countries. Journal of Neurology, Neurosurgery and Psychiatry 2000; 68: 137–143.

[107] Del Brutto OH, Rajshekhar V, White AC Jr, Tsang VC, Nash TE, Takayanagui OM, Schantz PM, Evans CA, Flisser A, Correa D, Botero D, Allan JC, Sarti E, Gonzalez AE, Gilman RH, Garcia HH. Proposed diagnostic criteria for neurocysticercosis. Neurology 2001; 57: 177–183.

[108] Dorny P, Brandt J, Zoli A, Geerts S. Immunodiagnostic tools for human and porcine cysticercosis. Acta Tropica 2003; 87: 79–86.

[109] Del Brutto OH. Neurocysticercosis. Seminars in Neurology 2005; 25: 243–251.

[110] Winkler AS, Willingham AL, Sikasunge CS, Schmutzhard E. Epilepsy and neurocysticercosis in sub-Saharan Africa. The Middle European Journal of Medicine 2009e; 121(suppl 3): 3–12.

[111] Abraham R, Livramento JA, Leite CDA, Pardini AX, Vaz AJ, Machado Lidos R. Neurocysticercosis: relationship between *Taenia* antigen levels in CSF and MRI. Arquivos de Neuropsiquiatrica 2010; 68: 7–11.

[112] Praet N, Rodriguez-Hidalgo R, Speybroeck N, Ahounou S, Benitez-Ortiz W, Berkvens D, Hul AV, Barrionuevo-Samaniego M, Saegerman C, Dorny P. Infection with versus exposure to *Taenia solium*: what do serological test results tell us? American Journal of Tropical Medicine and Hygiene 2010; 83: 413–415.

[113] Almeida CR, Ojopi EP, Nunes CM, Machado LR, Takayanagui OM, Livramento JA, Abraham R, Gattaz WF, Vaz AJ, Dias-Neto E. *Taenia solium* DNA is present in cerebrospinal fluid of neurocysticercosis patients and can be used for diagnosis. European Archives of Psychiatry and Clinical Neurosciences 2006; 56: 307–310.

[114] Hernández M, Gonzalez LM, Fleury A, Saenz B, Parkhouse RM, Harrison LJ, Garate T, Sciutto E. Neurocysticercosis: detection of *Taenia solium* DNA in human cerebrospinal fluid using a semi-nested PCR based on HDP2. Annals of Tropical Medicine and Parasitology 2008; 102: 317–323.

[115] Chang KH, Han MH. MRI of CNS parasitic disease. Journal of Magnetic Resonance Imaging 1998; 8: 297–307.

[116] Del Brutto OH, Wadia NH, Dumas M, Cruz M, Tsang VCW, Schantz PM. Proposal of diagnostic criteria for human cysticercosis and neurocysticercosis. Journal of the Neurological Sciences 1996; 142: 1–6.

[117] Nash TE, Garcia HH. Diagnosis and treatment of neurocysticercosis. Nature Reviews Neurology 2011; 7: 584–94.

[118] Del Brutto OH, Roos KL, Coffey CS, Garcia HH. Meta-analysis: Cysticidal drugs for neurocysticercosis: albendazole and praziquantel. Annals of Internal Medicine 2006; 145: 43–51.

[119] Corona T, Lugo R, Medina R, Sotelo J. Single-day praziquantel therapy for neurocysticercosis. New England Journal of Medicine 1996; 334: 125.

[120] Pretell EJ, Garcia HH, Gilman RH, Saavedra H, Martinez M; The Cysticercosis Working Group in Peru. Failure of one-day praziquantel treatment in patients with multiple neurocysticercosis lesions. Clinical Neurology and Neurosurgery 2001; 103: 175–177.

[121] Nash TE, Mahanty S, Garcia HH; Cysticercosis Group in Peru. Corticosteroid use in neurocysticercosis. Expert Review of Neurotherapeutics 2011; 11: 1175–1183.

[122] Mall RK, Agarwal A, Garg RK, Kar AW, Shukla R. Short course of prednisolone in Indian patients with solitary cysticercus granuloma and new onset seizures. Epilepsia 2003; 44: 1397–1401.

[123] Garg RK, Potluri N, Kar AM, Singh MK, Shukla R, Agrawal A, Verma R. Short course of prednisolone in patients with cysticercus granuloma: a double blind placebo controlled trial. Journal of Infection 2006; 53: 65–69.

[124] Prakash S, Garg RK, Kar AM, Shukla R, Agarwal A, Verma R, Singh MK. Intravenous methyl prednisolone in patients with solitary cysticercus granuloma: a random evaluation. Seizure 2006; 15; 328–323.

[125] Kishore D, Misra S. A short course of oral prednisolone on disappearance of lesion and seizure recurrence in patients of solitary cysticercus granuloma with single small enhancing CT lesion: an open label randomized prospective study. Journal of the Association of Physicians of India 2007; 55: 419–424.

[126] Carpio A. Neuroimaging in Neurocysticercosis. 2012. http//emedicine.medscape.com/article/1168784-differential Last accessed July 2012

[127] Gonzalez AE, Gauci CG, Barber D, Gilman RH, Tsang VC, Garcia HH, Verastegui M, Lightowlers MW. Short report: vaccination of pigs to control human neurocysticercosis. American Journal of Tropical Medicine and Hygiene 2005; 72: 837–839.

[128] Pawlowski ZS. Control of neurocysticercosis by routine medical and veterinary services. Transactions of the Royal Society of Tropical Medicine and Hygiene 2008; 102: 228–232.

[129] Fisher RS, van Emde Boas W, Blume W, Elger C, Genton P, Lee P, Engel Jr J. Epileptic seizures and epilepsy: definitions proposed by the International League Against Epilepsy (ILAE) and the International Bureau for Epilepsy (IBE). Epilepsia 2005; 46: 470–472.

[130] Lossius MI, Hessen E, Mowinckel P, Stavem K, Erikssen J, Gulbrandsen P, Gjerstad L. Consequences of antiepileptic drug withdrawal: a randomized, double-blind study (Akershus Study). Epilepsia 2008; 49: 455–463.

[131] Gabriël S, Blocher J, Dorny P, Abatih E, Schmutzhard E, Ombay M, Mathias B, Winkler AS. Added value of antigen ELISA in the diagnosis of neurocysticercosis in resource poor settings. PLoS Neglected Tropical Diseases 2012, in print

[132] Nakano A, Yamasaki R, Miyazaki S, Horiuchi N, Kunishige M, Mitsui T. Beneficial effect of steroid pulse therapy on acute viral encephalitis. European Neurology 2003; 50: 225–229.

[133] Ramachandran TS 2008. Tuberculous meningitis. http://emedicine.medscape.com/article/1166190-overview Last accessed August 2012

[134] Garcia HH, Pretell EJ, Gilman RH, Martinez SM, Moulton LH, Del Brutto OH, Herrera G, Evans CA, Gonzalez AE; Cysticercosis Working Group in Peru. A trial of antiparasitic treatment to reduce the rate of seizures due to cerebral cysticercosis. New England Journal of Medicine 2004; 350: 249–258.

[135] Das K, Mondal GP, Banerjee M, Mukherjee BB, Singh OP. Role of antiparasitic therapy for seizures and resolution of lesions in neurocysticercosis patients: an 8 year randomized study. Journal of Clinical Neuroscience 2007; 14: 1172–1177.

Surgical Treatment of Neurocysticercosis-Related Epilepsy

Alejandro L. Escalaya and Jorge G. Burneo

Additional information is available at the end of the chapter

http://dx.doi.org/10.5772/54275

1. Introduction

Seizures are the most frequent clinical manifestation associated with neurocysticercosis (NCC) [1]. But, not all patients with NCC and seizures will develop epilepsy [2)]. Nearly 85% of patients with a single NCC in transitional or degenerative phase have a good seizure outcome following resolution of the lesion, and antiepileptic drugs (AEDs) withdrawal [3)]. Patients with residual calcifications and those with both recurrent seizures and multiple cysts before treatment with albendazole have the highest rate of relapse after complete disappearance of the cysts and withdrawal of AEDs [4]. Cerebral calcifications are a common finding in persons with seizures or epilepsy in endemic populations [5], and perilesional edema is associated with episodic seizure activity in patients with calcified NCC [6]. However, a high rate of negative correlations between the electroclinical localization and the topography of intracranial calcification has been reported [7], and an irritative zone in the temporal lobe is more relevant in determining the severity and frequency of seizures, than the number and location of calcifications [8].

Drug-resistant epilepsy (DRE) is now defined as "failure of two adequate trials, appropriately chosen and tolerated AEDs schedules (whether as monotherapy or in combination) to achieve sustained seizure freedom" [9]. NCC is an uncommon cause of DRE, even in endemic regions [10]. Perilesional gliosis (best visualized on magnetization transfer spin-echo magnetic resonance imaging), may cause seizures that could be difficult to control with antiepileptic drugs (AEDs) in patients with a solitary cysticercal cyst in the brain [11, 12].

Epilepsy surgery is highly effective in selected patients with DRE, has durable benefits, and improves quality of life [13]. The standard presurgical evaluation should encompass careful history and physical examination, interictal electroencephalography (EEG) including sleep, prolonged video EEG monitoring, magnetic resonance imaging (MRI) with specific

INTECH
open science | open minds

© 2013 Escalaya and Burneo, licensee InTech. This is a paper distributed under the terms of the Creative Commons Attribution License (http://creativecommons.org/licenses/by/3.0), which permits unrestricted use, distribution, and reproduction in any medium, provided the original work is properly cited.

sequences, and neuropsychological assessment. In some cases, invasive monitoring with intracranially-placed electrodes is needed for the purpose of seizure localization. Epilepsy surgery as a treatment of DRE due to NCC has been uncommonly reported.

2. Epilepsy surgery and NCC

Rassi Neto et al. [14], in 1998, reported three cases of patients with DRE associated to calcified neurocysticercotic lesions in the temporal lobe. Two of them had MRI imaging, and one of the studies showed perilesional edema. In all cases, the epileptiform focus was demonstrated by EEG. The patients were submitted to removal of the lesion with use of perioperative electrocorticogram, also rendering possible removal of the irritative perilesional focus. In all the cases, the histologic examination showed NCC. However, the authors did not report complete histological description. Out-patient follow-up was approximately 30 months. Two patients were seizure-free and one patient presented an improvement of 95% in seizure frequency.

Chung et al. [15], in 1998, reported a 47-year-old man with intractable temporal lobe epilepsy. Computed tomography (CT) and MRI imaging showed a calcification in the region of the left medial temporal lobe, and atrophy of the hippocampal head portion. Interictal EEG and prolonged video-EEG monitoring were compatible with left temporal lobe epilepsy. The patient underwent standard left temporal lobectomy. Histologic examination revealed degenerated cysticercus and scolex, with the surrounded hippocampus showing a fascia dentada with neuronal loss and gliosis. He was seizure-free for two years after the first postoperative day.

Ooi et al. [16], in 2011, presented a 23-year-old male with recurrent focal seizures despite continued treatment with AED. CT and MRI imaging showed a calcified lesion with surrounding edema in the right frontal lobe that waxed and waned over time. After extensive presurgical evaluation, including mapping of the seizure focus to the right frontal lobe, the lesion was excised. The histological description was available. The capsule, around a degenerated cysticercus, contained marked mononuclear infiltrates that extended to adjacent brain, which showed marked astrocytosis, microgliosis, and inflammatory perivascular infiltrates. The patient was seizure-free for a period of 2 years while on AEDs until he presented again with seizures associated with perilesional edema around the one cyst in the left frontal lobe that had evolved into a calcified granuloma.

Based on these cases published in the literature, it appears important to presurgically identify the presence of perilesional gliosis (around the cysticercotic lesion), as this appeared to be an important predictor of seizure freedom following surgery. This would indicate the important role of gliosis in the generation of seizures, which are particularly difficult to treat in this group of patients. The technique of magnetization transfer spin-echo magnetic resonance imaging is useful for this purpose, as well as the use of electrocorticography when possible, which would allow delineating the epileptogenic tissue.

3. Epilepsy surgery in NCC and coexistence of other lesions

The association of NCC with hippocampal sclerosis (HS) has been reported in developing countries [17, 18]. In a cross-sectional study of 512 patients with DRE, 54.8% of them had HS, and 37% of them presented with HS plus NCC [19]. The mechanism of this association is not clarified. First, NCC might work as an initial precipitating injury leading to HS [20]. Second, the occurrence of NCC lesions in association with HS, or *vice versa*, may be merely coincidental [21]. Finally, both diseases might share common predisposing factors [10].

Leite et al. [21], in Brazil, determined the clinical and pathologic findings of 30 patients with HS and compared them with 32 patients with HS and calcified cysticercotic lesions (CCL) from an epilepsy surgery program. Preoperative data localized the focus to the anterior temporal region and patients were referred for a standardized en-bloc resection including 2 to 3 cm of the hippocampus. In three patients, a CCL ipsilateral to the atrophic hippocampus was located within the margins of resection and removed. The mean follow-up was 29.7 months. The percentage of patients with very good seizure control was similar in both groups. 81.2% patients in the HS + CCL group and 76.6% in the HS group had seizure-free outcome ($p = 0.90$]. No differences were found between the 2 groups in regards to age at seizure onset, hippocampal cell densities, or fascia dentata neo-Timm's staining patterns. Accordingly, their findings indicate that there is no need for removal of CCL in order to achieve good postsurgical seizure control in this set of patients.

Chandra et al. [22], in India, presented a series of 28 DRE cases resulting from post-infectious etiologies requiring surgery. All patients underwent a complete epilepsy presurgical evaluation. The criteria used to define infection-related DRE included absence of other potential etiologies preceding the infection as a cause of epilepsy. This was determined by reviewing the clinical history and MRI/CT scans performed at the time of onset of initial infection (the authors did not report if this initial MRI scan was with a special epilepsy protocol). The mean duration of epilepsy prior to surgery was 8.2 ± 2.1 years. Patients were followed after surgery for an average of 14.2 months. The pathologies included NCC in six cases. Four of the five cases with NCC in the temporal lobe, had HS. Histology of one of these cases showed evidence of early HS (not detected earlier on MRI, but with significant spike activity in electrocorticography). Free-seizure outcome was seen in all six cases.

In our center, one patient with DRE NCC-related epilepsy was assessed for possible epilepsy surgery. He was a 39 year-old man who had a previous history of a single, non-febrile, generalized tonic–clonic seizure at age of 5. At age of 13, he began to experience recurrent seizures consisting of fear, followed by loss of awareness associated with unusual movement of the hands. He then would scream, run and have forceful eye deviation to the left. Postictal confusion and aggressiveness were reported. The episodes were lasting from two to five minutes and they would occur one to two times a month. Once a year, those events would be followed by a secondarily generalized tonic-clonic seizure. He had an unclear history of central nervous system infection at the age of two years and some developmental delay. He had been treated with three different AEDs before he was referred to our epilepsy program. He was a Mexican Mennonite, who immigrated to Canada at the age of 6 years, with frequent travels to his country of origin. The CT scan and the MRI study revealed right HS as well as 3 extratemporal calcified cysticerci (Figure 1). Initial presurgical evaluation indicated possible frontal epilepsy (Figure 2), but subsequent placement of intracranial electrodes identified that seizures arose from the right mesial temporal lobe (Figure 3). He underwent a right temporal lobectomy and has been seizure free for over 2 years.

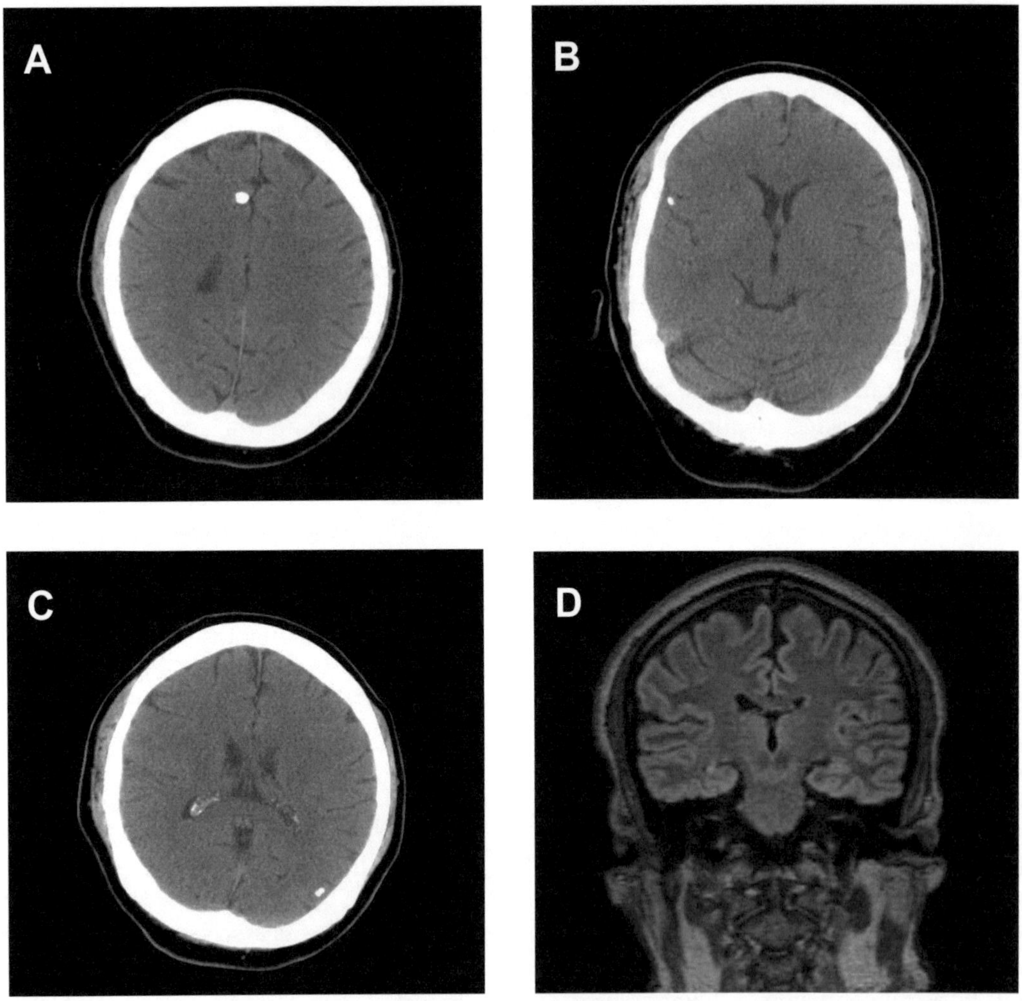

Figure 1. Preoperative imaging studies in one patient with drug resistant epilepsy. (A, B and C) Serial CT scan of the patient showing 3 extratemporal calcified cysticerci. (D) MRI fluid-attenuated inversion recovery (FLAIR) reveals a focal high signal intensity lesion in the right mesial temporal region and minimal atrophy of the hippocampus support hippocampal sclerosis.

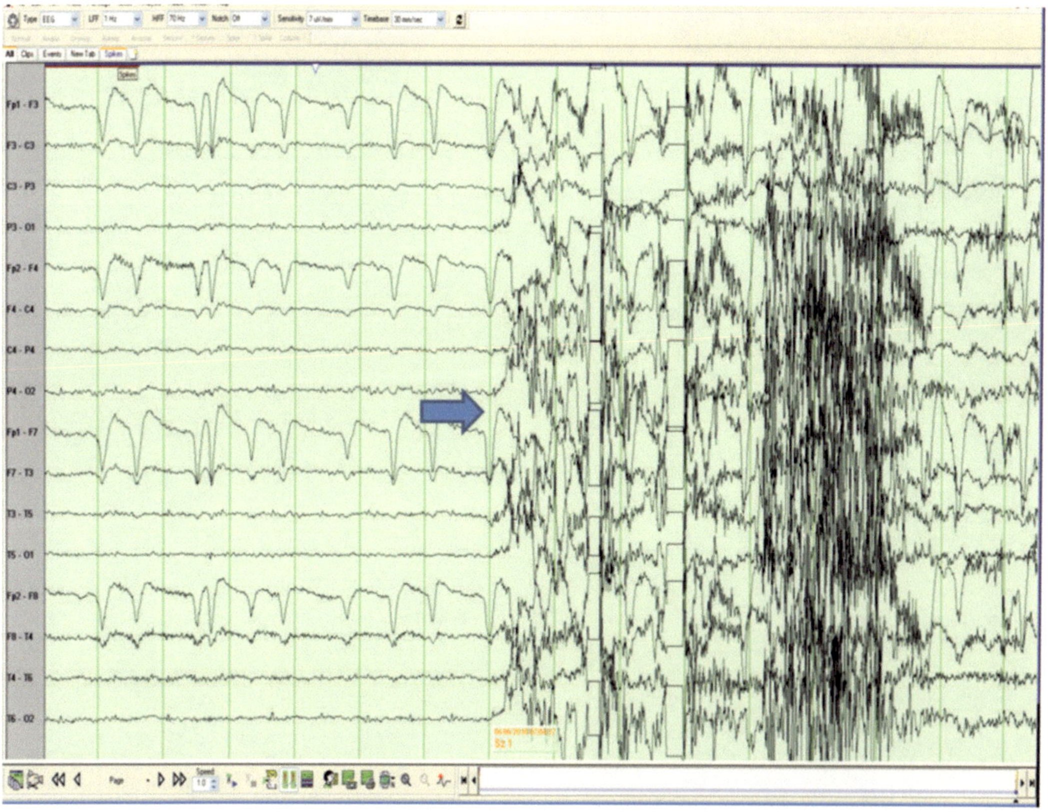

Figure 2. Initial presurgical evaluation in one patient with drug resistant epilepsy with right hippocampal sclerosis and three extratemporal calcified cysticerci. Video electroencephalography monitoring was obscured by movement and muscle artifact (arrow), but the semiology of the seizures captured on video, were concerning for a possible extratemporal lobe focus, despite the initial symptom of fear.

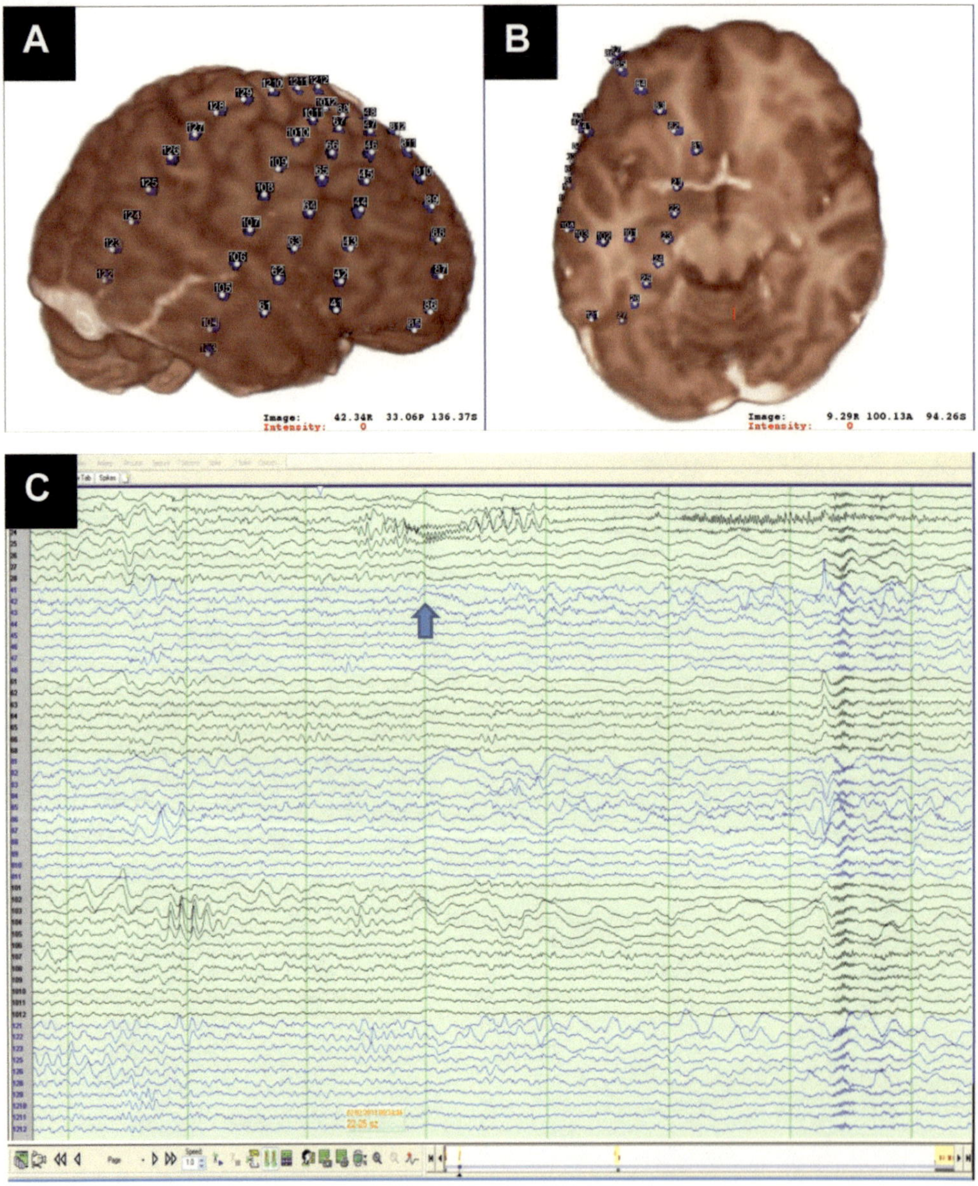

Figure 3. Presurgical evaluation in one patient with drug resistant epilepsy with right hippocampal sclerosis and three extratemporal calcified cysticerci. (A and B) Localization of the intracranial electrodes. (C) Invasive recordings show an ictal onset from the mesial right temporal lobe.

4. Conclusions

Epilepsy surgery in NCC is rare but effective. Patient with DRE and NCC should be referred for consideration of epilepsy surgery. The presurgical evaluation is essential and extensive investigations at experienced centers may also be required. NCC itself is not necessarily the epileptogenic lesion in this set of patients. The association of NCC and HS is rather frequent, further studies are necessary to clarify the mechanisms of this association.

Author details

Alejandro L Escalaya and Jorge G Burneo*
Epilepsy Program, Western University, London, Ontario, Canada

5. References

[1] Carabin H, Ndimubanzi PC, Budke CM, Nguyen H, Qian Y, Cowan LD, et al. Clinical manifestations associated with neurocysticercosis: a systematic review. PLoS neglected tropical diseases. 2011;5(5):e1152.
[2] Carpio A, Escobar A, Hauser WA. Cysticercosis and epilepsy: A critical review. Epilepsia. 1998;39(10):1025-40.
[3] Rajshekhar V, Jeyaseelan L. Seizure outcome in patients with a solitary cerebral cysticercus granuloma. Neurology. 2004;62(12):2236-40.
[4] Del Brutto OH. Prognostic factors for seizure recurrence after withdrawal of antiepileptic drugs in patients with neurocysticercosis. Neurology. 1994;44(9):1706-9.
[5] Nash TE, Del Brutto OH, Butman JA, Corona T, Delgado-Escueta A, Duron RM, et al. Calcific neurocysticercosis and epileptogenesis. Neurology. 2004;62(11):1934-8.
[6] Nash TE, Pretell EJ, Lescano AG, Bustos JA, Gilman RH, Gonzalez AE, et al. Perilesional brain oedema and seizure activity in patients with calcified neurocysticercosis: a prospective cohort and nested case-control study. The Lancet Neurology. 2008;7(12):1099-105.
[7] Cukiert A, Puglia P, Scapolan HB, Vilela MM, Marino Junior R. Congruence of the topography of intracranial calcifications and epileptic foci. Arq Neuropsiquiatr. 1994;52(3):289-94.
[8] Kowacs PA, Rogacheski E, Muzzio J, Werneck LC. The role of the irritative zone and of the number and distribution of calcifications in the severity of epilepsy associated with intracranial calcifications.[Erratum appears in Arq Neuropsiquiatr. 2007 Mar;65(1):182]. Arq Neuropsiquiatr. 2006;64(4):905-11.
[9] Kwan P, Arzimanoglou A, Berg AT, Brodie MJ, Allen Hauser W, Mathern G, et al. Definition of drug resistant epilepsy: Consensus proposal by the ad hoc Task Force of the ILAE Commission on Therapeutic Strategies. Epilepsia. 2010;51(6):1069-77.
[10] Velasco TR, Zanello PA, Dalmagro CL, Araujo D, Jr., Santos AC, Bianchin MM, et al. Calcified cysticercotic lesions and intractable epilepsy: a cross sectional study of 512 patients. J Neurol Neurosurg Psychiatry. 2006;77(4):485-8.
[11] Pradhan S, Kathuria MK, Gupta RK. Perilesional gliosis and seizure outcome: A study based on magnetization transfer magnetic resonance imaging in patients with neurocysticercosis. Annals of Neurology. 2000;48(2):181-7.

* Corresponding Author

[12] de Souza A, Nalini A, Kovoor JME, Yeshraj G, Siddalingaiah HS, Thennarasu K. Perilesional gliosis around solitary cerebral parenchymal cysticerci and long-term seizure outcome: a prospective study using serial magnetization transfer imaging. Epilepsia. 2011;52(10):1918-27.

[13] Wiebe S, Jette N. Epilepsy surgery utilization: who, when, where, and why? Current Opinion in Neurology. 2012;25(2):187-93.

[14] Rassi Neto A, Centeno RS, Ferraz F. Tratamento cirúrgico da epilepsia associada à neurocisticercose. J bras neurocir. 1998;9(3):99-102.

[15] Chung CK, Lee SK, Chi JG. Temporal lobe epilepsy caused by intrahippocampal calcified cysticercus: a case report. Journal of Korean medical science. 1998;13(4):445-8.

[16] Ooi WW, Wijemanne S, Thomas CB, Quezado M, Brown CR, Nash TE. Short report: A calcified Taenia solium granuloma associated with recurrent perilesional edema causing refractory seizures: Histopathological features. American Journal of Tropical Medicine and Hygiene. 2011;85(3):460-3.

[17] Bianchin MM, Velasco TR, Takayanagui OM, Sakamoto AC. Neurocysticercosis, mesial temporal lobe epilepsy, and hippocampal sclerosis: An association largely ignored. Lancet Neurology. 2006;5(1):20-1.

[18] Singla M, Singh P, Kaushal S, Bansal R, Singh G. Hippocampal sclerosis in association with neurocysticercosis. Epileptic Disorders. 2007;9(3):292-9.

[19] Bianchin MM, Velasco TR, Wichert-Ana L, Takayanagui OM, Leite JP, Sakamoto AC. How frequent is the association of neurocysticercosis and mesial temporal lobe epilepsy with hippocampal sclerosis? Epilepsia. 2010;51(11):2359-60.

[20] Rathore CT, B. ; Kesavadas, C. ; Radhakrishnan, K. Calcified neurocysticercosis lesions and hippocampal sclerosis: Potential dual pathology? Epilepsia. 2012;53(4):e60-e2.

[21] Leite JP, Terra-Bustamante VC, Fernandes RMF, Santos AC, Chimelli L, Sakamoto AC, et al. Calcified neurocysticercotic lesions and postsurgery seizure control in temporal lobe epilepsy. Neurology. 2000;55(10):1485-91.

[22] Chandra PS, Bal C, Garg A, Gaikwad S, Prasad K, Sharma BS, et al. Surgery for medically intractable epilepsy due to postinfectious etiologies. Epilepsia. 2010;51(6):1097-100.

Chapter 14

Extraparenchymal Neurocysticercosis

Kelesidis Theodoros

Additional information is available at the end of the chapter

http://dx.doi.org/10.5772/48801

1. Introduction

Neurocysticercosis (NCC) is the most common disease causing cystic lesions in the central nervous system, especially in developing and tropical countries (1-5). Although neurocysticercosis is pleomorphic in its presentation, extraparenchymal neurocysticercosis may be challenging to diagnose and treat. With increasing globalization and international travel, NCC is now being reported from many developed countries such as the USA, UK and many European countries. Neurologists and neuroradiologists in these countries are often unaware of the pre-/post-treatment radiographic patterns of extraparenchymal NCC and the potentially poor prognosis if not correctly diagnosed and managed. Herein, we review the literature on extraparenchymal neurocysticercosis as a cause of meningitis and hydrochephalus and we discuss challenges in diagnosis and management of these cases.

2. Definition

Extraparenchymal neurocysticercosis (NCC) is defined as neurocysticercosis involving the subarachnoid, meningeal and intraventricular space (1;6;7). Thus, the clinical manifestations of extraparenchymal NCC range from asymptomatic lesions to meningitis and hydrocephalus (1;6;7).

3. Epidemiology of extraparenchymal NCC

Neurocysticercosis is the most common parasitic infestation of the central nervous system worldwide (1;4-7;11;12). Extraparenchymal NCC is frequently seen in Latin American countries whereas it is less common in the Indian subcontinent. Genetic differences in *T. solium* cysticerci have been reported from different countries (15) and may contribute towards the clinical variations across countries. These variations are perhaps due to complex interactions between the host, parasite and environmental factors (13;16-18). Cysticercal meningitis, although reported to constitute 42-48% of cases in Latin American case-series of

INTECH
open science | open minds

© 2013 Theodoros, licensee InTech. This is a paper distributed under the terms of the Creative Commons Attribution License (http://creativecommons.org/licenses/by/3.0), which permits unrestricted use, distribution, and reproduction in any medium, provided the original work is properly cited.

[10] Mosser P, Schmutzhard E, Winkler AS. The pattern of epileptic seizures in rural Tanzania. Journal of the Neurological Sciences 2007; 258: 33–38.
[11] Winkler AS, Mosser P, Schmutzhard E. Neurological disorders in rural Africa: a systematic approach. Tropical Doctor 2009a; 39: 102–104.
[12] Winkler AS, Kerschbaumsteiner K, Stelzhammer B, Meindl M, Kaaya J, Schmutzhard E. Prevalence, incidence and clinical characteristics of epilepsy – a community-based door-to-door study in northern Tanzania. Epilepsia 2009b; 50: 2310–2313.
[13] Tekle-Haimanot R. The pattern of epilepsy in Ethiopia: analysis of 468 cases. Ethiopian Medical Journal 1984; 22: 113–118.
[14] Tekle-Haimanot R, Abebe M, Gebre-Mariam A, Forsgren L, Heijbel J, Holmgren G, Ekstedt J. Community-based study of neurological disorders in rural Central Ethiopia. Neuroepidemiology 1990; 9: 263–277.
[15] Osuntokun BO, Adeuja AO, Nottidge VA, Bademosi O, Olumide A, Ige O, Yaria F, Bolis CL, Schoenberg BS. Prevalence of the epilepsies in Nigerian Africans: a community-based study. Epilepsia 1987; 28: 272–79.
[16] Birbeck G. Neurologic disease in a rural Zambian hospital. Tropical Doctor 2001a; 31: 82–85.
[17] Birbeck G. Seizures in rural Zambia. Epilepsia 2001b; 41: 277–281.
[18] Birbeck G, Kalichi EMN. Epilepsy prevalence in rural Zambia: a door-to-door survey. Tropical Medicine and International Health 2004; 9: 92–95.
[19] Dent W, Helbok R, Matuja WBP, Scheunemann S, Schmutzhard E. Prevalence of active epilepsy in a rural area in South Tanzania: a door-to-door survey. Epilepsia 2005; 46: 1963–1969.
[20] International League Against Epilepsy (ILAE). Commission on Classification and Terminology of the International League Against Epilepsy. Proposal for revised clinical and electroencephalographic classification of epileptic seizures. Epilepsia 1981; 22: 489–501.
[21] International League Against Epilepsy (ILAE). Commission on Classification and Terminology of the International League Against Epilepsy. Proposal for classification of epilepsies and epileptic syndromes. Epilepsia 1985; 26: 268–278.
[22] International League Against Epilepsy (ILAE). Commission on Classification and Terminology of the International League Against Epilepsy. Proposal for revised classification of epilepsies and epileptic syndromes. Epilepsia 1989; 30: 389–399.
[23] World Health Organization 2001. The world health report 2001. http://www.who.int/whr/2001/en/whr01_en.pdf Last accessed July 2012
[24] Birbeck GL. Revising and refining the epilepsy classification system: Priorities from a developing world perspective. Epilepsia 2012; 53(Suppl 2):18–21.
[25] Winkler AS, Schaffert M, Schmutzhard E. Epilepsy in resource poor countries — suggestion of an adjusted classification. Epilepsia 2007; 48: 1029–1030.
[26] Winkler AS, Schaffert M, Schmutzhard E. The pattern of epilepsy in a rural African hospital – an approach adapted to local circumstances. Tropical Doctor 2009c; 39: 44–47.
[27] Fröscher W, Vassella F, Hufnagel A, editors. Die Epilepsien. Stuttgart: Schattauer; 2004.
[28] Reutens DC, Berkovic SF. Idiopathic generalized epilepsy of adolescence: are the syndromes clinically distinct? Neurology 1995; 45: 1469–1476.

NC, is somewhat uncommon with <8% of cases having meningitis among adult patients (6-9;19). Extraparenchymal NCC is also of emerging importance in developed countries (11;20). This increase likely includes extraparenchymal cases, and a recent study reported an overall frequency of subarachnoid cysts in 2%, ventricular cysts in 6%, and hydrocephalus in 16% of NCC cases (11). These cases represented almost one-third of NCC in a medical center in New Mexico (21). Intraventricular NCC, the presence of *Taenia solium* cysts in the cerebral ventricular system, occurs in 7–30% of patients with NCC (10;21-23).Thus, extraparenchymal NCC is probably more frequent than previously thought (14;18).

4. Pathogenesis of extraparenchymal NCC

4.1. Subarachnoid NCC

The disease occurs when humans ingest eggs of *Taenia solium* from contaminated food (1). Brain parenchyma is most likely seeded through hematogenous dissemination and the ventricular system, subarachnoid space, and basal cisterns are then seeded via the choroid plexus (1). When cysts lodge outside the brain parenchyma (extraparenchymal NCC), they tend to grow irregularly depending on the space available and usually elicit a strong inflammatory response. Subarachnoid cysts can also grow abnormally as a membranous and/or cystic mass called racemose cysticercosis (7). Occasionally the cysts enlarge considerably, become racemose without scolices and cause mass effects. Cysticercus racemose is characterized by larger size (4–12 cm), absence of scolex and a variable appearance. Cysticercus racemosus is a form multilobular grape-like cluster without scolex thought to be a *forme fruste* of cysticercus cellulosae (24), most frequently located in the basal cisterns, Sylvian fissure, or ventricles (10;21-23).These cysts continually grow compared with intraparenchymal NCC and commonly result in basilar arachnoiditis (7) with inflammation and fibrosis in and around critical structures, causing meningeal inflammation, hydrocephalus due to CSF outflow obstruction, or cerebrovascular complications (10;21-23). The cyst often tends to migrate to the fourth ventricle because of gravity and CSF flow patterns (10;21-23). Although neurocysticerci undergo four stages of involution: vesicular, colloidal, granulovacuvolar and calcific, this evolution does not occur in the intraventricular or the subarachnoid forms (or racemose type) of NCC (25).

4.2. Cysticercal meningitis

"Racemose" cysticercosis is associated with an intense inflammatory reaction and progressive thickening of the leptomeninges at the base of the brain. Signs of meningitis, cranial nerve palsy and cerebral infarcts secondary to vasculitis may also develop (26). In approximately 50–60% of the cases, there is an obstruction of the CSF circulation, resulting in progressive intracranial hypertension and hydrocephalus and mortality of over 20% of cases (26). When hydrocephalus secondary to cysticercotic meningitis is present, the mortality rate is high (50%) and most patients die within 2 years after CSF shunting(4). Therefore, basal cisternal locations are considered to be malignant forms of NCC (26).

4.3. Intraventricular NCC

Hydrocephalus can result either because of direct obstruction of cerebrospinal fluid (CSF) pathways by intraventricular cysts or secondary to inflammatory obstruction. Intraventricular neurocysticercal cysts occur singly or in multiples and frequently coexist with parenchymal and sub-arachnoid cysts (10;21-23). Intracranial hypertension is a common manifestation of extraparenhymal NCC and the increased intracranial pressure can be from the mass effect of a giant subarachnoid cyst (27), or from obstructive hydrocephalus produced by direct obstruction of the ventricular system by a cyst (28), distortion of ventricular CSF pathways (29), or blockage of CSF pathways within the subarachnoid space from the inflammatory reaction (28). However, a cyst in the fourth ventricle tends to be solitary, without accompanying parenchymal cysts (10;21-23).

4.4. Extramedullary cysticercosis

Involvement of the spinal cord is rare, accounting for 1–5% of all cases of NCC (30;31). Spinal NCC may be intramedullary or extramedullary (intradural or extradural); however these forms are rare, and most disease involves the subarachnoid spaces, which may result from direct CSF dissemination (30;31). It has been suggested that small, or developing larvae present in the subarachnoid space settle to the basal cisterns by way of gravity and then further descend into the subarachnoid spaces of the lower parts of the spine including the lumbosacral space where they find adequate room to grow and develop (30;31). Many of the pathologic descriptions of cysticerci recovered from the spinal canal have a racemose morphology, which consists of membranous cells that proliferate, which may cause seeding of the spine from the base of the brain and subsequent growth (30;31). Cervical involvement consists mostly of unilocular or multilocular cystic forms, primarily due to direct extension of cysts located in the basal subarachnoid cisterns (30;31). Conversely, lumbosacral involvement has a more varied picture including multilocular cystic lesions causing spinal displacement or flattening, and clumping or displacement of the nerve roots most likely due to adhesive arachnoiditis (30;31). Clinical signs can be caused by direct compression of the spinal cord and/or roots by cysticerci or, indirectly, by the inflammatory reaction, including progressive paraparesis and sphincter disturbances.

4.5. Orbital neurocysticercosis

Ocular cysticercosis is caused by the growth of the larvae of Taenia solium within the ocular tissues and the cysts may be located in descending order of frequency, subretinal space (35%), vitreous (22%), conjunctiva (22%), anterior segment (5%) and orbit (1%)(32). The extraocular muscle form is the most common type of orbital cysticercosis (33-35). In the ocular form, the most favored sites are the vitreous and the subretinal space whereas the inferior rectus and the medial rectus are the most common extraocular muscles involved (33-35). Intraocular cysticercosis is predominant in the Western countries, whereas extraocular is more common in the Indian population and several authors have attributed geographic and environmental factors to this difference (33-35). The continuation of the retina with the optic nerve allows direct communication of the subarachnoid space with subretinal space but it remains unclear whether subretinal NCC can be considered another form of subarachnoid NCC (33-35).

There is lack of understanding of the pathophysiology of extraparenchymal NCC. Circulating antigen detection assays could help establish if living parasites are still present after apparent radiographic cyst regression, providing an indication to continue or reuse antiparasitic treatment (36). It is unclear whether chronic inflammation in extraparenchymal NCC is due to continuous cyst degeneration, or continuous antigen release from dead parasitic tissues (37). Newer mechanisms are being explored to understand the complex neuropathology and heterogeneity of NCC.

5. Clinical manifestations of extraparenchymal NCC

The clinical and radiologic manifestations of NCC are pleomorphic. Epilepsy, present in both intraparenchymal and extraparenchymal NCC, focal neurological signs, and headache are the most common clinical manifestations of the disease (1;38). Focal neurological signs that vary according to the size, number and location of the parasites have been described in up to 20% patients with neurocysticercosis (1;38). Pyramidal tract signs predominate, but sensory deficits, involuntary movements, and signs of brainstem dysfunction, may occur in some patients (1;38). These manifestations usually follow a subacute or chronic course resembling that of a brain tumor and are most often seen in patients with large subarachnoid cysts compressing the brain parenchyma (1;38). Thus, several varieties of NCC have been recognized depending upon the number, location, and evolutionary stage of the cysticerci in the human brain (39).

Extraparenchymal NCC occurs mainly in young adult males and is uncommon in children (38;40). The patients typically present with subacute or chronic intracranial hypertension from mass effect or hydrocephalus; chronic meningitis characterized by lack of meningeal signs of exam, often due to chronicity of symptoms , a mild-to-moderate CSF lymphocytic pleocytosis and moderate-high increase in protein; radiographic hydrocephalus with or without obvious cysts; radiographic presence of cysts in the ventricles or subarachnoid space and protracted clinical or radiographic course after antiparasitic treatment (8;21). Stroke can occur secondary to vasculitis caused by inflammatory occlusion of the arteries at the base of the brain secondary to arachnoiditis (4;5;12).

Hydrocephalus develops in approximately 30% of all patients with NCC because of obstruction by intraventricular or subarachnoid lesions (10;21-23). Intraventricular NCC can cause non-communicating hydrocephalus by obstructing the CSF pathway and communicating hydrocephalus by development of ependymitis (10;21-23). Abrupt permanent obstruction can cause sudden death due to brain herniation (10;21-23). Life-threatening acute intermittent hydrocephalus (Brunn syndrome)(41) can occur due to cyst-inducing intermittent CSF obstruction from a ball-valve mechanism (10;22). Overall, extraparenchymal NCC has a more aggressive behavior and a higher morbidity and mortality rate than parenchymal form (10;21-23). Presence of sub-arachnoid cysts can cause chronic cysticercal meningitis. Cysticercal meningitis (CM) is characterized by inflammatory cerebrospinal fluid (CSF) and negative bacterial and fungal cultures (8). There have been no systematic studies of CM. In a recent study of patients with CM these patients often had intracranial hypertension, meningeal signs, CSF hypoglycorrachia, positive CSF results in an enzyme-linked immunosorbent assay (ELISA) for cysticercal antigens, negative CSF cultures for bacteria, fungi, and mycobacteria and longer clinical course of NCC (8). The management of the chronic inflammation and the complications caused by this meningitis are usually very difficult, and the mortality rate can be up to 33% (10;21-23). It is likely that CM is often not identified and its correct identification may reduce morbidity and risks of unnecessary surgery in patients with chronic neurocysticercosis and CSF shunts (10;21-23).

6. Diagnosis of extraparenchymal NCC

The diagnosis of NCC is often made based on presence of lesion highly suggestive of neurocysticercosis on neuroimaging study , positive serum immunoassay for the detection of anticysticercal antibodies , positive CSF immunoassay for detection of anticysticercal antibodies and epidemiologic criteria including individual coming from an area where cysticercosis is endemic (1).These diagnostic criteria have been stratified in four categories—absolute, major, minor, and epidemiological- on the basis of their individual diagnostic strength(1). Based on a previous consensus, the absolute criterion for the diagnosis of neurocysticercosis that is being considered as pathognomonic of this disease is the detection of a scolex inside a cyst by CT or MRI although, *C. racemosus* doesn't have a scolex (1).

6.1. Clinical presentation

Extraparenchymal NCC is associated with a local inflammatory response with high protein concentration and cell counts in the CSF (8). Clinical manifestations and CSF findings are similar to the more common tuberculous meningitis, (8;23) and other forms of chronic meningitis including chronic HIV- associated meningitis (42;43) since the CSF findings consist of pleocytosis (usually lymphocytic but frequently polymorphonuclear) , reduced glucose and elevated protein(8). In one series of cysticercal meningoencephalitis, confusion with tubercular meningitis was present in 61.5% cases (7;8). An important differentiating feature with these other forms of chronic meningitis is the presence of eosinophils in the CSF (7;8) which is usually seen only in the initial phases of the illness (8;21). However, this staining of the CSF is not routinely done in most places (8;23). Although the suspicion of NCC as the cause of chronic meningitis is increased when CSF eosinophils are found, CSF eosinophils (above 5%) occur in only 15% of patients (21). It is often a common practice to attribute chronic meningitis and hydrocephalus to tubercular meningitis in the presence of appropriate epidemiologic history and treat empirically by shunting and anti-tubercular therapy. Thus, an astute clinical acumen is required to make the diagnosis of CM.

6.2. Imaging

Both computed tomography (CT) and magnetic resonance imaging (MRI) are indispensable tools for diagnosis and characterization of NCC (38;44;45); CT is superior for diagnosis of racemose cysticercosis, brain granulomas and calcifications, which are the most frequent finding of NCC, and may be missed by MRI (38;44;45). However, neuroimaging findings of extraparenchymal cysticerci are subtle and are usually not seen by CT. Thus, MRI is more useful than CT for diagnosis of ocular, ventricular, and subarachnoid cysticercosis and for analysis of the inflammatory reaction that accompanies most cases of active NCC (38;44;45).

Neuroimaging findings are variable depending on the stage of the infection. The first stage, described as the larval tissue invasion phase, is not normally imaged owing to lack of symptoms at this very early stage (1;46). During the vesicular stage, cysts and scolex, the "mouth" of the tapeworm that is lined with suckers and hooks, are both imaged without enhancement. However, as observed in one study(47) in which imaging was performed regularly to follow anticysticercal therapy, this phase appears as a localized focus of edema on T2-weighted images and displays nodular tissue enhancement following the administration of gadopentetate dimeglumine (1;46).

The second stage (the vesicular stage) describes the formation of a cyst that encircles the scolex (1;46). These cysts are thin walled, contain clear fluid and are typically 1-2 cm. On imaging, the cyst fluid parallels cerebrospinal fluid intensity. The scolex is approximately 2–4 mm and appears as a mural nodule that is isointense with brain parenchyma (48). The lesion is antigenically inert and therefore does not induce an inflammatory reaction or circumferential edema (49).

During the third stage (the colloidal stage) the parasite dies, and as a result the cysticercus becomes nonviable (1;46). As the scolex dies, the cyst fluid transforms into a colloidal suspension containing protein solutes (1;46) and on MRI imaging this results in T1 shortening while the scolex and cyst capsule are decreased in T2 signal intensity. The surrounding edema suggests that the parasite is in its colloidal state, and, therefore, enhancement of the capsule and scolex will occur avidly. In addition, the proteinaceous nature of the cyst fluid during involution of the cysticercus is appears as hypointense central T1 signal to white matter but hyperintense to cerebrospinal fluid and appears markedly hyperintense on T2-weighted images (1;46). At CT, cystic contents increase in attenuation (50). Thus, in the colloidal vesicular stage, ring enhancement and edema are appreciated by both CT and MRI imagings (1;46).

The fourth stage (the nodular granular stage) represents the degeneration of the cysticercus. The edema begins to subside gradually, the contents begin to mineralize and the cyst involutes. Thus, the lesion becomes isointense with brain parenchyma on T1-weighted MR images and hypointense on T2-weighted MR images. At CT, a thick nodular ring continues to enhance and the lesion becomes isoattenuating (51).

The final stage is the calcified stage, which describes complete involution of the lesion with continued mineralization. The calcifications are obvious at CT as small areas of hypointensity (1) and show susceptibility at MR imaging, particularly on gradient-echo images (47). However MRI is not the imaging modality of choice for calcified NCC (47). Also, in the nodular calcified stage, when the cystic lesion is mineralized and shrunken and a nonenhanced CT scan is diagnostic, enhancement is unusual (51). The granular nodular phase is characterized by decreased ring enhancement and edema, along with the calcification of cysts (46).

Subarachnoid (racemose) neurocysticercosis usually infiltrates the basal cisterns and sylvian fissure and has different imaging findings compared to parenchymal NCC. Common neuroimaging findings to suspect the diagnosis include hydrocephalus (with or without obvious cysts), cysts obstructing CSF pathways or freely floating inside ventricles, cysts in the basal subarachnoid cisterns, migrating cysts across the cerebral aqueduct, and ependymitis or arachnoiditis (21). The most common CT finding in subarachnoid NCC is hydrocephalus (1;9). Because the cyst membrane is thin and the fluid is isodense with the cerebrospinal fluid, uninflamed extraparenchymal cysticerci are usually not visible on computed tomography scanning and may only reveal subtle, indirect findings on MRI (9). Therefore, neuroimaging may reveal hydrocephalus without noticeable cysts (1;9).

6.3. Laboratory tests for diagnosis of NCC

Taenia antibodies detected by methods such as Western Blot is considered as a major criterion whereas the positive serologic test in the CSF is listed as a minor criterion (19).The development of numerous serodiagnostic tests using different parasitic antigens is indicative of the fact that none of them are 100% sensitive and specific. For multiple lesions, the enzyme-linked immunoelectrotransfer blot (EITB) assay using purified glycoprotein antigens from *T. solium* cysticerci was reported to be highly specific (100%) and nearly 98% sensitive (4;5;12). The sensitivity was less for single lesions (52)and for calcified lesions (2;2;53-56). A comparative study of enzyme-linked immunosorbent assay (ELISA) and dot-blot assay in children found that both were more sensitive in cases with multiple brain lesions (100%) than in those with a single lesion (87%) (5). The sensitivity of antibody detecting EITB assays is not better with the use of CSF samples as compared with serum samples (55). Detection of circulating cysticercosis antigens using ELISA has a modest sensitivity especially for parenchymal lesions. The antigen detecting ELISA has a better sensitivity with the use of CSF samples as compared with serum samples. However, ELISA has less sensitivity as compared with EITB for serum as well as CSF samples, for both intraparenchymal and extraparenchymal NCC (55;57-59).

It has been suggested that the use of excretory secretory (ES) antigens, rather than somatic antigens might improve the serodiagnosis of cases with vesicular stages of the parasite (60;61). The use of ES antigens for the detection of antibodies in serum was found to be more useful than that in urine in patients with enhancing lesions (62). Three ES peptides were reported to have high sensitivity and specificity in both serum and CSF reactivity; (60;61). It has been suggested that synthetic peptide selected by phage display may be useful in the immunodiagnosis of NCC (63;64).

Polymerase chain reaction (PCR) in CSF has also been used for the diagnosis of neurocysticercosis but is not widely available (19). However, extensive and comprehensive revision of the diagnostic criteria of neurocysticercosis, especially of extraparenchymal neurocysticercosis is mandatory according to many recent publications (2;8-11).

7. Treatment

There is still no consensus regarding optimal treatment strategies in patients with extraparenchymal NCC (10;21-23). Various therapeutic modalities include antihelminthic medication, microneurosurgical removal, ventriculoperitoneal shunting, and endoscopic management (8).

7.1. Medical therapy

Although parenchymal cysts have historically been treated quite effectively with antihelminthics such as praziquantel and albendazole, medical therapy alone is not favored for extraparenchymal NCC because of the limited efficacy in such cases, and a risk of developing acute hydrocephalus during the clinical treatment period (10;21-23). Good results for antiparasitic treatment with different albendazole and praziquantel regiments for extraparenchymal NCC including orbital, spinal , intraventricular and subarachnoid NCC, and even for giant cysts have been reported (57;65-69) although resistance has been reported by some (13;16;17). However, although treatment with antihelminthic medication such as albendazole has been shown to improve outcome in live, cystic parenchymal cysticercosis, the benefits of antihelminthic treatment in patients with solitary cystic lesion remain uncertain (70). While it is generally accepted that both praziquantel and albendazole are effective in destroying viable cysts, their use in cases with enhancing lesions has been debated as these lesions are considered to represent degenerating cysts, many of which resolve spontaneously (4;5;12). Thus, the decision whether antiparasitic treatment should be used in these cases is always a clinical decision and should be made on an individual basis.

Antihelminthic agents hasten the evolution of intraventricular viable cysts, which may trigger an inflammatory response similar to that seen with the natural history of the parasite (25). This may result in long-term sequelae (1;6;9;71). Extraparenchymal cysts may regress only after long term and multiple antiparasitic courses (1;6;9;71). The optimal treatment to prevent chronic inflammation is unknown due the lack of understanding of its pathophysiology and lack of controlled trials to help guide management. Likewise, controversy exists regarding the use of corticosteroids, alone or in combination with antihelminthic drugs (1;6;70;71). At a previous consensus meeting, experts agreed that no single treatment approach could be advocated and that management options varied according to the type of clinical presentation (9). However, intraventricular neurocysticercosis has a risk of ependymitis in those treated with anthelminthics such as albendazole and praziquantel regiments. Thus these agents should be used with caution in cases with extraparenchymal NCC as any increase in the inflammatory response may lead to the development of infarct; pretreatment with steroids and management of intracranial hypertension is warranted and surgical evaluation is often needed prior to medical treatment (8).

7.2. Surgical therapy

In patients presenting with acute hydrocephalus, surgery is the only option (10;21-23). Neurosurgical procedures for NCC are still part of the armamentarium when treating this disease and good results for open craniotomy and rigid endoscopic surgery in patients with intraventricular and subarachnoid NCC have been reported (72;73). Infratentorial intraventricular cysts have been treated with open surgery for excision whereas it is generally suggested that supratentorial cysts, due to not only location but also the need to often treat hydrocephalus in these patients, be removed endoscopically (74). Ependymitis, confirmed by neuroimaging is a relative contraindication for surgical removal of the cysts (10;21-23).

Ventriculoperitoneal CSF shunting is burdened by a high shunt dysfunction rate which leads to worsening obstruction of CSF flow and increased intracranial pressure, risk of infection and thus high mortality rates. Microneurosurgical approaches can be technically demanding and associated with various complications (10;21-23). For these reasons, endoscopic approaches for intraventricular neurocysticercosis have been described in recent years and often allow for cyst removal and hydrocephalus treatment, freeing the patient from shunt procedures (75;76).

Although the literature regarding the use of endoscopic management of intraventricular NCC is scarce, this modality has shown encouraging results in the treatment of intraventricular NCC (10;21-23). In a recent comparative study of 140 patients from Mexico with intraventricular NCC, traditional treatment with albendazole and steroid had similar outcome versus neuroendoscopic surgery in terms of survival, hospitalization (23). However, almost all patients with traditional treatment remained with at least one shunt whereas most of the patients from the neuroendoscopic surgery series did not have any shunts (23). Thus, the neuroendoscopic approach to intraventricular neurocysticercal cysts is safe and effective and offers the additional benefit of avoiding shunt placement (10;21-23). At centres having the required expertise, this should be the treatment of choice. Traditional treatment is a second option where the endoscopic procedure is not available. However, endoscopic cyst excision can be difficult and hazardous in patients with severe ependymitis and dense adhesions and intraventricular bleeding could also report (10;21-23). Thus, despite its many advantages, neuroendoscopy has some limitations even when performed by experienced hands.

Regarding subarachnoid NCC, there are no controlled trials on the management of this form of extraparenchymal NCC (1;6;71). In a series of patients treated with only CSF diversion, 50% died at a median follow-up of 8 years and 11 months (2). More recently, case series using anti-parasitic drugs, corticosteroids, and shunting for hydrocephalus have been associated with an improved prognosis compared with older studies (1;2;6;71).Thus, most experts consider subarachnoid NCC a clear indication for anti-parasitic therapy (2).

However, the optimal dose and duration of anti-parasitic therapy for subarachnoid cysticercosis has not been established (2). In the largest cases series, Proaño and others treated 33 patients with giant cysticerci with albendazole (15 mg/kg/day) for 4 weeks and most patients required several courses of anti-parasitic therapy (23). However, with controversy in the literature in the optimal management of this condition and without further evidence-based guidelines to help management of extraparenchymal NCC, the decision of the total dose and duration of antiparasitic and steroid therapy must be made on a case by case basis.

8. Conclusion

Extraparenchymal NCC may be a more common form of NCC than previously thought and is often difficult to diagnose, more complex to treat, and carries a graver prognosis. The clinical course is protracted and difficult to cure. Different medical (anthelmintics, steroids), surgical (cyst excision, CSF diversion), or medical-surgical approaches have been reported but not adequately studied. Because clinicians in developed countries often unfamiliar with NCC as a cause of chronic meningitis, chronic ventriculitis, or hydrocephalus without obvious cysts, the diagnosis of extraparenchymal NCC often depends on the correct interpretation of neuroimaging which may miss the diagnosis. Thus, extraparenchymal NCC should always be considered by clinicians and radiologists in the differential diagnosis of chronic meningitis and hydrocephalus.

Author details

Kelesidis Theodoros
Department of Medicine, Division of Infectious Diseases, David Geffen School of Medicine at UCLA, Los Angeles, California, USA

9. References

[1] Del Brutto OH. Neurocysticercosis. Semin Neurol 2005; 25(3):243-251.

[2] Garcia HH, Del Brutto OH, Nash TE, White AC, Jr., Tsang VC, Gilman RH. New concepts in the diagnosis and management of neurocysticercosis (Taenia solium). Am J Trop Med Hyg 2005; 72(1):3-9.

[3] Naumov YN, Bahjat KS, Gausling R, Abraham R, Exley MA, Koezuka Y et al. Activation of CD1d-restricted T cells protects NOD mice from developing diabetes by regulating dendritic cell subsets. Proc Natl Acad Sci U S A 2001; 98(24):13838-13843.

[4] Atluri SR, Singhi P, Khandelwal N, Malla N. Neurocysticercosis immunodiagnosis using Taenia solium cysticerci crude soluble extract, excretory secretory and lower molecular mass antigens in serum and urine samples of Indian children. Acta Trop 2009; 110(1):22-27.

[5] Mandal J, Singhi PD, Khandelwal N, Malla N. Evaluation of ELISA and dot blots for the serodiagnosis of neurocysticercosis, in children found to have single or multiple enhancing lesions in computerized tomographic scans of the brain. Ann Trop Med Parasitol 2006; 100(1):39-48.

[6] Cardenas G, Carrillo-Mezo R, Jung H, Sciutto E, Hernandez JL, Fleury A. Subarachnoidal Neurocysticercosis non-responsive to cysticidal drugs: a case series. BMC Neurol 2010; 10:16.

[7] Del Brutto OH. Meningeal cysticercosis. Singh G, Prabhakar S, eds. Taenia solium Cysticercosis: From Basic to Clinical Science. Oxford, United Kingdom: CABI Publishing, 177-188. 2002.

[8] Cardenas G, Jung H, Rios C, Fleury A, Soto-Hernandez JL. Severe cysticercal meningitis: clinical and imaging characteristics. Am J Trop Med Hyg 2010; 82(1):121-125.

[9] Garcia HH, Evans CA, Nash TE, Takayanagui OM, White AC, Jr., Botero D et al. Current consensus guidelines for treatment of neurocysticercosis. Clin Microbiol Rev 2002; 15(4):747-756.

[10] Kalra V, Mishra D, Suri A, Seth R, Garg A. Intraventricular neurocysticercosis. Indian J Pediatr 2009; 76(4):420-423.

[11] Wallin MT, Kurtzke JF. Neurocysticercosis in the United States: review of an important emerging infection. Neurology 2004; 63(9):1559-1564.

[12] Singhi P. Neurocysticercosis. Ther Adv Neurol Disord 2011; 4(2):67-81.

[13] Cardenas G, Carrillo-Mezo R, Jung H, Sciutto E, Hernandez JL, Fleury A. Subarachnoidal Neurocysticercosis non-responsive to cysticidal drugs: a case series. BMC Neurol 2010; 10:16.

[14] Bluml S, Kirchberger S, Bochkov VN, Kronke G, Stuhlmeier K, Majdic O et al. Oxidized phospholipids negatively regulate dendritic cell maturation induced by TLRs and CD40. J Immunol 2005; 175(1):501-508.

[15] Maravilla P, Gonzalez-Guzman R, Zuniga G, Peniche A, Dominguez-Alpizar JL, Reyes-Montes R et al. Genetic polymorphism in Taenia solium cysticerci recovered from experimental infections in pigs. Infect Genet Evol 2008; 8(2):213-216.

[16] Cardenas G, Jung H, Rios C, Fleury A, Soto-Hernandez JL. Severe cysticercal meningitis: clinical and imaging characteristics. Am J Trop Med Hyg 2010; 82(1):121-125.

[17] Fleury A, Hernandez M, Avila M, Cardenas G, Bobes RJ, Huerta M et al. Detection of HP10 antigen in serum for diagnosis and follow-up of subarachnoidal and intraventricular human neurocysticercosis. J Neurol Neurosurg Psychiatry 2007; 78(9):970-974.

[18] Fleury A, Escobar A, Fragoso G, Sciutto E, Larralde C. Clinical heterogeneity of human neurocysticercosis results from complex interactions among parasite, host and environmental factors. Trans R Soc Trop Med Hyg 2010; 104(4):243-250.

[19] Michelet L, Fleury A, Sciutto E, Kendjo E, Fragoso G, Paris L et al. Human neurocysticercosis: Comparison of different diagnostic tests in cerebrospinal fluid. J Clin Microbiol 2011; 49(1):195-200.

[20] Ong S, Talan DA, Moran GJ, Mower W, Newdow M, Tsang VC et al. Neurocysticercosis in radiographically imaged seizure patients in U.S. emergency departments. Emerg Infect Dis 2002; 8(6):608-613.

[21] Figueroa JJ, Davis LE, Magalhaes A. Extraparenchymal Neurocysticercosis in Albuquerque, New Mexico. J Neuroimaging 2011; 21(1):38-43.

[22] Goel RK, Ahmad FU, Vellimana AK, Suri A, Chandra PS, Kumar R et al. Endoscopic management of intraventricular neurocysticercosis. J Clin Neurosci 2008; 15(10):1096-1101.

[23] Proano JV, Torres-Corzo J, Rodriguez-Della VR, Guizar-Sahagun G, Rangel-Castilla L. Intraventricular and subarachnoid basal cisterns neurocysticercosis: a comparative study between traditional treatment versus neuroendoscopic surgery. Childs Nerv Syst 2009; 25(11):1467-1475.

[24] Ghosh D, Dubey TN, Prabhakar S. Brain parenchymal, subarachnoid racemose, and intraventricular cysticercosis in an Indian man. Postgrad Med J 1999; 75(881):164-166.

[25] Suri A, Goel RK, Ahmad FU, Vellimana AK, Sharma BS, Mahapatra AK. Transventricular, transaqueductal scope-in-scope endoscopic excision of fourth ventricular neurocysticercosis: a series of 13 cases and a review. J Neurosurg Pediatr 2008; 1(1):35-39.

[26] Brenchley JM, Price DA, Schacker TW, Asher TE, Silvestri G, Rao S et al. Microbial translocation is a cause of systemic immune activation in chronic HIV infection. Nat Med 2006; 12(12):1365-1371.

[27] Proano JV, Madrazo I, Avelar F, Lopez-Felix B, Diaz G, Grijalva I. Medical treatment for neurocysticercosis characterized by giant subarachnoid cysts. N Engl J Med 2001; 345(12):879-885.

[28] Estanol B, Kleriga E, Loyo M, Mateos H, Lombardo L, Gordon F et al. Mechanisms of hydrocephalus in cerebral cysticercosis: implications for therapy. Neurosurgery 1983; 13(2):119-123.

[29] Lobato RD, Lamas E, Portillo JM, Roger R, Esparza J, Rivas JJ et al. Hydrocephalus in cerebral cysticercosis. Pathogenic and therapeutic considerations. J Neurosurg 1981; 55(5):786-793.

[30] Callacondo D, Garcia HH, Gonzales I, Escalante D, Nash TE. High frequency of spinal involvement in patients with basal subarachnoid neurocysticercosis. Neurology 2012; 78(18):1394-1400.

[31] De Souza QL, Filho AP, Callegaro D, De Faria LL. Intramedullary cysticercosis. Case report, literature review and comments on pathogenesis. J Neurol Sci 1975; 26(1):61-70.

[32] Kruger-Leite E, Jalkh AE, Quiroz H, Schepens CL. Intraocular cysticercosis. Am J Ophthalmol 1985; 99(3):252-257.
[33] Rath S, Honavar SG, Naik M, Anand R, Agarwal B, Krishnaiah S et al. Orbital cysticercosis: clinical manifestations, diagnosis, management, and outcome. Ophthalmology 2010; 117(3):600-5, 605.
[34] Sekhar GC, Lemke BN. Orbital cysticercosis. Ophthalmology 1997; 104(10):1599-1604.
[35] Natarajan S, Malpani A, Kumar NP, Dutta B. Management of intraocular cysticercosis. Graefes Arch Clin Exp Ophthalmol 1999; 237(10):812-814.
[36] Fleury A, Hernandez M, Avila M, Cardenas G, Bobes RJ, Huerta M et al. Detection of HP10 antigen in serum for diagnosis and follow-up of subarachnoidal and intraventricular human neurocysticercosis. J Neurol Neurosurg Psychiatry 2007; 78(9):970-974.
[37] Nash TE, Singh G, White AC, Rajshekhar V, Loeb JA, Proano JV et al. Treatment of neurocysticercosis: current status and future research needs. Neurology 2006; 67(7):1120-1127.
[38] Del Brutto OH. Neurocysticercosis: a review. ScientificWorldJournal 2012; 2012:159821.
[39] Del Brutto OH. Single parenchymal brain cysticercus in the acute encephalitic phase: definition of a distinct form of neurocysticercosis with a benign prognosis. J Neurol Neurosurg Psychiatry 1995; 58(2):247-249.
[40] Kelesidis T, Tsiodras S. Extraparenchymal neurocysticercosis in the United States: a case report. J Med Case Reports 2011; 5:359.
[41] Giorgi JV, Hultin LE, McKeating JA, Johnson TD, Owens B, Jacobson LP et al. Shorter survival in advanced human immunodeficiency virus type 1 infection is more closely associated with T lymphocyte activation than with plasma virus burden or virus chemokine coreceptor usage. J Infect Dis 1999; 179(4):859-870.
[42] Hollander H, McGuire D, Burack JH. Diagnostic lumbar puncture in HIV-infected patients: analysis of 138 cases. Am J Med 1994; 96(3):223-228.
[43] Marshall DW, Brey RL, Cahill WT, Houk RW, Zajac RA, Boswell RN. Spectrum of cerebrospinal fluid findings in various stages of human immunodeficiency virus infection. Arch Neurol 1988; 45(9):954-958.
[44] Del Brutto OH. Neurocysticercosis. Semin Neurol 2005; 25(3):243-251.
[45] Salgado P, Rojas R, Sotelo J. Cysticercosis. Clinical classification based on imaging studies. Arch Intern Med 1997; 157(17):1991-1997.
[46] do Amaral LL, Ferreira RM, da Rocha AJ, Ferreira NP. Neurocysticercosis: evaluation with advanced magnetic resonance techniques and atypical forms. Top Magn Reson Imaging 2005; 16(2):127-144.
[47] Teitelbaum GP, Otto RJ, Lin M, Watanabe AT, Stull MA, Manz HJ et al. MR imaging of neurocysticercosis. AJR Am J Roentgenol 1989; 153(4):857-866.

[48] Barry M, Kaldjian LC. Neurocysticercosis. Semin Neurol 1993; 13(2):131-143.

[49] Lotz J, Hewlett R, Alheit B, Bowen R. Neurocysticercosis: correlative pathomorphology and MR imaging. Neuroradiology 1988; 30(1):35-41.

[50] Suss RA, Maravilla KR, Thompson J. MR imaging of intracranial cysticercosis: comparison with CT and anatomopathologic features. AJNR Am J Neuroradiol 1986; 7(2):235-242.

[51] Chang KH, Lee JH, Han MH, Han MC. The role of contrast-enhanced MR imaging in the diagnosis of neurocysticercosis. AJNR Am J Neuroradiol 1991; 12(3):509-512.

[52] Blake GJ, Rifai N, Buring JE, Ridker PM. Blood pressure, C-reactive protein, and risk of future cardiovascular events. Circulation 2003; 108(24):2993-2999.

[53] Garcia HH, Evans CA, Nash TE, Takayanagui OM, White AC, Jr., Botero D et al. Current consensus guidelines for treatment of neurocysticercosis. Clin Microbiol Rev 2002; 15(4):747-756.

[54] Ong S, Talan DA, Moran GJ, Mower W, Newdow M, Tsang VC et al. Neurocysticercosis in radiographically imaged seizure patients in U.S. emergency departments. Emerg Infect Dis 2002; 8(6):608-613.

[55] Rodriguez S, Dorny P, Tsang VC, Pretell EJ, Brandt J, Lescano AG et al. Detection of Taenia solium antigens and anti-T. solium antibodies in paired serum and cerebrospinal fluid samples from patients with intraparenchymal or extraparenchymal neurocysticercosis. J Infect Dis 2009; 199(9):1345-1352.

[56] Tsang VC, Brand JA, Boyer AE. An enzyme-linked immunoelectrotransfer blot assay and glycoprotein antigens for diagnosing human cysticercosis (Taenia solium). J Infect Dis 1989; 159(1):50-59.

[57] Proano JV, Torres-Corzo J, Rodriguez-Della VR, Guizar-Sahagun G, Rangel-Castilla L. Intraventricular and subarachnoid basal cisterns neurocysticercosis: a comparative study between traditional treatment versus neuroendoscopic surgery. Childs Nerv Syst 2009; 25(11):1467-1475.

[58] Torres-Corzo JG, Tapia-Perez JH, Vecchia RR, Chalita-Williams JC, Sanchez-Aguilar M, Sanchez-Rodriguez JJ. Endoscopic management of hydrocephalus due to neurocysticercosis. Clin Neurol Neurosurg 2010; 112(1):11-16.

[59] Rodriguez S, Dorny P, Tsang VC, Pretell EJ, Brandt J, Lescano AG et al. Detection of Taenia solium antigens and anti-T. solium antibodies in paired serum and cerebrospinal fluid samples from patients with intraparenchymal or extraparenchymal neurocysticercosis. J Infect Dis 2009; 199(9):1345-1352.

[60] Sahu PS, Parija SC, Narayan SK, Kumar D. Evaluation of an IgG-ELISA strategy using Taenia solium metacestode somatic and excretory-secretory antigens for diagnosis of neurocysticercosis revealing biological stage of the larvae. Acta Trop 2009; 110(1):38-45.

[61] Sahu PS, Parija SC, Jayachandran S. Antibody specific to 43kDa excretory-secretory antigenic peptide of Taenia solium metacestode as a potential diagnostic marker in human neurocysticercosis. Acta Trop 2010; 115(3):257-261.

[62] Atluri SR, Singhi P, Khandelwal N, Malla N. Neurocysticercosis immunodiagnosis using Taenia solium cysticerci crude soluble extract, excretory secretory and lower molecular mass antigens in serum and urine samples of Indian children. Acta Trop 2009; 110(1):22-27.

[63] Hell RC, Amim P, de Andrade HM, de Avila RA, Felicori L, Oliveira AG et al. Immunodiagnosis of human neurocysticercosis using a synthetic peptide selected by phage-display. Clin Immunol 2009; 131(1):129-138.

[64] Hellerstein MK, McCune JM. T cell turnover in HIV-1 disease. Immunity 1997; 7(5):583-589.

[65] Nash TE, Singh G, White AC, Rajshekhar V, Loeb JA, Proano JV et al. Treatment of neurocysticercosis: current status and future research needs. Neurology 2006; 67(7):1120-1127.

[66] Proano JV, Madrazo I, Avelar F, Lopez-Felix B, Diaz G, Grijalva I. Medical treatment for neurocysticercosis characterized by giant subarachnoid cysts. N Engl J Med 2001; 345(12):879-885.

[67] Proano JV, Madrazo I, Garcia L, Garcia-Torres E, Correa D. Albendazole and praziquantel treatment in neurocysticercosis of the fourth ventricle. J Neurosurg 1997; 87(1):29-33.

[68] Agapejev S, Da Silva MD, Ueda AK. Severe forms of neurocysticercosis: treatment with albendazole. Arq Neuropsiquiatr 1996; 54(1):82-93.

[69] Del Brutto OH, Sotelo J, Aguirre R, Diaz-Calderon E, Alarcon TA. Albendazole therapy for giant subarachnoid cysticerci. Arch Neurol 1992; 49(5):535-538.

[70] Singh G, Rajshekhar V, Murthy JM, Prabhakar S, Modi M, Khandelwal N et al. A diagnostic and therapeutic scheme for a solitary cysticercus granuloma. Neurology 2010; 75(24):2236-2245.

[71] Del Brutto OH, Roos KL, Coffey CS, Garcia HH. Meta-analysis: Cysticidal drugs for neurocysticercosis: albendazole and praziquantel. Ann Intern Med 2006; 145(1):43-51.

[72] Colli BO, Martelli N, Assirati JA, Jr., Machado HR, de Vergueiro FS. Results of surgical treatment of neurocysticercosis in 69 cases. J Neurosurg 1986; 65(3):309-315.

[73] Madrazo I, Garcia-Renteria JA, Sandoval M, Lopez Vega FJ. Intraventricular cysticercosis. Neurosurgery 1983; 12(2):148-152.

[74] Psarros TG, Krumerman J, Coimbra C. Endoscopic management of supratentorial ventricular neurocysticercosis: case series and review of the literature. Minim Invasive Neurosurg 2003; 46(6):331-334.

[75] Bergsneider M. Endoscopic removal of cysticercal cysts within the fourth ventricle. Technical note. J Neurosurg 1999; 91(2):340-345.

[76] Rangel-Castilla L, Serpa JA, Gopinath SP, Graviss EA, Diaz-Marchan P, White AC, Jr. Contemporary neurosurgical approaches to neurocysticercosis. Am J Trop Med Hyg 2009; 80(3):373-378.